Practical Pelvic Floor Ultrasonography

S. Abbas Shobeiri

Editor

Practical Pelvic Floor Ultrasonography

A Multicompartmental Approach
to 2D/3D/4D Ultrasonography
of Pelvic Floor

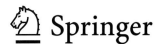 Springer

Editor
S. Abbas Shobeiri, M.D.
Female Pelvic Medicine & Reconstructive Surgery
The University of Oklahoma Health Sciences Center
Oklahoma City, OK, USA

ISBN 978-1-4614-8425-7   ISBN 978-1-4614-8426-4 (eBook)
DOI 10.1007/978-1-4614-8426-4
Springer New York Heidelberg Dordrecht London

Library of Congress Control Number: 2013950169

Springer is part of Springer Science+Business Media (www.springer.com)

This book is dedicated to the four chambers of my heart: Eileen, Sara, Sophie, and Susan who have been mentally, spiritually, emotionally, and physically PRESENT in my life.

Preface

Imaging currently plays a limited role in the clinical investigation of pelvic floor disorders. The most promising modality to date has been magnetic resonance imaging. But MRI has limitations due to cost and access. Ultrasonography, on the other hand, is part of general practice in obstetrics and gynecology, urology, and colorectal surgery. Translabial or transperineal ultrasound imaging was popularized by extensive publications by H.P. Dietz. "The Atlas of Pelvic Floor Ultrasound" published in 2007 introduced transperineal modality to a larger audience. Endoanal imaging of the anorectal area has been the gold standard in colorectal surgery for the past 20 years. "Benign Anorectal Diseases" by Giulio Santoro, M.D. in 2006 is perhaps one of the better books on the subject of endoanal imaging. 3D Endovaginal pelvic floor imaging is gaining in popularity [1–4]; however, it is limited by the fact that true dynamic imaging is hindered by the presence of vaginal or anal transducer. It is generally agreed that different ultrasound routes visualize different structures better, but because the pelvic floor functions as a unit, a multicompartmental approach may be preferred [3]. A book that has addressed all three modalities has been "Pelvic Floor Disorders" by Giulio Santoro, M.D. However, there is a need for a more focused book that purely describes complimentary use of transperineal, endovaginal, and endoanal ultrasound imaging.

The current book "Practical Pelvic Floor Ultrasonography" is the most up-to-date, state-of-the-art review of current literature which provides an introduction to pelvic floor imaging as well as a resource to be used during initial and more advanced practice.

The book stresses understanding of pelvic floor anatomy [5, 6], as without a thorough understanding of the anatomy, the sonographer will be at a loss what they are visualizing. To assure that there is no doubt about the identity of the structures visualized, our group pioneered 3D endovaginal imaging of the pelvic floor structures in 2006 and published the results in early 2009 [7, 8]. We have collaborated with researchers across the world [3, 8] to refine the techniques. We have conducted annual workshops at the International Continence Society (ICS) and the International Urogynecological Association (IUGA) to disseminate our knowledge of comprehensive pelvic floor ultrasonography to international physicians. We have coached interested researchers and as such, currently, there is an explosion of manuscripts submitted utilizing comprehensive approach.

Ultrasound techniques are minimally invasive and easily available for pelvic floor imaging. Recent developments such as 3D/4D imaging have increased their competitiveness. By the end of this book we hope the reader gains competence in performing transperineal, endovaginal, and endoanal 3D/4D ultrasound evaluation of the pelvic floor including anal sphincter and levator ani complex. After reading this book, the reader should have a basic understanding of how to perform a transperineal, an endovaginal, and an endoanal pelvic floor ultrasound.

Dramatic improvement in 3D and 4D ultrasound imaging has allowed greater insight into the complex anatomy of the pelvic floor and its pathological modifications. Obstetric events leading to fecal and urinary incontinence in women, the development of pelvic organ prolapse, and the mechanism of voiding dysfunction and obstructed defecation can now be accurately assessed, which is essential for appropriate treatment decision making.

Obstetrical events leading to pelvic floor disorders in females, the relationship between periurethral structures, levator ani muscles and anorectal support, and mechanisms of urinary incontinence, fecal incontinence, pelvic organ prolapse, and obstructed defecation syndrome can now be easily evaluated. Due to improvements in the diagnosis of these disorders, new forms of treatments have been developed with better outcome for patients. New 3D/4D transperineal, 3D endoanal, and 3D endovaginal ultrasonographic and magnetic resonance imaging techniques have given better insight into the complex anatomy of the pelvic floor. Ultrasound has replaced other modalities as the main imaging modality for the diagnosis of pelvic floor disorders in women. 3D/4D transperineal imaging, 3D endovaginal imaging, and 3D endoanal imaging are each well established as individual modalities for visualization of pelvic floor. Since pelvic floor structures function as a unit there is consensus that 3D/4D transperineal imaging can give the most valuable data for overall functional imaging of the pelvic floor while 3D endovaginal and 3D endoanal imaging can provide the most information on the static structural integrity of the muscles. Information obtained from two or more of these modalities can provide additive or complementary data. "Practical Pelvic Floor Ultrasonography" provides an introduction to 3D/4D comprehensive pelvic floor ultrasonography as a cost-effective modality as well as a resource to be used during more advanced practice.

In recognition of the pelvic floor disorders and its squeal on the quality of life of women, the authors have compiled the practical evidence-based book that will aid as a resource for practitioners with an interest in the imaging, diagnosis, and treatment of pelvic floor dysfunction. The book is meant to be concise, evidence-based, and practical for the first-time users and confers technical capability to the reader. Concise textual information from acknowledged experts is complemented by high-quality diagrams and images to provide a thorough update of this rapidly evolving field. Measurement protocols are introduced in the respective chapters and case reviews will be demonstrated at the conclusion.

With luxurious number of well-marked pictures, readers will gain a clear understanding of the fundamental principles and techniques of 3D/4D comprehensive pelvic floor ultrasonography as well as of the normal anatomy of the pelvic floor and its modification in various benign pelvic floor disorders. The book provides a rich practical resource, written in a simple step-by-step approach for a novice in the use of ultrasound in pelvic floor imaging.

Oklahoma City, OK, USA   S. Abbas Shobeiri, M.D.

References

1. Santoro G, Wieczorek A, Shobeiri S, Mueller E, Pilat J, Stankiewicz A, et al. Interobserver and interdisciplinary reproducibility of 3D endovaginal ultrasound assessment of pelvic floor anatomy. Int Urogynecol J. 2010;22:53–9.
2. Quiroz LH, Shobeiri SA, Nihira MA. Three-dimensional ultrasound imaging for diagnosis of urethrovaginal fistula. Int Urogynecol J. 2010;21:1031–3. PubMed PMID: 20069418.
3. Santoro GA, Wieczorek AP, Dietz HP, Mellgren A, Sultan AH, Shobeiri SA, et al. State of the art: an integrated approach to pelvic floor ultrasonography. Ultrasound Obstet Gynecol. 2011;37:381–96.
4. Shobeiri SA, White D, Quiroz LH, Nihira MA. Anterior and posterior compartment 3D endovaginal ultrasound anatomy based on direct histologic comparison. Int Urogynecol J. 2012;23(8):1047–53. PubMed PMID: 22402641. Epub DOI 10.1007/s00192-012-1721-3. [English].
5. Shobeiri SA, Chesson RR, Gasser RF. The internal innervation and morphology of the human female levator ani muscle. Am J Obstet Gynecol. 2008;199(6):686. e1–e6.
6. Shobeiri SA, Elkins TE, KA T. Comparison of sacrospinous ligament, sacrotuberous ligament, and 0 polypropylene suture tensile strength. J Pelvic Surg. 2000;6:261–7.
7. Shobeiri SA, Leclaire E, Nihira MA, Quiroz LH, O'Donoghue D. Appearance of the levator ani muscle subdivisions in endovaginal three-dimensional ultrasonography. Obstet Gynecol. 2009;114:66–72. PubMed PMID: 19546760.
8. Santoro GA, Wieczorek AP, Stankiewicz A, Wozniak MM, Bogusiewicz M, Rechberger T. High-resolution three-dimensional endovaginal ultrasonography in the assessment of pelvic floor anatomy: a preliminary study. Int Urogynecol J Pelvic Floor Dysfunct. 2009;20(10):1213–22. PubMed PMID: 19533007. [English].

Contents

Contributors

G. Willy Davila Section of Urogynecology and Reconstructive Pelvic Surgery, Department of Gynecology, Cleveland Clinic Florida, Weston, FL, USA

Aparna Hegde Founder, Delhi Pelvic Health Institute, Former IUGA fellow, Cleveland Clinic, Florida, FL, USA

Jittima B. Manonai Department of Obstetrics and Gynecology, Faculty of Medicine Ramathibodi Hospital, Ratchathewi, Bangkok, Thailand

Sthela Murad-Regadas Department of Surgery, School of Medicine of the Federal University of Ceará, Fortaleza, Ceara, Brazil

Head Pelvic Floor Unit, Clinical Hospital, Federal, University of Ceará, Fortaleza, Ceará, Brazil

Lieschen H. Quiroz Department of Obstetrics and Gynecology, The University of Oklahoma Health Sciences Center, Oklahoma City, OK, USA

Ghazaleh Rostaminia Female Pelvic Medicine and Reconstructive Surgery, The University of Oklahoma Health Sciences Center, Oklahoma, USA

Giulio A. Santoro Head Pelvic Floor Unit, 3rd Division of Surgery, Regional Hospital, Treviso, Italy

S. Abbas Shobeiri Female Pelvic Medicine and Reconstructive Surgery, The University of Oklahoma Health Sciences Center, Oklahoma , USA

Milena Weinstein Department of Obstetrics and Gynecology, Massachusetts General Hospital, Boston, MA, USA

Dena E. White Department of Obstetrics and Gynecology, Section of Female Pelvic Medicine and Reconstructive Surgery, The University of Oklahoma Health Sciences Center, Oklahoma City, OK, USA

Andrzej Pawel Wieczorek Department of Pediatric Radiology, Medical University of Lublin, Lublin, Poland

Magdalena Maria Wozniak Department of Pediatric Radiology, Medical University of Lublin, Lublin, Poland

Pelvic Floor Anatomy

S. Abbas Shobeiri

Learning Objectives
1. Conceptualize pelvic organ support
2. Become familiarize with room analogy and suspension bridge analogy of pelvic organ support
3. Understand the intricate anatomy of the levator ani subdivisions
4. Understand the role of endopelvic fascia and connective tissue for pelvic organ support

1.1 Introduction

Pelvic floor disorders, including urinary incontinence, fecal incontinence, and pelvic organ prolapse (POP) represent a major public health issue in the United States [1]. Pelvic floor disorders, including POP and urinary incontinence, are debilitating conditions where 24 % of adult women have at least one pelvic floor disorder [2] which results in surgery in 1 of 9 women [3]. In the United states the National Center for Health Statistics estimates 400,000 operations per year are performed for pelvic floor dysfunction each year with 300,000 occurring in the inpatient setting [4]. A study in

S.A. Shobeiri, M.D. (✉)
Female Pelvic Medicine and Reconstructive Surgery, The University of Oklahoma Health Sciences Center, WP 2410, 920 Stanton L. Young Blvd., Oklahoma City, OK 73104, USA
e-mail: Abbas-Shobeiri@ouhsc.edu

Australian women found that the lifetime risk of surgery for POP in the general female population was 19 % [5]. In an Austrian study an estimation of the frequency for post-hysterectomy vault prolapse requiring surgical repair was between 6 and 8 % [6]. A single vaginal birth has been shown to significantly increase the odds of prolapse (OR 9.73, 95 % CI 2.68–35.35). Additional vaginal births were not associated with a significant increase in the odds of prolapse [7].

It is forecasted that the number of American women with at least one pelvic floor disorder will increase from 28.1 million in 2010 to 43.8 million in 2050. During this time period, the number of women with UI will increase 55 % from 18.3 million to 28.4 million. For fecal incontinence, the number of affected women will increase 59 % from 10.6 to 16.8 million, and the number of women with POP will increase 46 % from 3.3 to 4.9 million. The highest projections for 2050 estimate that 58.2 million women in the United States will have at least one pelvic floor disorder, 41.3 million with UI, 25.3 million with fecal incontinence, and 9.2 million with POP. This forecast has important public health implications. Understanding the causes of pelvic floor disorders is in its infancy. But what is known is that prolapse arises because of injuries and deterioration of the muscles, nerves, and connective tissue that support and control normal pelvic function. This chapter focuses on the *functional* anatomy of the pelvic floor in women and how the anterior, posterior, apical, and lateral compartments are supported.

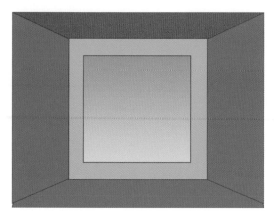

Fig. 1.1 Room analogy © SHOBEIRI 2013

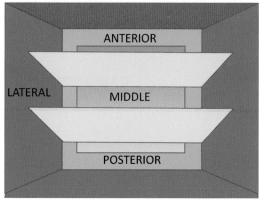

Fig. 1.3 Room analogy with anterior, middle, posterior compartments, and the lateral walls marked © SHOBEIRI 2013

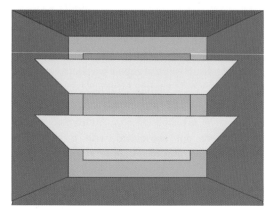

Fig. 1.2 Room analogy with three compartments separated © SHOBEIRI 2013

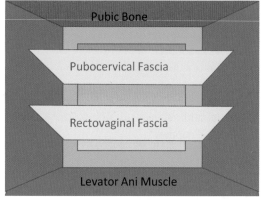

Fig. 1.4 Room analogy; pubocervical fibromuscularis and rectovaginal fascia separating the three compartments © SHOBEIRI 2013

1.1.1 Support of the Pelvic Organs: Conceptual Overview

The pelvic organs rely on (1) their connective tissue attachments to the pelvic walls and (2) support from the levator ani muscles that are under neuronal control from the peripheral and central nervous systems. In this chapter, the term "pelvic floor" is used broadly to include all the structures supporting the pelvic cavity rather than the restricted use of this term to refer to the levator ani group of muscles.

To convey the pelvic floor supportive structures to the reader, we can use the "room analogy." Using this analogy, the reader can conceptualize the pelvic floor hiatus as the door out of this room (Fig. 1.1). Using this very simplified analogy, if you view the pelvic floor hiatus from where the

sacrum is, the door frame for this room is the perineal membrane, the walls and the floor the levator ani muscle, and the ceiling the pubic bone. However, the pelvic floor is separated into three compartments (Fig. 1.2). We arbitrarily call these anterior, middle, posterior, and lateral compartments (Fig. 1.3). The tissue separating the anterior and middle compartments is pubocervical fibromuscularis or pubocervical fascia. The tissue separating the middle and posterior compartments is rectovaginal fibromuscularis or rectovaginal fascia (Fig. 1.4). The pubocervical fibromuscularis and the rectovaginal septum are attached laterally to the levator ani muscle with thickening of adventitia in this area. Anatomically, the endopelvic fascia refers to the areolar connective tissue that surrounds the

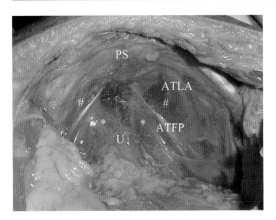

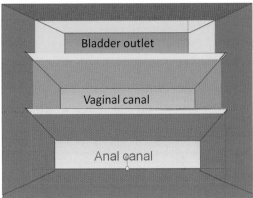

Fig. 1.5 Retropubic anatomy showing points of attachments of the ATLA and the ATFP. The urethra sits on the hammock like pubocervical fibromuscularis. # denotes the levator ani attachment to the obturator internus muscle © SHOBEIRI 2013

Fig. 1.7 Room analogy; three compartments separation © SHOBEIRI 2013

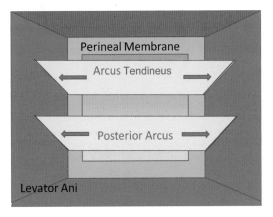

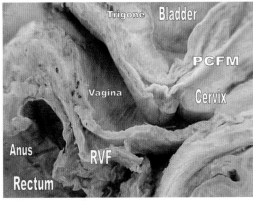

Fig. 1.6 Room analogy; the line of attachment of the pubocervical fascia to the levator ani is arcus tendineus fascia pelvis. The line of attachment of the rectovaginal fascia to the levator ani is the posterior arcus. Both are shown as *red lines* © SHOBEIRI 2013

Fig. 1.8 Midsagittal anatomy of an intact cadaveric specimen demonstrating the three different compartments © SHOBEIRI 2013

vagina. It continues down the length of the vagina as loose areolar tissue surrounding the pelvic viscera. Histologic examination has shown that the vagina is made up of three layers—epithelium, muscularis, and adventitia [8, 9]. The adventitial layer is loose areolar connective tissue made up of collagen and elastin and form the vaginal tube. Therefore the tissue that surgeons call fascia at the time of surgery is best described as fibromuscularis since it is a mixture of muscularis and adventitia.

Anteriorly, pubocervical fibromuscularis is attached to the levator ani using arcus tendineus fascia pelvis (Fig. 1.5). Posterior attachment of rec-

tovaginal septum to the levator ani is poorly understood but we will refer to it as the posterior arcus (Fig. 1.6) [10]. The anterior compartment is home to the urethra and the lower part of the bladder. The middle compartment is the vagina, and the posterior compartment is home to anorectum (Fig. 1.7). This analogy is not far from reality. When one looks at the pelvic floor structures, the three compartments are clearly separated as described (Fig. 1.8). Compartmentalization of the pelvic floor has lead to different medical specialties looking at that specific compartment and paying less attention to the whole pelvic floor (Fig. 1.9).

If one looks at the middle compartment from the side, he or she can appreciate different levels of support as described by DeLancey and colleagues [11] (Fig. 1.10). Looking at these supportive

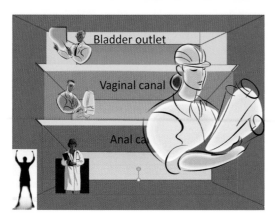

Fig. 1.9 Room analogy; each area or compartment may be managed by a different specialist. There is a great need for one specialty that understands the interaction between different compartments and manages them concurrently as much as possible © SHOBEIRI 2013

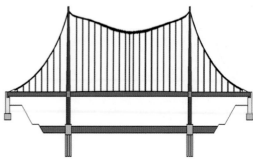

Fig. 1.11 Suspension bridge analogy; the depiction of a normal bridge © SHOBEIRI 2013

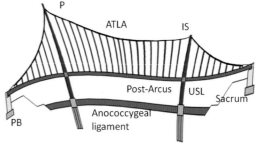

Fig. 1.12 Suspension bridge analogy; the depiction of a suspension bridge adapted to human female pelvic floor structures. The *red* masts are the ischial spine and the pubis. The *blue lines* are the levator ani fibers. The *green line* is the uterosacral ligaments continuous with the posterior arcus line. The anococcygeal ligament provides anchoring point for the posterior structures © SHOBEIRI 2013

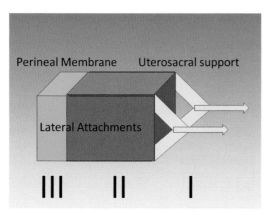

Fig. 1.10 Room analogy; level one support are provided by the uterosacral-cardinal ligament complex which keep the room upright. These are demonstrated as the *yellow arrows*. The level II supports are provided by the lateral tendineus attachments drawn as *red lines*. The level III support is provided by perineal membrane which is the *green area* © SHOBEIRI 2013

structures from the sagittal view exposes the connective tissue elements that keep the room standing. Generally, a "suspension bridge" analogy is useful for to describing these structures (Fig. 1.11). Although in room analogy, the anterior, middle, and posterior compartments house the pelvic organs; in reality, the pelvic organs are part of the pelvic floor and play an important supportive role through their connections with structures, such as the cardinal and uterosacral

ligaments. Adapting this suspension bridge to human body, perineal body and the sacrum become the two anchoring points of the bridge. Perineal membrane (DeLancey Level III) and the uterosacral ligaments (DeLancey Level I) form the two masts of the suspension bridge (Fig. 1.12). The lateral wires are the levator ani muscles of the lateral wall (Fig. 1.13) and the attachments of the vagina to the levator ani muscles laterally in the mid part of the vagina forms Delancey's Level II support. The levator ani muscles and the interconnecting fibromuscular structures support bladder and urethra anteriorly, vaginal canal in the middle, and anorectal structures posteriorly (Fig. 1.14).

Like a room or a suspension bridge, the pelvic floor is subjected to loads that should be appropriate

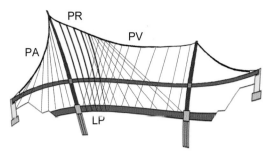

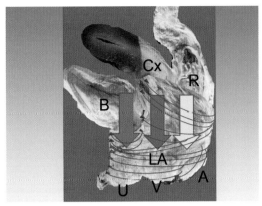

Fig. 1.13 Suspension bridge analogy; the depiction of a suspension bridge adapted to human female pelvic floor structures. The levator ani fibers have intricate and overlapping paths. The puboanalis (PA) and puboperinealis form some of the supportive structures of the perineum. The puborectalis (PR) fibers form the sling behind the rectum. Pubovisceralis (PV) is a collective term we have applied here to the iliococcygeus and pubococcygeous fibers. The levator plate (LP) is formed by overlapping of the PV and PR fibers © SHOBEIRI 2013

Fig. 1.15 Right lateral standing anatomic depiction of the three compartments exposed to intraabdominal pressure which results in activation of the muscles to prevent prolapse or urinary and fecal incontinence. *B* bladder, *Cx* cervix, *R* rectum, *LA* levator ani, *U* urethra, *V* vagina, *A* anus © SHOBEIRI 2013

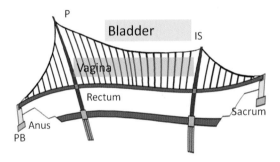

Fig. 1.14 Suspension bridge analogy; the depiction of different compartments of pelvic floor © SHOBEIRI 2013

(Fig. 1.16). Pubococcygeus is a functional unit of the iliococcygeus and these two collectively are known as the pubovisceralis muscle. The relationship of these muscles to each other is interesting as they criss cross in different angles to each other (Figs. 1.17 and 1.18).

1.2 Practical Anatomy and Prolapse

1.2.1 Overview

for its design. Should these loads exceed what the pelvic floor is capable of handling there would be failure in one or multiple supportive elements. Pelvic floor is not a static structure. The levator ani works in concert with the ligamentous structures to withstand intraabdominal pressure that could predispose to POP and urinary or fecal incontinence during daily activities (Fig. 1.15). The lower end of the pelvic floor is held closed by the pelvic floor muscles, preventing prolapse by constricting the base. The spatial relationship of the organs and the pelvic floor are important. Pelvic support is a combination of constriction, suspension, and structural geometry.

The levator ani muscle has puboperinealis, puboanalis, pubovaginalis, puborectalis, pubococcygeus, and iliococcygeus subdivisions

Level I support is composed of the uterosacral and cardinal ligaments which form the support of the uterus and upper 1/3 of the vagina. Stretching and failure of level I can result in pure apical prolapse of the uterus or an enterocele formation. At Level II, there are direct lateral attachments of the pubocervical fibromuscularis and rectovaginal fibromuscularis to the lateral compartments formed by the levator ani muscles. The variations of defects in this level will be described in the following sections. In the Level III the vaginal wall is anteriorly fused with the urethra, posteriorly with the perineal body. Levator ani muscles in this area are poorly described, but mostly consist of fibrous sheets that envelop the lateral aspects of the vaginal introitus.

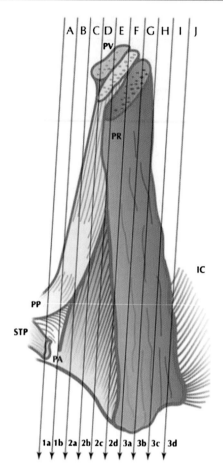

Fig. 1.16 The relative position of levator ani subdivisions during ultrasound imaging. *IC* iliococcygeus, *PP* puboperinealis, *STP* superficial transverse perinei, *PA* puboanalis. Illustration: John Yanson. *Shobeiri. Ultrasonography Validation. Obstet Gynecol 2009*

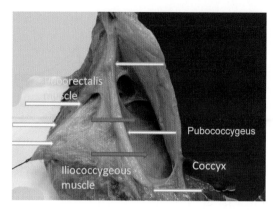

Fig. 1.17 Right hemipelvis of a fresh frozen pelvis showing the overlapping of the levator ani subdivisions fibers. The *orange arrows*: puborectalis; the *blue arrows*: iliococcygeus; the *white arrows*: pubococcygeus. Note the relationship between the iliococcygeus and pubococcygeus fibers. © SHOBEIRI 2013

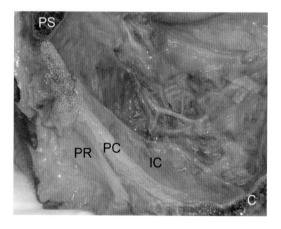

Fig. 1.18 Right hemipelvis of a fresh frozen pelvis with the organs removed. The puborectalis (PR), iliococcygeus (IC), and pubococcygeus (PC) form the lateral sidewall. Note the relationship between the iliococcygeus and pubococcygeus fibers. © SHOBEIRI 2013

1.2.2 Apical Segment

While level I cardinal and uterosacral ligaments can be surgically identified supporting the cervix and the upper 1/3 of the vagina [12, 13], as they fan out toward the sacrum and laterally, they become a mixture of connective tissue, blood vessels, nerves, smooth muscle, and adipose tissue. The uterosacral ligaments act like rubber bands in that they may lengthen with initial Valsalva, but resist any further lengthening at a critical point in which they have to return to their comfortable length or break (Fig. 1.19). Level I and levator ani muscles are interdependent. Intact

levator ani muscles moderate the tension placed on the level I support structures and intact level I support lessen the pressure imposed from above on the pelvic floor.

1.2.3 Anterior Compartment

Anterior compartment support depends on the integrity of vaginal muscularis and adventitia and their connections to the arcus tendineus fascia

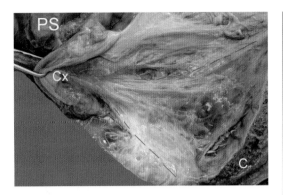

Fig. 1.19 Right hemipelvis of a fresh frozen pelvis showing the uterosacral fibers. The borders of the ligament are shown in *dotted line*. *Cx* cervix, *C* coccyx, *PS* pubic symphysis. © SHOBEIRI 2013

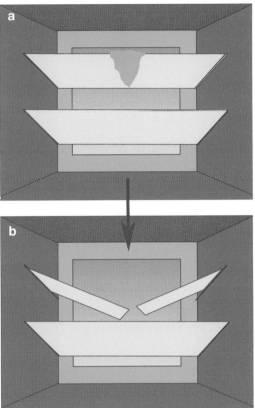

Fig. 1.20 Room analogy; (**a**): an occult pubocervical fibromuscularis defect can result in an overt cystocele (**b**). © SHOBEIRI 2013

pelvis. The arcus tendineus fascia pelvis is at one end connected to the lower sixth of the pubic bone, 1–2 cm lateral to the midline, and at the other end to the ischial spine. A simple case of a distension cystocele could result from a defect in pubocervical fibromuscularis (Fig. 1.20a, b)

The anterior wall fascial attachments to the arcus tendineus fascia pelvis have been called the paravaginal fascial attachments by Richardson et al. [14]. Detachment of arcus tendineus from the levator ani is associated with stress incontinence and anterior prolapse. The detachment can be unilateral (Fig. 1.21) or bilateral (Fig. 1.22) causing a displacement cystocele. In addition, the defect can be complete or incomplete. The surgeon who performs an anterior repair on Fig. 1.22 in reality worsens the underlying disease process. The upper portions of the anterior vaginal wall can prolapse due to lack of Level I support and failure of uterosacral-cardinal complex. Over time this failure may lead to increased load in the paravaginal area and failure of level II paravaginal support. A study of 71 women with anterior compartment prolapse has shown that paravaginal defect usually results from a detachment of the arcus tendineus fascia pelvis from the ischial spine, and rarely from the pubic bone [15]. Resuspension of the vaginal apex at the time of surgery in addition to paravaginal or anterior colporrhaphy may help to return the anterior wall to

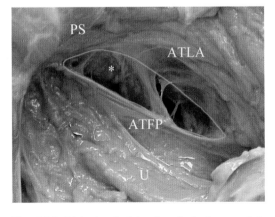

Fig. 1.21 Right hemipelvis of a fresh frozen pelvis showing a paravaginal defect repair outlined in *green* © SHOBEIRI 2013

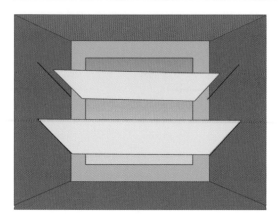

Fig. 1.22 Room analogy; bilateral detachment of the pubocervical fibromuscularis can result in a cystocele © SHOBEIRI 2013

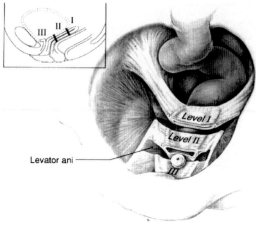

Fig. 1.24 Three levels of support. DeLancey. AJOG 1992

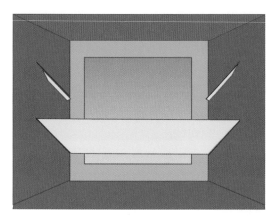

Fig. 1.23 Room analogy; absence or severe deficiency of the pubocervical fibromuscularis can result in a cystocele © SHOBEIRI 2013

a more normal position or at least prevent future failures. Another scenario that the surgeon faces is the lack of any tangible fibromuscular tissue in the anterior compartment (Fig. 1.23). Plication of the available tissue may cause vaginal narrowing and dyspareunia. The knowledge of this condition is essential as it will require bridging of the anterior compartment with autologous fascia lata graft [16] or other commercially available tissue augmentation.

Various grading systems such as Pelvic Organ Prolapse Quantification (POPQ) system [17] used to describe prolapse do not take into account the underlying cause of the prolapse.

Different clinical and imaging based modalities have been used to pinpoint the location of defect. MRI holds promise in this regard, although good studies investigating validation of this technique compared to physical examination are lacking.

1.2.4 Perineal Membrane (Urogenital Diaphragm)

A critical but perhaps underappreciated part of pelvic floor support is the perineal membrane as it forms the level III part of Delancey support (Fig. 1.24) and one of the anchoring points in the suspension bridge analogy. The tissue that spans the anterior part of the pelvic outlet, below the levator ani muscles, there is a dense triangular membrane was called the urogenital diaphragm. However this layer is not a single muscle layer with a double layer of fascia ("diaphragm"), but rather a set of connective tissues that surround the urethra, the term perineal membrane has been used more recently to reflect its true nature [18]. The perineal membrane is a single connective tissue membrane, with muscle lying immediately above. The perineal membrane lies at the level of the hymen and attaches the urethra, vagina, and perineal body to the ischiopubic rami.

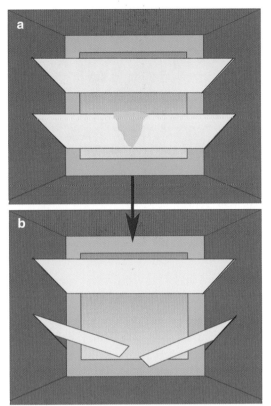

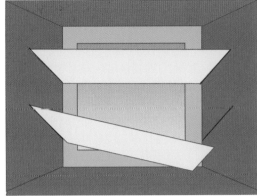

Fig. 1.26 Room analogy; right lateral detachment of the rectovaginal septum can result in a rectocele © SHOBEIRI 2013

Fig. 1.25 Room analogy; (**a**): an occult rectovaginal defect can result in an overt rectocele (**b**). © SHOBEIRI 2013

1.2.5 Posterior Compartment and Perineal Membrane

The posterior compartment is bound to perineal body and the perineal membrane caudad (level III), paracolpium and the uterosacral ligaments cephalad (level I), and the posterior arcus connected to the levator ani laterally (Level II). As in the anterior compartment, a simple defect in rectovaginal fibromuscularis (Fig. 1.25) can cause a distention rectocele. A defect in the posterior arcus is associated with a pararectal defect that can be unilateral (Fig. 1.26) or bilateral (Fig. 1.27). Such defects need to be differentiated from total loss of rectovaginal fibromuscularis which may require augmentation of the compartment with autologous or cadaveric tissue. At times, the separation of the posterior arcus may

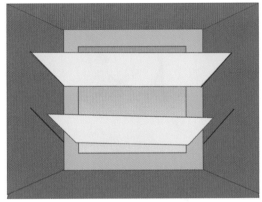

Fig. 1.27 Room analogy; bilateral detachment of the rectovaginal septum can result in a rectocele © SHOBEIRI 2013

be apical and may require reattachment of the posterior arcus to the uterosacral ligament or the iliococcygeal muscle.

The fibers of the perineal membrane connect through the perineal body thereby providing a layer that resists downward descent of the rectum. A separate level I support does not exist for anterior and posterior compartments. In the room analogy used in this chapter, the perineal membrane is analogous to the door frame. If the bottom of the door frame is missing (Fig. 1.28), then the resistance to downward descent is lost and a

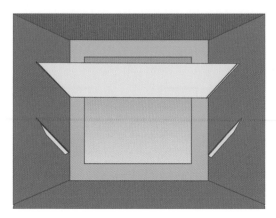

Fig. 1.28 Room analogy; Absence or severe deficiency of rectovaginal fascia can result in a rectocele. © SHOBEIRI 2013

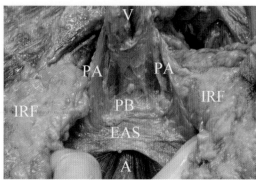

Fig. 1.30 Perineal dissection in a fresh frozen pelvis shows the relationship of the external anal sphincter (EAS) to the perineal body (PB) and the puboanalis/puboperinealis complex. IRF denotes the ischiorectal fat. © SHOBEIRI 2013

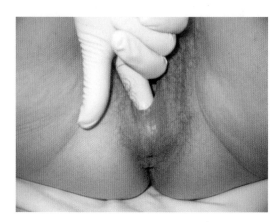

Fig. 1.29 A perineocele in a patient with need to splint to have bowel movement © SHOBEIRI 2013

perineocele develops. This situation can be elusive as the clinical diagnosis is made by realizing the patient's need to splint very close to the vaginal opening in order to have a bowel movement and the physical examination may reveal an elongated or "empty" perineal body (Fig. 1.29). Reattachment of the separated structures during perineorrhaphy corrects this defect and is a mainstay of reconstructive surgery. Because the puboperinealis muscles are intimately connected with the cranial surface of the perineal membranes, this reattachment also restores the mus-

cles to a more normal position under the pelvic organs in a location where they can provide support.

Three anal canal muscular structures that contribute to fecal continence are the internal anal sphincter (IAS), the external anal sphincter (EAS), and the levator plate. The EAS is made up of voluntary muscle that encompasses the anal canal. It is described as having three parts: (1) The deep part is integral with the puborectalis. Posteriorly there is some ligamentous attachment. Anteriorly some fibers are circular. (2) The superficial part has a very broad attachment to the underside of the coccyx via the anococcygeal ligament. Anteriorly there is a division into circular fibers and a decussation to the superficial transverse perinei. (3) The subcutaneous part lies below the IAS.

The IAS always extends cephalad to the EAS for a distance of more than 1–2 cm. The internal sphincter lies consistently between the external sphincter and the anal mucosa, extending below the dentate line by 1 cm. Normally, the EAS begins below the IAS [19].

The muscle fibers from the puboanalis portion of the levator ani become fibroelastic as they extend caudally to merge with the conjoined longitudinal layer (CLL) that is inserted between the external and IASs (Fig. 1.30) [20]. The CLL

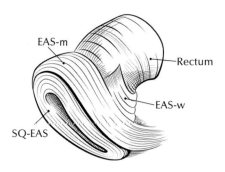

Fig. 1.31 Drawing of EAS subdivisions. Anterior portion of model is to the *left*, posterior to the *right*. Notice decussation of fibers toward the coccyx posteriorly. The main body of the EAS also has a concentric portion posteriorly that is not shown in this view. *EAS-M* main body of EAS, *EAS-W* winged portion of EAS, *SQ-EAS* subcutaneous EAS

Table 1.1 International standardized terminology

	Origin/insertion
Puboperinealis (PP)	Pubis/perineal body
Pubovaginalis (PV)	Pubis/vaginal wall at the level of the mid-urethra
Puboanalis (PA)	Pubis/intersphincteric groove between internal and external anal sphincter to end in the anal skin
Puborectalis (PR)	Pubis/forms sling behind the rectum
Iliococcygeus (IC)	Tendinous arch of the levator ani/ the two sides fuse in the iliococcygeal raphe
Pubococcygeus (PC)	Pubic symphysis to superficial part of anococcygeal ligament

Divisions of the levator ani muscles

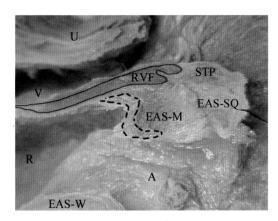

Fig. 1.32 Perineal dissection in a cadaveric specimen shows the relationship of the subcutaneous external anal sphincter (EAS-SQ) to the main portion of EAS, the winged portion of EAS, and the superficial transverse perinei (STP). The internal anal sphincter is marked with the *dotted line*. The rectovaginal fascia is marked with RVF © SHOBEIRI 2013

fibers and the puboanalis fibers cannot be palpated clinically. However, the puboperinealis fibers which medially located can be palpated as a distinct band of fibers joining the perineal body (Fig. 1.31).

Per MRI studies done by Hsu and colleagues, the EAS includes a subcutaneous portion (EAS-SQ) (Fig. 1.31), a visibly separate deeper portion (EAS-M) and a lateral portion that has lateral winged projections (EAS-W). The EAS-SQ is the distinct part of the EAS (Fig. 1.32). A clear separation does not exist between concentric portion of EAS-M and the winged EAS-W. The EAS-W fibers have differing fiber directions than the other portions, forming an open "U-shaped" configuration which cannot be visualized in midsagittal view except in the posterior anus. These fibers are contiguous with the EAS but visibly separate from the levator plate muscles, whose fibers they parallel [21].

1.2.6 Lateral Compartment and the Levator Ani Muscles

It is generally accepted that the levator ani muscles and the associated fascial layer surround pelvic organs like funnel to form the pelvic diaphragm [22]. Given that we employ concepts such as pelvic floor spasm, levator spasm, and pelvic floor weakness, understanding the basic concepts of pelvic floor musculature is essential to formulate a clinical opinion. The area posterior to the pubic bone is dense with bands of intertwined levator ani muscles which defy conventional description of the levator ani being consisted of puborectalis, pubococcygeus, and iliococcygeus. The anatomy of distal subdivisions of the levator ani muscle was further described in a study by Kearney et al. [23]. The origins and insertions of these muscles as well as their characteristic anatomical relations are shown in Table 1.1 and Fig. 1.16. Using a nomenclature based on the attachment points, the lesser known subdivisions of the levator ani muscles, the muscles posterior to the pubic bone are identified as pubovaginalis, puboanalis, and puboperinealis. The pubovaginalis is poorly described, but may be analogous to the urethrovaginal ligaments. The puboanalis originates from behind the pubic bone as a thin band and inserts around the anus into the longitudinal ligaments. Puboperinealis which is most often 0.5 cm in diameter originates from the pubic bone and inserts into the perineal body. The four major components of the levator ani muscle; the iliococcygeus forms a thin, relatively flat, horizontal shelf that spans the potential gap from one pelvic sidewall to the other. The pubococcygeus muscle travels from the tip of the coccyx to the pubic bone (Fig. 1.17) while the puborectalis muscle originates from the anterior portion of the perineal membrane and the pubic bone to form a sling behind the rectum, the puboperinealis, and puboanalis are thin broad complex muscles poorly described that attach to the perineal body and anus to stabilize the perineal region.

Margulies and colleagues showed excellent reliability and reproducibility of visualizing major portions of the levator ani with magnetic resonance imaging in nulliparous volunteers [24]. Because puboanalis, pubovaginalis, and puboperinealis are small, they are proven hard to visualize by magnetic resonance imaging. However, these muscles are seen well with 3D endovaginal ultrasonography [25].

The shortest distance between the pubic symphysis and the levator plate is the minimal levator hiatus. This is different from the urogenital hiatus which bounded anteriorly by the pubic bones, laterally by levator ani muscles, and posteriorly by the perineal body and EAS. The baseline tonic activity of the levator ani muscle keeps the minimal levator hiatus closed by compressing the urethra, vagina, and rectum against the pubic bone as they exit through this opening [26]. The levator ani fibers converge behind the rectum to form the levator plate. With contraction, the levator plate elevates to form a horizontal shelf over which pelvic organs rest. The deficiency of

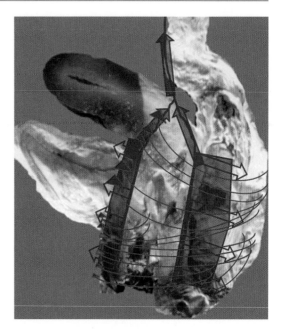

Fig. 1.33 Right lateral standing anatomic depiction of the levator ani muscle and uterosacral-cardinal complex interaction © SHOBEIRI 2013

any portion of the levator ani results in weakening of the levator plate and descensus of pelvic organs [27].

1.2.7 Endopelvic Fascia and Levator Ani Interactions

The levator ani muscles and the endopelvic fascia work as a unit to provide pelvic organ support. If the muscles maintain normal tone, the ligaments of the endopelvic fascia will have little tension on them even with increases in abdominal pressure (Fig. 1.33). If the muscles are damaged by a tear or complete separation from their attachments, the pelvic floor sags downward overtime and the organs are pushed through the urogenital hiatus (Fig. 1.34a, b). In such cases the ligaments and the endopelvic fascia will assume the majority of the pelvic floor load until they fail as well. Different varieties of levator ani injury can cause different interesting types of clinical defects. A partial defect and

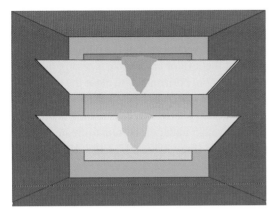

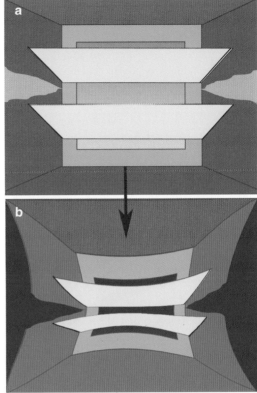

Fig. 1.34 Room analogy; The clinical presentation of a combined cystocele/rectocele may have varied pathophisiologies. Depicted to the left is a cystocele/rectocele due to pubocervical and rectovaginal fibromuscularis defects. (**a**): bilateral levator ani tears may or may not result in prolapse or incontinence initially, but over time the other supportive structures will decompensate resulting in pelvic floor laxity (**b**) © SHOBEIRI 2013

separation of the pubovisceralis muscles will result in a displacement cystocele (Fig. 1.35a, b). However, the clinician may not be able to distinguish if this is a displacement cystocele due to paravaginal defect and arcus tendineus separation or due to muscle loss. The consequences of this lack of recognition can be that the surgeon may elect to do an anterior repair and by placating the pubocervical fibromuscularis make the lateral defect worse. The lack of basic information about the levator ani status may account for varied results in the anterior repair studies. Additionally, in an attempted paravaginal repair, the surgeon may realize that there is no muscle to attach the arcus tendenious to. A partial defect as in Fig. 1.35a is subjected

to excessive forces and may progress over time to involve the apical and posterior compartments as well (Fig. 1.35b). How fast this occurs depends on the strength of the patient's connective tissue. One woman with injured muscles may have strong connective tissue that compensates and never develops prolapse while another woman with even less muscle injury but weaker connective tissue may develop prolapse with aging. There are instances of catastrophic injury during childbirth during which complete muscle loss occurs and the patient presents with a displacement cystocele, rectocele, and varied types of incontinence (Fig. 1.36a, b). This scenario is different with patients who have a defect in pubocervical and rectovaginal fibromuscularis

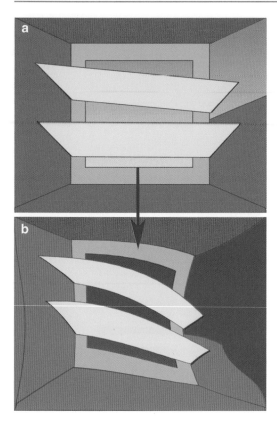

Fig. 1.35 Room analogy; (**a**): unilateral levator ani tears may or may not result in prolapse or incontinence initially, but over time the other supportive structures will decompensate resulting in pelvic floor laxity (**b**) © SHOBEIRI 2013

(Fig. 1.37) which develop into a distention cystocele and rectocele over time. A cystocele and rectocele repair that can be used for the latter case will worsen the first patient's condition that has levator damage.

1.2.8 The Levator Plate

The levtor plate has varied definitions and is viewed differently by different sources. On one hand, Hsu and colleagues' modeling views it as a flap valve that requires the dorsal traction of the uterosacral ligaments, and to some extent the cardinal ligaments, to hold the cervix back in the

hollow of the sacrum. The measurement obtained is called the levator plate angle (LPA). It also requires the ventral pull of the pubovisceral portions of the levator ani muscle to swing the levator plate more horizontally to close the urogenital hiatus. From our point of view, the levator plate is the point that pubovisceralis and the puborectalis come together under the rectum to create the anorectal angle (Figs. 1.13, 1.17, and 1.18). We measure the movement of the levator plate relative to the pubic bone by a measurement called Levator Plate Descent Angle (LPDA) [28]. LPA and LPDA likely measure different functions. LPDA change has been correlated with levator ani deficiency (Fig. 1.38).

1.2.9 Nerves

There are two main nerves that supply the pelvic floor:

1. The pudendal nerve supplies the urethral and anal sphincters and perineal muscles. The pudendal nerve originates from S2 to S4 foramina runs through Alcock's canal which is caudal to the levator ani muscles. The pudendal nerve has three branches: the clitoral, perineal, and inferior hemorrhoidal which innervate the clitoris, the perineal musculature, inner perineal skin, and the EAS respectively [20]. The blockade of the pudendal nerve decreases resting and squeeze pressures in the vagina and rectum, increases the length of the urogenital hiatus, and decreases EMG activity of the puborectalis muscle [29].

2. The levator ani nerve innervates the major musculature that supports the pelvic floor. The levator ani nerve originates from S3 to S5 foramina, runs inside of the pelvis on the cranial surface of the levator ani muscle and provides the innervation to all the subdivisions of the muscle.

Motor nerves to the IAS are derived from (1) L5-presacral plexus sympathetic fibers and (2) S2-4 parasympathetic fibers of the pelvic splanchnic nerve. The levator ani muscle often

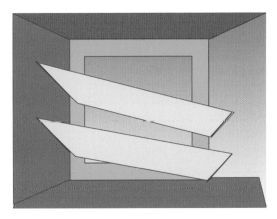

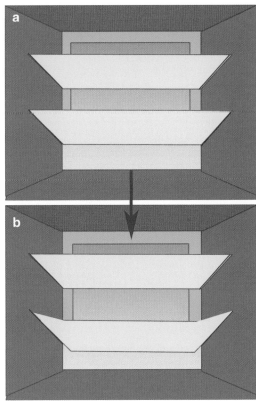

Fig. 1.36 Room analogy; Obstetrics injuries can be catastrophic or subtle. To the left is a complete right unilateral levator ani detachment (avulsion). To the right is injury to the perineal support (the missing green part of the door frame) (**a**), which may result in sliding of the rectovaginal fascia and a clinical perineocele, (**b**). © SHOBEIRI 2013

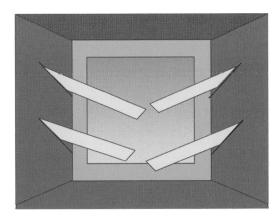

Fig. 1.37 Room analogy; multicompartmental defect: pubocervical fibromuscularis and rectovaginal septum defects © SHOBEIRI 2013

has a dual somatic innervation with the levator ani nerve as its constant and main neuronal supply [20, 30].

1.3 Summary

The knowledge of pelvic floor anatomy and function is essential for effective ultrasound imaging of pelvic floor pathologies. With advancing ultrasound technology, new ultrasound techniques have increased our ability to detect pelvic floor defects and helped us gain insight into pathophysiology of pelvic floor disorders.

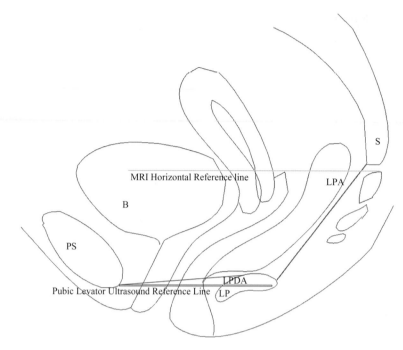

Fig. 1.38 Drawing of the levator plate angle (LPA) vs. the levator plate descent angle obtained by 3D endovaginal ultrasound. © SHOBEIRI 2013. The levator plate position relative to the PLURAL is shown. A normal LPDA relative to the reference line (PLURAL) is normally 15 degrees. B: bladder, LP: levator plate, LPA: levator plate angle obtained by MRI, LPDA: levator plate descent angle obtained by 3D endovaginal ultrasound, PLURAL: Pubic Levator plate Ultrasound Reference Assessment Line, PS: Pubic symphysis, S: Sacrum/coccyx

References

1. Landefeld SC, Bowers BJ, Feld AD, et al. NIH State-of-the Science Conference Statement on Prevention of Fecal and Urinary Incontinence in Adults. NIH consensus and state-of-the-science statements. 2007; 24(1):1–37. PubMed PMID: 5667460.
2. Nygaard I, Barber MD, Burgio KL, Kenton K, Meikle S, Schaffer J, et al. Prevalence of symptomatic pelvic floor disorders in US women. JAMA. 2008; 300(11):1311–6. PubMed PMID: 18799443. Pubmed Central PMCID: Source: NLM. NIHMS219469. Source: NLM. PMC2918416. English.
3. Olsen AL, Smith VJ, Bergstrom JO, Colling JC, Clark AL. Epidemiology of surgically managed pelvic organ prolapse and urinary incontinence. Obstet Gynecol. 1997;89(4):501–6. PubMed PMID: 9083302. English.
4. Boyles SH, Weber AM, Meyn L. Procedures for pelvic organ prolapse in the United States, 1979–1997. Am J Obstet Gynecol. 2003;188(1):108–15. PubMed PMID: 12548203. Epub 2003/01/28. eng.
5. Smith FJ, Holman CDAJ, Moorin RE, Tsokos N. Lifetime risk of undergoing surgery for pelvic organ prolapse. Obstet Gynecol. 2010;116(5):1096–100. PubMed PMID: 20966694. English.
6. Aigmueller T, Dungl A, Hinterholzer S, Geiss I, Riss P. An estimation of the frequency of surgery for posthysterectomy vault prolapse. Int Urogynecol J. 2010;21(3):299–302. PubMed PMID: 19936593. English.
7. Quiroz LH, Munoz A, Shippey SH, Gutman RE, Handa VL. Vaginal parity and pelvic organ prolapse. J Reprod Med. 2010;55(3–4):93–8. PubMed PMID: 20506667. English.
8. Ricci JV, Thom CH. The myth of a surgically useful fascia in vaginal plastic reconstructions. Q Rev Surg Obstet Gynecol. 1954;11:253.
9. Gitsch E, Palmrich AH. Operative anatomie. Berlin: De Gruyter; 1977.
10. Albright T, Gehrich A, Davis G, Sabi F, Buller J. Arcus tendineus fascia pelvis: a further understanding. Am J Obstet Gynecol. 2005;193(3):677–81.
11. DeLancey JO. Anatomic aspects of vaginal eversion after hysterectomy. Am J Obstet Gynecol. 1992;166: 1717–28.
12. Campbell RM. The anatomy and histology of the sacro-uterine ligaments. Am J Obstet Gynecol. 1950;59:1.

13. Range RL, Woodburne RT. The gross and microscopic anatomy of the transverse cervical ligaments. Am J Obstet Gynecol. 1964;90:460.

14. Richardson AC, Edmonds PB, Williams NL. Treatment of stress urinary incontinence due to paravaginal fascial defect. Obstet Gynecol. 1981;57(3):357–62. PubMed PMID: 7465150. English.

15. DeLancey J. Fascial and muscular abnormalities in women with urethral hypermobility and anterior vaginal wall prolapse. Am J Obstet Gynecol. 2002;187(1):93–8.

16. Chesson RR, Schlossberg SM, Elkins TE, Menefee S, McCammon K, Franco N, et al. The use of fascia lata graft for correction of severe or recurrent anterior vaginal wall defects. J Pelvic Surg. 1999;5(2):96–103.

17. Bump RC, Mattiasson A, Bo K, Brubaker LP, DeLancey JO, Klarskov P, et al. The standardization of terminology of female pelvic organ prolapse and pelvic floor dysfunction. Am J Obstet Gynecol. 1996;175(1):10–7. PubMed PMID: 8694033. Epub 1996/07/01. eng.

18. Oelrich T. The striated urogenital sphincter muscle in the female. Anat Rec. 1983;205:223–32.

19. DeLancey JO, Toglia MR, Perucchini D. Internal and external anal sphincter anatomy as it relates to midline obstetric lacerations. Obstet Gynecol. 1997;90:924.

20. Shobeiri SA, Chesson RR, Gasser RF. The internal innervation and morphology of the human female levator ani muscle. Am J Obstet Gynecol. 2008;199(6):686.e1–e6.

21. Hsu Y, Fenner DE, Weadock WJ, DeLancey JOL. Magnetic resonance imaging and 3-dimensional analysis of external anal sphincter anatomy. Obstet Gynecol. 2005;106(6):1259–65. PubMed PMID: 16319250. Pubmed Central PMCID: Source: NLM. NIHMS10240. Source: NLM. PMC1479222.

22. Lawson JO. Pelvic anatomy. I. Pelvic floor muscles. Ann R Coll Surg Engl. 1974;54:244.

23. Kearney R, Sawhney R, DeLancey JOL. Levator ani muscle anatomy evaluated by origin-insertion Pairs. Obstet Gynecol. 2004;104(1):168–73.

24. Margulies RU, Hsu Y, Kearney R, Stein T, Umek WH, DeLancey JOL. Appearance of the levator ani muscle subdivisions in magnetic resonance images. Obstet Gynecol. 2006;107(5):1064–9. PubMed PMID: 16648412. Pubmed Central PMCID: Source: NLM. NIHMS10237. Source: NLM. PMC1479224.

25. Shobeiri SA, Leclaire E, Nihira MA, Quiroz LH, O'Donoghue D. Appearance of the levator ani muscle subdivisions in endovaginal three-dimensional ultrasonography. Obstet Gynecol. 2009;114:66–72. PubMed PMID: 19546760.

26. Taverner D. An electromyographic study of the normal function of the external anal sphincter and pelvic diaphragm. Dis Colon Rectum. 1959;2:153.

27. Nichols DH, Milley PS, Randall CL. Significance of restoration of normal vaginal depth and axis. Obstet Gynecol. 1970;36:251.

28. Shobeiri SA, Rostaminia G, White DE, Quiroz LH. The determinants of minimal levator hiatus and their relationship to the puborectalis muscle and the levator plate. BJOG. 2012. doi:10.1111/1471-0528.12055

29. Guaderrama NM, Liu J, Nager CW, Pretorius DH, Sheean G, Kassab G, et al. Evidence for the innervation of pelvic floor muscles by the pudendal nerve. Obstet Gynecol. 2005;106(4):774–81. PubMed PMID: 16199635. English.

30. Wallner C, van Wissen J, Maas CP, Dabhoiwala N, DeRuiter MC, Lamers WH. The contribution of the levator ani nerve and the pudendal nerve to the innervation of the levator ani muscles; a study in human fetuses. Eur Urol. 2008;54:1136.

2D/3D Endovaginal and Endoanal Instrumentation and Techniques

2

S. Abbas Shobeiri

Learning Objectives
1. Understand the pelvic floor ultrasound instrumentation and techniques
2. Appreciate the capabilities and limitations of ultrasound equipment
3. Become familiarized with systems for performing meaningful 2D/3D endovaginal and endoanal ultrasound imaging and techniques
4. Learn how to use pelvic floor ultrasonography to make accurate and comprehensive diagnoses and guide therapeutic decisions

2.1 Introduction

Varying pelvic floor disorders require varying degrees of imaging for proper management. The pelvic floor is a complex structure functionally and anatomically. Muscles, nerves, and connective tissue all play a role in its proper functioning. Therefore, many factors, including birth-related trauma and age, play a role in pelvic floor dysfunctions. Despite much progress in the diagnosis of pelvic floor dysfunction, general practitioners in women's health are often not fully aware of the potential of pelvic floor ultrasonography. Although physical examination, cystoscopy, and urodynamics are main stays of pelvic floor diagnosis, cheap, simple, noninvasive 2D, 3D, or 4D office ultrasound is not in widespread use. It can be important to view all compartments of the pelvic floor in order to (1) find the causes of dysfunction, (2) plan treatment, and (3) evaluate outcomes. More and more clinical studies are reporting the value of a thorough pelvic floor ultrasound examination that includes endovaginal and endoanal as well as transperineal imaging. The benefits of high-resolution 3D imaging of pelvic floor structures are also being increasingly recognized. Ultrasound allows fast, multicompartmental assessment, facilitating optimal patient throughput. It allows for high-resolution assessment of the morphology and function of the different parts of the pelvic floor. It facilitates observation of the entire pelvic floor with minimal disruption to the natural condition of the structures. Preoperative evaluation may reveal more in-depth information about the nature of incontinence. It may help the practitioner visualize the position and mobility of the bladder neck and urethra, in combination with maneuvers like squeeze and Valsalva. To evaluate prolapse, cystocele, rectocele, and enterocele, postoperative evaluation may help ensure that corrective devices, such as tension-free vaginal tape (TVT) or mesh implants, are properly placed. The value of anal sphincter ultrasonography to

S.A. Shobeiri, M.D. (✉)
Female Pelvic Medicine and Reconstructive Surgery,
The University of Oklahoma Health Sciences Center,
WP 2410, 920 Stanton L. Young Blvd., Oklahoma
City, OK 73104, USA
e-mail: Abbas-shobeiri@ouhsc.edu

S.A. Shobeiri (ed.), *Practical Pelvic Floor Ultrasonography: A Multicompartmental Approach to 2D/3D/4D Ultrasonography of Pelvic Floor*, DOI 10.1007/978-1-4614-8426-4_2, © Springer Science+Business Media New York 2014

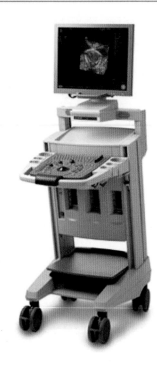

Fig. 2.1 A Pro Focus UltraView scanner

Table 2.1 UltraView specifications

Imaging modes: B, M, color Doppler, power Doppler, pulsed wave Doppler, tissue harmonic, contrast imaging

Features and options: vector flow imaging (VFI), 3D professional, 360° probe support, DICOM, HistoScanning™, remote control, 3 array connectors

Display: 19″ LCD flat monitor

Dimensions (approx): system height, 1,475–1,565 mm/58–62 in.; width, 525 mm/21 in.; depth, 765 mm/30 in.

Weight: 70 kg/154 lb

detect and evaluate anal sphincter tears and perianal fistulas is well established [1].

2.2 2D Transperineal and 3D Endovaginal and Endoanal Ultrasound Imaging

A fair amount of information can be obtained with an abdominal 2D concave probe that is placed on the perineum [2]. Additional information can be obtained by endovaginal and endoanal imaging. Analogic's BK Pro Focus UltraView (Fig. 2.1, Table 2.1) and Flex Focus are suited for this purpose. These systems offer high performance with efficiency and speed, a high-resolution

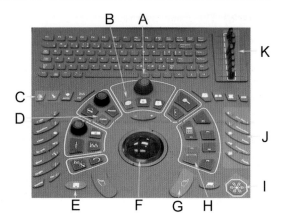

Fig. 2.2 The Pro Focus UltraView 2202 console. A: The general toggle control which amplifies or mutes the signal all across the screen. B: The most important button. Once your machine has your desired setting, the 3D button starts and stops scanning. C: For ID input and probe selection, D: for color Doppler, E: save button saves a video clip of specified duration or if the screen is frozen, an image is captured. F: Your mouse, G: the mouse click, H: for distance measurements, I: freeze button, J: buttons used for changing the depth of scanning, frequency, width, resolution, and range, K: the toggle buttons control selective amplification or muting of signals on the screen © SHOBEIRI 2013

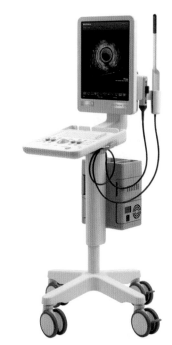

Fig. 2.3 A Flex Focus machine

19″ monitor, and a sensitive color Doppler with superb spatial resolution and sensitivity. The UltraView system (Fig. 2.2) has all the features

Table 2.2 Flex Focus specifications

Imaging modes: B, M, color Doppler, PW Doppler, tissue harmonic
Features and options: 3D 360° probe, DICOM, BK power pack
Display: 19″ LCD flat monitor
Dimensions (approx): system height, 1,350–1,602 mm/53–63 in.; keyboard height, 745–1,055 mm/29–41.5 in.; body width, 350 mm/14 in.; depth, 610 mm/24 in.
Weight: 49 kg/108 lb (excluding probes and printer), 7 kg/15 lb (imaging unit only)

Table 2.3 8802 probe specifications

8802 specifications	
Frequency range	4.3–6.0 MHz
Focal range (typical)	6–114 mm
Contact surface	52 × 8 mm
Disinfection	Immersion, sterile covers are available
Physical data (length × width)	100 × 60 mm
Weight (approx)	150 g (approx)

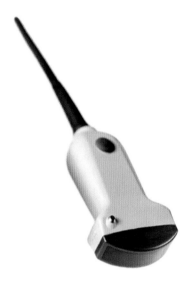

Fig. 2.4 8802 probe

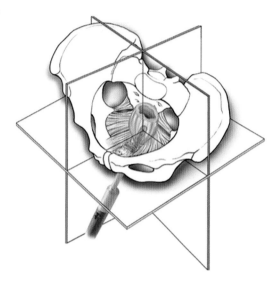

Fig. 2.5 *x*, *y*, *z* planes

such as HistoScanning™ capabilities, while Flex Focus (Fig. 2.3, Table 2.2) has a small footprint—fits in the tightest spaces—4 h plug-free imaging, innovative and easy to use, smooth, sealed keyboard for easy cleaning and disinfection. The ultrasound machine comes with state-of-the-art probes. Although there are probes for multiple principles, there are only two or three probes needed for pelvic floor imaging. These probes offer innovative design for access to all areas, advanced puncture guides, convenient one-button control, and easy sterilization and disinfection.

2.2.1   The 2D Probes

Although any available 2–8 MHz abdominal probe can be used for scanning of the pelvic floor, the images in this book are from a BK 8802 probe unless specified otherwise (Fig. 2.4, Table 2.3).

2.2.2   The 3D Endocavitary High-Resolution Probes

High-resolution 3D allows the automatic acquisition and construction of high-resolution data volumes by synthesis of a high number of parallel transaxial or radial 2D images, ensuring that true dimensions in all three *x*, *y*, and *z* planes are equivalent. The constructed data cube technique provides accurate distance, area, angle, and volume measurements. The volume rendering technique resulting from high-resolution 3D provides accurate visualization of the deeper structures. High-resolution endovaginal or endoanal anatomy can be obtained in 30–60 s. The scanned data set is also highly reproducible, with limited operator dependency. The probe can visualize all rectal wall layers; evaluate the radial, longitudinal extension of sphincter tears; and measure detailed pelvic floor architecture in all *x*, *y*, and *z* planes accurately (Fig. 2.5).

Table 2.4 2052 endocavitary 360° probe specifications

2052 specifications	
Frequency range	6–16 MHz
Focal range (typical)	Up to 50 mm
Sector angle	360°
Disinfection	Immersion
Physical data	Length: 542 mm
	Shaft length: 270 mm
	Handle width: 38.4 mm
	Shaft width: 17 mm
Weight (approx)	850 g (approx)

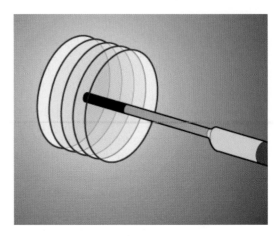

Fig. 2.7 2052 probe creates parallel axial images that are packaged to create a 3D volume

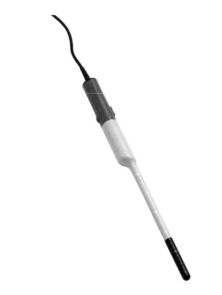

Fig. 2.6 2052 probe

2052 Endocavitary 360° Probe

The 2052 probe (Table 2.4, Fig. 2.6) has an internal automated motorized system that allows an acquisition of 300 aligned transaxial 2D images over a distance of 60 mm every 0.2 mm in 60 s, without any movement of the probe within the cavity (Fig. 2.7). The probe has buttons on the handle that allows manual control of the probe (Fig. 2.8). The set of 2D images is instantaneously reconstructed into a high-resolution 3D image for real-time manipulation and volume rendering. The 3D volume can also be archived for offline analysis on the ultrasonographic system or on PC with the help of dedicated 3D Viewer software. The main limitation of this probe is the total length of the probe of 54 cm.

Although the probe is also used by colorectal surgeons for staging of rectal tumors which necessitates the length, in pelvic floor imaging, the length may create anxiety for the patients. For pelvic floor imaging, the length requires keeping the hand in a stable position to avoid image distortion. From the methodological point of view, mechanical character of the probe does not allow to obtain the same resolution in all sections, only the axial section (the section of acquisition) has the best quality, and all other sections coming from post-processing of the 3D volume data set have lower resolution.

8848 Endocavitary Biplane Probe

Broad views of anterior and posterior compartments for functional and anatomical studies may be obtained using the 8848 probe (Table 2.5, Fig. 2.9). To obtain quick views of the anterior and posterior compartments, this probe can be rotated manually, but to obtain reproducible 180° 3D measurements, the 8848 probe can be installed on an external mover (Fig. 2.10). The probe has two buttons on the handle that allows for selection of axial or sagittal scanning. It provides detailed high-resolution biplane with 6.5 cm linear and convex views. One can obtain 3D volumes by manually rotating hand 180° when in sagittal mode or withdrawing the hand 6.5 cm when scanning the urethra or the rectum vaginally. However, these 3D volumes are not accurate if measurement

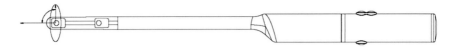

Fig. 2.8 The 2052 probe has two buttons on the handle anteriorly that allows manual pilot of the scanner elements within the probe. The button posteriorly activates the probe or freezes the image on the screen

Table 2.5 8848 180° probe specification

8848 specifications	
Frequency range	5–12 MHz
Focal range (typical)	3–60 mm
Frame rate/td>	>150
Disinfection	Immersion, STERIS SYSTEM 1*, STERIS SYSTEM 1E, STERRAD 50,100S and 200
Scanning modes	B,M, Doppler, BCFM, tissue harmonic imaging
Contact surface (overall)	Transverse: 127 mm², sagittal: 357 mm²
Image field (expanded)	180°(transverse)
Weight (approx)	250 g

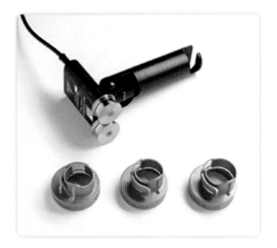

Fig. 2.10 The external mover elements for 8848 probe

Table 2.6 8838 endocavitary 360° probe specification

2D frequency (MHz)	12–6
Doppler frequency (MHz)	7.5–6.5
Tissue harmonic imaging frequency (MHz)	10
Contrast imaging frequency (MHz)	4
Image field	65 mm wide acoustic surface able to rotate 360°
2D penetration depth (mm)	82–85
Footprint (mm)	65 × 5.5

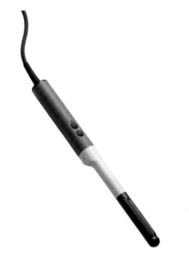

Fig. 2.9 8848 probe

of structures is the desired endpoint. To obtain consistent 3D volumes, a 3D mover needs to be utilized.

8838 Endocavitary 360° Probe

8838 is similar to 8848 probe, but all the mechanisms are internalized (Table 2.6, Fig. 2.11). The probe is world's first electronic probe for endovaginal and endoanal imaging with built-in high-resolution 3D capabilities. The probe has built-in linear array which rotates 360° inside the probe. The probe has no need for additional accessories or movers; no moving parts come in contact with the patient. The probe has capability for dynamic 2D (Fig. 2.12) and 3D scanning (Fig. 2.13). The probe has wide frequency range 12–6 MHz, with the same excellent imaging capabilities across all frequencies. Probe has a slim 16 mm (0.6) diameter for more comfortable

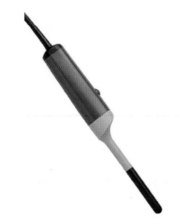

Fig. 2.11 8838 probe

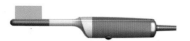

Fig. 2.12 8838 set at scanning at 12:00 o'clock position for dynamic imaging of the bladder

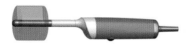

Fig. 2.13 The 8838 probe elements move within the shaft radially to create a 3D data volume

patient imaging with an easy grip to hold and manipulate. Unlike 2052 probe's long profile which was designed with staging of colorectal cancers in mind, the 8838 is short and less threatening to the patients.

The 8838 probe allows an acquisition of radial 2D images without any movement of the probe within the cavity. The set of 2D images is instantaneously reconstructed into a high-resolution 3D image for real-time manipulation and volume rendering. The 3D volume can also be archived for offline analysis using BK PC software.

2.2.3 BK 3D Viewer Software

The 3D volume can be used on the scanner, but the ease of use and functionality is better when the free software is installed on any PC (Fig. 2.14). The available functions are lined to the right, bottom, and the left side of the screen. One can scan any patient and export their data files to a CD, DVD, USB, external hard drive, or a server and then view them at any time, on any PC. This is akin to the virtual examination of the patient. The work can be saved and reproduced with ease. On the left side there is an "eye" icon where you can create "memory points." By clicking on the eye icon, you save the 3D view and find it easily

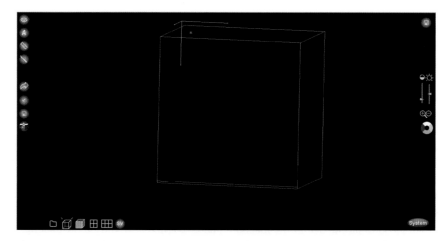

Fig. 2.14 The screen view of BK 3D software. The empty 3D wire frame is seen in the center with control icons all around it © SHOBEIRI 2013

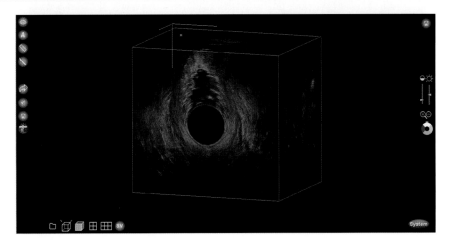

Fig. 2.15 The "eye icon" saves your screen shot and creates a menu of images of interest for future reference © SHOBEIRI 2013

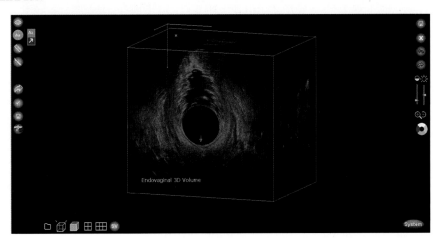

Fig. 2.16   The annotation and arrow icon allows for marking of the structures on the screen © SHOBEIRI 2013

for documentation or research purposes at a later time (Fig. 2.15). Below the "eye icon" is the annotation and arrow icon for writing and marking structures on the 3D volumes (Fig. 2.16). The third icon on the left is the measurement icon. You can obtain linear measurement, angle, area, and volume measurements. When in the measurement mode, additional icons appear on the upper right side that allows to undo or delete all your measurements (Fig. 2.17). The fourth icon on the upper left of the screen is the sculpting icon. One can cut the structures out (Fig. 2.18) or cut the inner structures (Fig. 2.19). Alternately, a structure could be isolated all together (Fig. 2.20). The next 4 icons on the middle left of

the screen are for taking snapshots, including the wire frame, removing the personal data, and saving the volumes (Fig. 2.14). On the right side of the screen, there are two icons for adjusting the brightness and the hue. There is also an icon for changing the volume color to soft yellow, blue, or green (Fig. 2.21). On the bottom of the screen, there are icons for opening files, obtaining rendered views (Fig. 2.22). Volume render mode is a technique for the analysis of the information inside 3D volume by digital enhancing individual voxels. It is currently one of the most advanced and computer-intensive rendering algorithm available for computed tomography and can also be applied to high-resolution 3D US data volume.

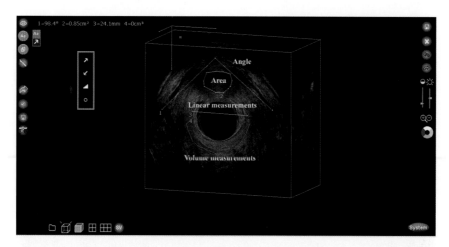

Fig. 2.17 The measurement icon allows very useful functions such as angle, area, linear, or area/volume measurements © SHOBEIRI 2013

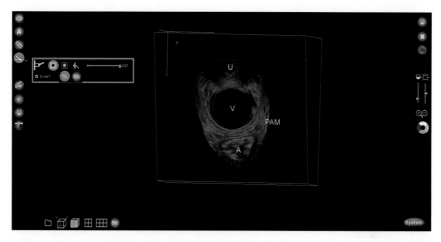

Fig. 2.18 The sculpting icon opens a window with multiple capabilities. Here the puboanalis muscle is isolated. *U* urethra, *V* vagina, *A* anus, *PAM* puboanalis muscle © SHOBEIRI 2013

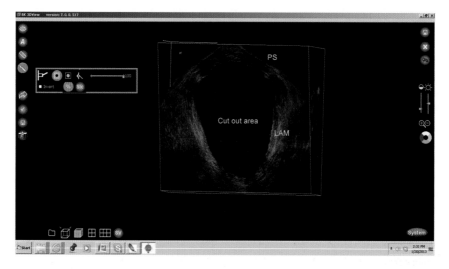

Fig. 2.19 The sculpting icon opens a window with multiple capabilities. Here the minimal levator hiatus is cut out leaving the surrounding levator ani muscles (LAM) © SHOBEIRI 2013

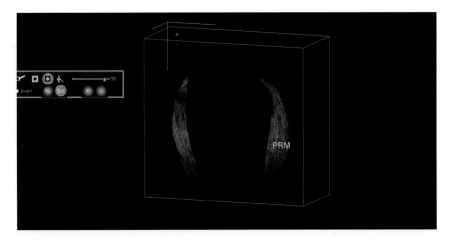

Fig. 2.20 The sculpting icon opens a window with multiple capabilities. Here everything but the puborectalis muscle (PRM) is cut out © SHOBEIRI 2013

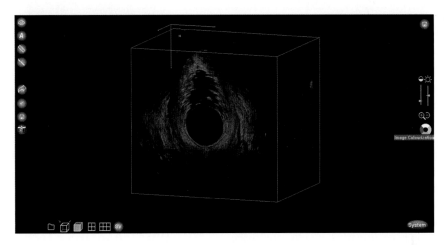

Fig. 2.21 The two icons on *upper right side* have toggle capabilities to adjust the brightness and the hue. The four-colored circle controls the desired color. Here the image is colored in *soft yellow* © SHOBEIRI 2013

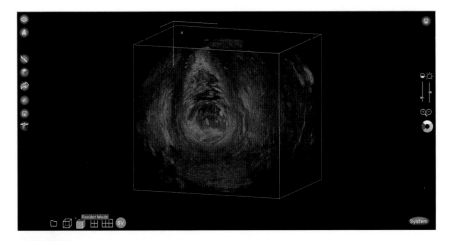

Fig. 2.22 The screen view of BK 3D software. The rendered endovaginal frame is seen in the center with control icons all around it. The icons on the *bottom left* of the screen from *left* to *right* are open file, normal view, rendered view, 4 shots, and 6 shots view © SHOBEIRI 2013

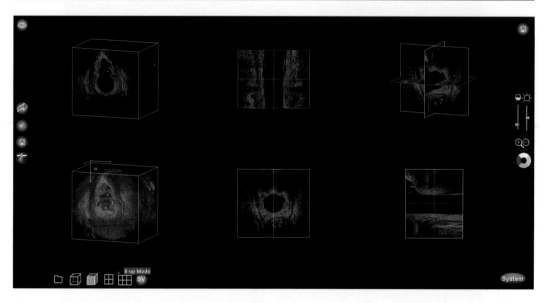

Fig. 2.23 The screen view of BK 3D software. The 6 shot view or the 6-up mode is a very useful tool as many functions can be carried out simultaneously © SHOBEIRI 2013

The typical ray-/beam-tracing algorithm sends a ray/beam from each point (pixel) of the viewing screen through the 3D space rendered. The beam passing through the volume data reaches the different elements (voxels) in the data set. Depending on the various render mode settings, the data from each voxel may be stored as a referral for the next voxel and further used in a filtering calculation, may be discarded, or may modify the existing value of the beam. The final displayed pixel color is computed from the color, transparency, and reflectivity of all the volumes and surfaces encountered by the beam. The weighted summation of these images produces the volume-rendered view. The render mode is useful for visualization of tapes and meshes that may seem isoechoic due to dense tissue ingrowth. The dark colors appear darker and the light colors appear lighter in rendered mode and anything in between has lesser intensity.

There are two icons that can give four or six concurrent views on the screen (Fig. 2.23). This is an interactive screen, and as the *x*, *y*, and *z* planes are moved on the upper right, all the other views adjust automatically to let the viewer know exactly what they are viewing. One important feature of BK 3D software is that analysis is not restricted to axial, coronal, and sagittal planes. The planes can be tilted

(Fig. 2.24) to follow the structures to their insertion points. This corrects for any operator error that may have occurred during acquisition. Multiple planes can be manipulated at once (Fig. 2.25).

2.3 Multicompartmental Ultrasonographic Techniques

2.3.1 Patient Positioning

During examination, the patient may be placed in the dorsal lithotomy, in the left lateral or in the prone position. The patient's positioning depends on cultural factors, local acceptable practices, physician's specialty, and equipment availability. In the United States urogynecologists perform pelvic examination in dorsal lithotomy position. At our institution, the pelvic floor ultrasound including endoanal examinations are performed in dorsal lithotomy position. This position allows symmetrical acquisition of ultrasound volumes regardless of being done endovaginally or endoanally [3, 4].

Imaging of the pelvic floor can be done in one or combination of the following five steps depending on the patient's presenting symptoms (Fig. 2.26).

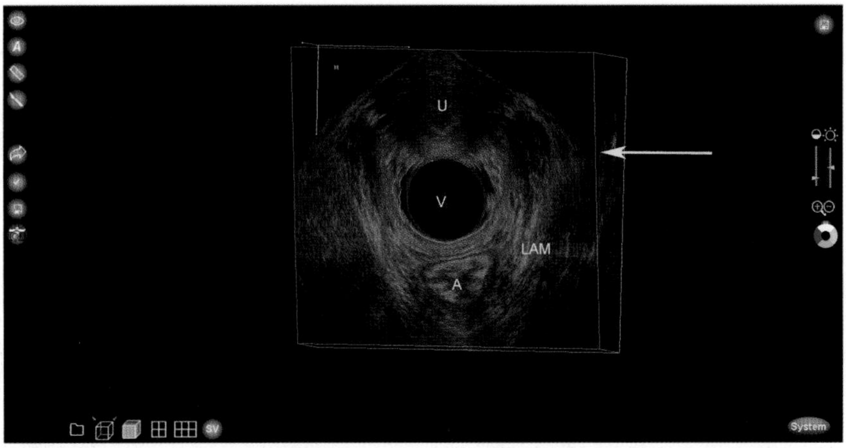

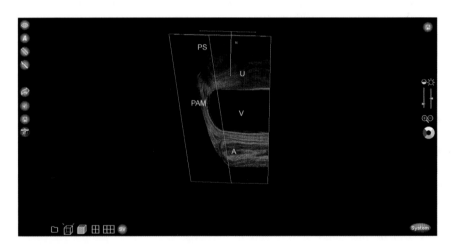

Fig. 2.24 One unique function of the BK software is the capability to twist the planes to follow the structure in axial, sagittal, or coronal planes. While twisting the planes the wire frame turns red to denote the action. The urethra (U), vagina (V), and the anus (A) are marked. The *yellow arrow* points to the tilting of the frame in axial view © SHOBEIRI 2013

Fig. 2.25 Multiple functions can be performed at once. Here the data volume that has been sculpted to cut out the puborectalis muscle and isolate the puboanalis muscle (PAM) is rotated in right midsagittal view to show the length of the urethra (U), vagina (V), and anus (A). PS is the pubic symphysis © SHOBEIRI 2013

2.3.2 2D Transperineal Functional Imaging

Indications: Enterocele, Rectocele, Cystocele, Mesh, Slings.

The probe surface is covered with gel and a nonpowdered glove or cover before it can be placed on the perineum between the labia. The symphysis pubis is seen anteriorly. Sequentially, the urethra, vagina, and the anal canal and the levator plate are seen anteriorly to posteriorly. A good-quality image contains both the symphysis pubis and the levator plate. The scanning is performed in the lithotomy position with a comfortable volume in the bladder. Generally if the patient is asked to empty her bladder, by the time scanning is started, sufficient volume is in the bladder to differentiate the structures. High bladder volume may prevent prolapse from manifesting itself. If needed, the patient can be asked to stand up for scanning.

Bladder neck descent (BND) can be measured in rest and maximum Valsalva; however, no definition of normal exists. Although funneling may be

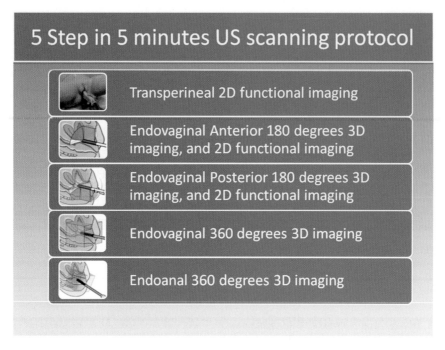

Fig. 2.26 Five steps for performing pelvic floor ultrasound © SHOBEIRI 2013

seen during ultrasonography, no clear ultrasound definition is available.

Transperineal ultrasound is most useful for indirect assessment of pelvic floor function. Measuring the distance from the symphysis pubis to the levator plate gives the anterior posterior (AP) measurement of the minimal levator hiatus which can be measured at rest and in Valsalva.

Different forms of cystocele can be identified, but the cervix is difficult to appreciate due to its hypoechoic nature. The imaging is very useful posteriorly as a high rectocele can be differentiated from a sigmoidocele and a low rectocele from a perineocele.

The patient is asked to empty the bladder. By the time you start imaging, she will have enough urine in the bladder to make the bladder hypoechoic. You can use a glove or an unlubricated ultrasound gel-filled condom/probe cover. Place ample water-soluble gel on the probe and place on the perineum or between the labia while paying attention to the screen (Fig. 2.27). The probe is placed on the perineum

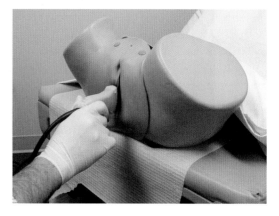

Fig. 2.27 The patient position and the 8802 probe position during transperineal scanning © SHOBEIRI 2013

and between the labia (Fig. 2.28) such that the image on the screen appears as if the patient is standing up facing the right side of the screen (Fig. 2.29). General guidelines for the settings are shown in Table 2.7. You can obtain measurements with resting, Valsalva and squeeze for the distance from the edge of the pubic symphysis to the edge of the levator plate that

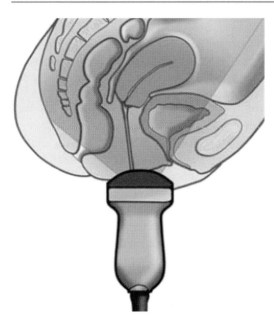

Fig. 2.28 This view demonstrates Incorrect positioning as the starting 2D field of view should include pubic symphysis anteriorly and the anorectal angle posteriorly. The field of view as demonstrated does not contain the pubic symphysis, and as such the distance from the edge of the pubic symphysis to the edge of the levator plate that creates the anorectal angle cannot be obtained. Depending on the patient's body habitus and pelvic floor laxity, the field of view may need to be made larger

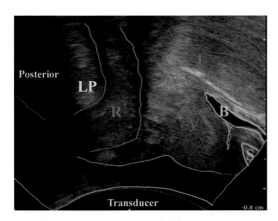

Fig. 2.29 This view demonstrates CORRECT positioning as the starting 2D field of view includes the pubic symphysis (S) anteriorly and the levator plate (LP) posteriorly. Also noted are the bladder (B), uterus (U), vagina (V), and anorectum (R) © SHOBEIRI 2013

Table 2.7 Describes the sample steps for performing transperineal 2D imaging using any abdominal probe

8802 transperineal imaging
Identify the 8802 transducer
Identify the probe orientation
Press the button on the side of the probe to activate the probe
Set the depth at 6.7 cm
Set the resolution at 1/32 Hz
Place the transducer on the perineal area and obtain sagittal view of the bladder, vagina, and the rectum (including the midsagittal view of pubic symphysis)
Adjust the gain
Ask the subject to cough or bear down to visualize the movement of anterior, apical, and posterior compartments
If you want the video clip of the action, press the DISK button which records the action for the past 10 s
Ask the subject to "squeeze vaginal muscles or perform Kegels" to visualize the movement of the levator plate
If you want the video clip of the action, press the DISK button which records the action for the past 10 s
In this example an 8802 probe is used

creates the anorectal angle. This has been shown to correlate well with levator function.

2.3.3   2D/3D Endovaginal Anterior Compartment Imaging

Indications: Voiding dysfunction, Enterocele, Cystocele, Location of mesh and slings, Anterior vaginal masses and cysts, Fistulas.

There are two BK probes available for this purpose, the 8848 (Fig. 2.30) and 8838 (Fig. 2.31). You can use an unlubricated ultrasound gel-filled condom/probe cover. Place ample water-soluble gel on the probe and place in the vagina (Fig. 2.32). 2D dynamic view of the urethra and bladder comes to view (Fig. 2.33). The measurement protocol for 8848 probe is in Table 2.8. Measurements of the urethral structures or any visible mesh or sling can be obtained (Fig. 2.34). Although bladder funneling can be visualized, this may be impeded by the presence of probe in the vagina [2, 5, 6].

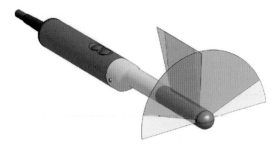

Fig. 2.30 8848 probe. Demonstrating 180° axial and sagittal planes

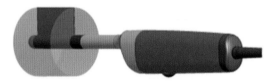

Fig. 2.31 8838 probe. Demonstrating the 360° rotation. The probe can be programmed to obtain 180° anterior or posterior 3D volume acquisition if this is desired

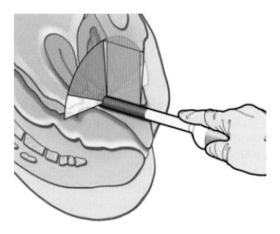

Fig. 2.32 8848 probe vaginal placement. The probe is generally advanced cephalad to the vesicourethral junction for image acquisition. Slight posterior pressure is desired when patient is prompted to cough or Valsalva

2.3.4   2D/3D Endovaginal Posterior Compartment Imaging

Indications: Defecatory dysfunction, Constipation, Intussusception, Sigmoidocele, Enterocele, Rectocele, Perineocele, Mesh, Posterior vaginal masses and cysts, Fistulas.

The same two BK probes, the 8848 and 8838, used for anterior imaging can be used for poste-

rior imaging as well. You can use an unlubricated ultrasound gel-filled condom/probe cover. Place ample water-soluble gel on the probe and place in the vagina (Fig. 2.35). 2D dynamic view of the anal canal and the levator plate comes to view (Fig. 2.36). The measurement protocol for 8848 probe is in Table 2.9. Measurements of the external anal sphincter, internal anal sphincter, and any visible mesh can be obtained (Fig. 2.37). If EAS and IAS are abnormal by endovaginal ultrasound, follow-up study by endoanal ultrasound should be performed if the patient has anal incontinence. Ask the patient to squeeze and Valsalva to visualize any high rectocele, enterocele, sigmoidocele, or intussusception. Visualization of a low rectocele may be impeded by the presence of probe in the vagina.

2.3.5   3D 360 Endovaginal Imaging

Indications: Mesh, Vaginal masses and cysts, Levator ani muscle subdivisions and defects.

3D endovaginal US may be performed with 2052 or 8838 probe or a radial electronic probe (type AR 54 AW, frequency: 5–10 MHz, Hitachi Medical Systems, Japan) to be discussed in chapter on emerging technologies. Since the Hitachi probe is withdrawn by hand, the measurements are not reliable (more about the Hitachi probe in emerging technology chapter).

Before the probe is inserted into the vagina, a gel-containing condom is placed over the probe. Any air bubbles are removed by squeezing the gel-filled condom downward (Fig. 2.38). Water-soluble lubricant is placed on the exterior of the cover, and the probe is advanced to the vesicourethral junction (Fig. 2.39). The probe should be inserted easily and gently (Fig. 2.40). If any pain is experienced, the procedure should be stopped.

Using 2052 probe, the pubic symphysis and the urethra are anterior, the levator ani lateral, and the anus posterior (Fig. 2.39). Generally starting the scanning from the vesicourethral junction will continue 6 cm caudad to include the perineal body (Fig. 2.41). The protocol for scanning with 2052 probe is in Table 2.10. In

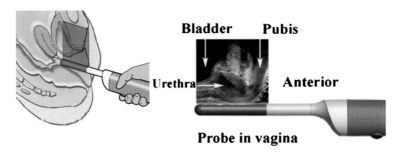

Fig. 2.33 Composite of anterior compartment imaging with 8838 probe. To the *right* the image as seen on the screen is demonstrated. The probe is advanced to the vesicourethral junction to visualize the full length of the urethra © SHOBEIRI 2013

Table 2.8 Describes the sample steps for performing endovaginal 2D/3D imaging using an 8848 probe

8848 endovaginal anterior imaging
Identify 8848 probe and attach the mechanical mover
Press the button on the probe to activate it
Confirm setting at 12 MHz
Insert the probe with the grooves on the transducer pointing anteriorly
Identify the depth on the upper right-hand side of the screen as 5.6 cm
Identify bladder, urethra, and the pubic symphysis
You can freeze the view and visualize periurethral structures and obtain urethral measurements
Press the probe posteriorly and ask the patient to Valsalva to visualize bladder neck funneling
Press the 3D button
Position the selection box on the screen to the desired area for 3D acquisition
Identify the resolution as 1/34 Hz
Identify the extent at 179°
Set spacing at every 0.3°
Acknowledge the time needed for scanning
Push the 3D button on the machine to activate probe rotation
This concludes 3D imaging of the anterior compartment

patients with perineal descensus, two overlapping 3D ultrasound volumes may need to be obtained. The 2052 probe generally obtains adequate images of the anterior and posterior compartment, but since the 2D images are in axial plane, dynamic imaging of the anterior and posterior compartments cannot be performed. Also, the sagittal images are less clear than the ones obtained by 8838.

Using 8838 probe, the bladder and the urethra are visualized in sagittal orientation on the screen. Advance the probe until vesicourethral junction is visualized and follow the protocol on Table 2.11. The probe rotates internally 360° (Fig. 2.42). Not only the 8838 probe obtains excellent views of anterior and posterior compartment, it has internalized rotational mechanism and is capable of dynamic imaging of anterior and posterior compartments. The levator ani appears different from that of 2052, and the views in axial view are pixelated. We run a protocol of imaging 360° every 0.55° in 30.8 s to obtain 655 frames. Again it is important to keep the hand and the elbow holding the probe steadied on a support such as own knees or a cushion while the other hand runs the controls on the console (Fig. 2.43). During endocavitary imaging the patients may be tempted to talk to alleviate their anxiety. It is important to calm the patients, let them know what is happening, and share with them that during scanning their talking and body movements may distort the desired image acquisition [4, 7].

2.3.6 3D 360 Endoanal Imaging

Indications: Perianal masses and cysts, Perianal fistulas, Anal sphincter injury.

3D endoanal US may be performed with 2052 or 8838 probes or a radial electronic probe (type AR 54 AW, frequency: 5–10 MHz, Hitachi Medical Systems, Japan) to be discussed in chapter on emerging technologies. Since the Hitachi probe is hand drawn, repeatable measurements may not be obtained.

Before the probe is inserted into the anus, a gel-containing condom is placed over the probe.

a

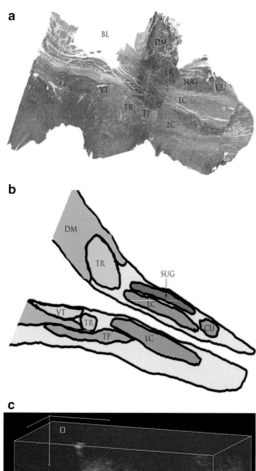

b

c

Fig. 2.34 The view of the *left side* of the anterior compartment: (**a**) histologic section, (**b**) drawing of the anterior compartment structures, and (**c**) the left sagittal view of the 3D EVUS cube with the structures marked. *BL* bladder, *CU* compressor urethra, *LCM* longitudinal and circular layer, *P* pubic bone, *PCF* pubocervical fascia, *SUG* striated urogenital sphincter, *TP* trigonal plate, *TR* trigonal ring, *U* urethra, *UT* uterus, *V* vagina, *VT* vesical trigone. From © Shobeiri, IUGJ

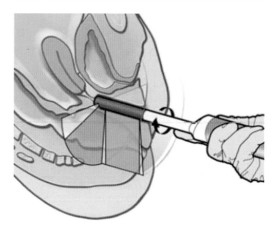

Fig. 2.35 8848 probe vaginal placement. The probe is generally advanced until the perineal body is to the *right* of the screen prior to image acquisition. Slight anterior pressure is desired when patient is prompted to cough or Valsalva

Any air bubbles are removed by squeezing the gel-filled condom downward. Water-soluble lubricant is placed on the exterior of the condom. The probe should be inserted easily and gently. If any pain is experienced, the procedure should be stopped (Fig. 2.44). The probe is pushed to the cephalad edge of the levator plate and the 3D button is pushed on the console.

Using 2052 probe, the anterior aspect of the anal canal is superior (12 o'clock) on the screen, right lateral is left (9 o'clock), left lateral is right (3 o'clock), and posterior is inferior (6 o'clock). The length of recorded data should extend from the upper aspect of the "U"-shaped sling of the levator plate to the anal verge [8, 9].

Using 8838 probe, the probe is inserted until the perineal body is anterior and to the right of the screen. You will visualize the midsagittal view of the rectovaginal septum as you advance the probe (Fig. 2.40) and follow the protocol on Table 2.11. The 8838 probe obtains excellent views of the anal sphincter complex. However, since there are no axial reference points and also because the images appear rendered, it has a

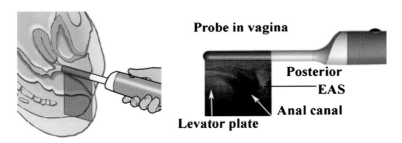

Fig. 2.36 Composite of posterior compartment imaging with 8838 probe. To the *right* the image as seen on the screen is demonstrated. The probe is advanced until the perineal body/EAS complex is visualized to the *right* of the screen © SHOBEIRI 2013

Table 2.9 Describes the sample steps for performing posterior compartment endovaginal 2D/3D imaging using an 8848 probe

8848 endovaginal posterior imaging
Identify 8848 probe and attach the mechanical mover
Press the button on the probe to activate it
Confirm setting at 12 MHz
Insert the probe with the grooves on the transducer pointing posteriorly
Identify the depth on the upper right-hand side of the screen as 4.9 cm
Identify external anal sphincter, internal anal sphincter, and the levator plate
Ask the patient to perform a Kegel to view levator plate movement
Ask patient to first perform Valsalva to view intussusception, rectocele, or inability to relax the levator plate
Press the 3D button
Position the selection box on the screen to the desired area for 3D acquisition
Identify the resolution as 1/34 Hz
Identify the extent at 179°
Set spacing at every 0.3°
Acknowledge the time needed for scanning
Push the 3D button on the machine to activate probe rotation
This concludes 3D imaging of the anterior compartment

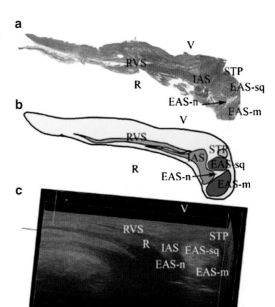

Fig. 2.37 The view of the *left side* of the posterior compartment: (**a**) histologic section, (**b**) drawing of the posterior compartment structures, and (**c**) the left sagittal view of the 3D EVUS volume with the structures marked. *EAS-m* external anal sphincter main section, *EAS-n* external anal sphincter notch, *EAS-sq* external anal sphincter subcutaneous section, *IAS* internal anal sphincter, *IAS-L* internal anal sphincter length, *IAS-T* internal anal sphincter thickness, *R* rectum, *RS* rectovaginal septum, *STP* superficial transverse perinei, *V* vagina. From © Shobeiri, IUGJ

Fig. 2.38 Application of
probe cover to a 2052
probe. Adequate removal
of air bubbles is manda-
tory. Ample gel is applied
to the outside of the cover
© SHOBEIRI 2013

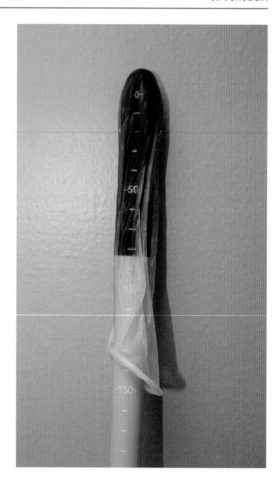

Fig. 2.39 2052 probe
vaginal placement. The
probe is generally advanced
until the vesicourethral
junction is viewed. Pressing
the 3D button will obtain a
serious of axial images
which will be packaged as a
3D volume

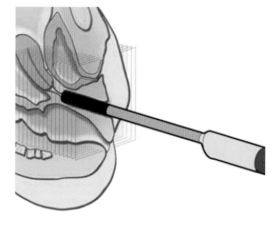

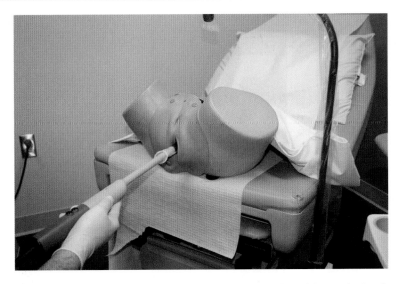

Fig. 2.40 Correct placement of an endovaginal probe. The hand is kept steady and the arm is placed on the knee or an elbow rest while the 3D volumes are being obtained © SHOBEIRI 2013

moderate learning curve. While with 2052 the axial images are displayed on the screen and the operator has an idea about the integrity of the anal complex, with 8838 the data volume has to be manipulated after data acquisition to obtain useful information. 8838s internalized rotational mechanism and good tissue penetration may visualize the entire levator ani muscle as long as there is no air in the rectum and if some gel is placed in the vagina (Fig. 2.45). However, if avulsion of the levator ani is the point of interest, an anal probe will place the operator further from the site of defect which is the site of the levator ani attachment to the pubic bone.

The levator ani also may appear different from that of 2052 and the views in axial view are pixelated. With either 2052 or 8838 probe used endoanally, the images appear similar (Fig. 2.46) (in publication).

2.4   Summary

Ultrasound visualization of pelvic floor structures requires a multicompartmental approach. Knowledge of anatomy, functionality of different probes, and capabilities of ultrasound machine used is essential for acquisition of meaningful images.

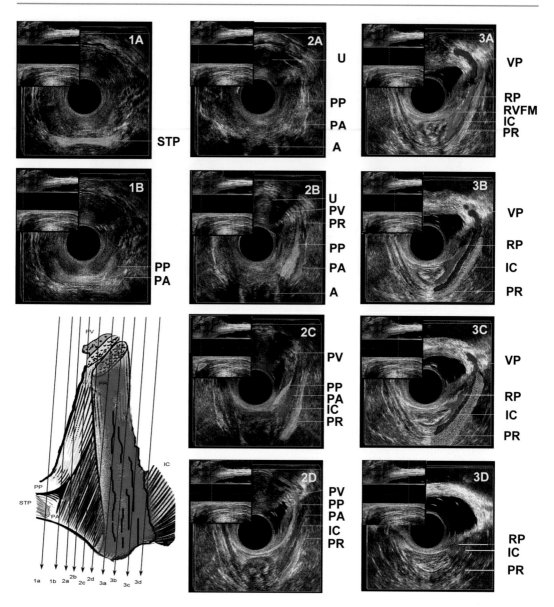

Fig. 2.41 Levator ani subdivisions seen at different levels. Midline structures are identified in lateral views with corresponding colors in the picture inserts at the *upper left* corner of the ultrasound images at each level. The relative position of levator ani subdivisions during ultrasound imaging: levels 1A–3D are identified in the figure insert. The *green vertical line* in the insert corresponds to the relative position in the vagina where the image is obtained. (**a**) Level 1A: at 0 cm, the first muscle seen is superficial transverse perinei (STP) (*green*) with mixed echogenicity. (**b**) Level 1B: immediately cephalad to superficial transverse perinei is puboperinealis (PP) (*yellow*) that can be traced to pubic bone (PB) with manipulation of 3D volume. It comes in at a 45° angle as a mixed echoic band to join the perineal body. Lateral to it, the puboanalis (PA) is seen as a hypoechoic triangle (*pink*). (**c**) Level 2A: this level marks the attachment of the muscles to the pubic

arch. The external urethral meatus (U) is visible (*dark red*). Puboperinealis and puboanalis insertions are highlighted. The anus (A) is marked. (**d**) Level 2B: (PV) pubovaginalis (*blue*) and (PR) puborectalis (*mustard*) insertion come to view. The urethra and the bladder are outlined (*red*) in the lateral view. (**e**) Level 2C: the heart-shape vaginal sulcus (outlined in *red*) marks the pubovaginalis insertion. (IC) Iliococcygeus fibers (*red*) come into view. Perineal body is outlined in the lateral view. (**f**) Level 2D: puboanalis is starting to thin out. Puborectalis is seen in the lateral view. (**g**) Level 3A: puboperinealis and puboanalis become obscure. Anatomically, puboanalis becomes a thick fibromuscularis layer forming a tendineus sheet, rectal pillar (RP). Perivesical venous plexus (VP) are prominent (*purple*). Rectovaginal fibromuscularis (RVFM) is shown (*green*) in sagittal view as a continuous mixed echogenic structure approaching the perineal body

Table 2.10 Describes the sample steps for performing endovaginal 3D imaging of the pelvic floor using a 2052 probe

2052 endovaginal 360° imaging
Identify the 2052 transducer
Set the depth at 3.9 cm
Press the button on the probe to activate the transducer
Press the 3D button
Insert the probe to the 5–6 cm mark at the hymenal level
Visualize the vesicourethral junction
Identify the extent as 60 mm and the spacing at 0.2 mm
Confirm the time required for scanning
Press the 3D button
Maximize the box to be scanned to the desired position
Press the 3D button
Keep your hand steady and level while performing the ultrasound imaging

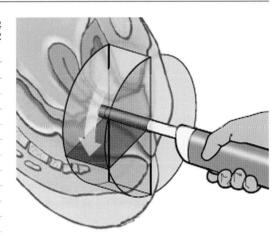

Fig. 2.42 8838 probe vaginal placement. The probe is generally advanced until the vesicourethral junction is viewed. Pressing the 3D button will obtain radial images of the pelvic floor which will be packaged as a 3D volume

Table 2.11 Describes the sample steps for performing endovaginal anterior, posterior, and lateral 3D imaging of the pelvic floor using an 8838 probe

8838 endovaginal anterior, posterior, lateral imaging
Identify 8838 probe
Press the button on the probe to activate it
Identify the depth on the upper right-hand side of the screen as 5.6 cm
Identify bladder, urethra, and the pubic symphysis and withdraw the probe until vesicourethral junction is visible to the left side of the screen
Set imaging for every 0.55°
Set the rotation at 360°
Press the 3D button
Position the selection box on the screen to the desired area for 3D acquisition
Acknowledge the time needed for scanning
Push the 3D button on the machine to activate probe rotation
Keep the hand steady and level while performing the ultrasound imaging
If the patient has perineal descensus, the perineal body may not be included in your 3D volume. Withdraw the probe slightly and redo the steps
This concludes 3D imaging of the anterior, posterior, and lateral compartments

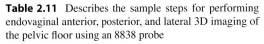

Fig. 2.41 (continued) and laterally attaching to RP. (h) Level 3B: rectal pillar (orange) is easily seen. The iliococcygeus becomes prominent and widens. (i) Level 3C: the iliococcygeus widens further and inserts into arcus tendineus fascia pelvis (ATFP). (j) Level 3D: puborectalis and fade out of view. Puborectalis (mustard) and iliococcygeus (red) are outlined in the lateral view showing their entire course. Adapted from © Shobeiri, Obstet and Gynecol 2009

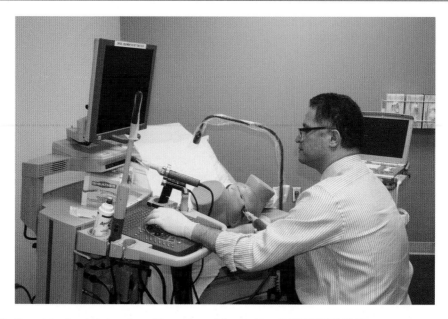

Fig. 2.43 Correct two handed operation of the probe and the machine © SHOBEIRI 2013

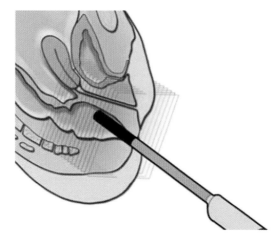

Fig. 2.44 Advancement of an endoanal probe requires initial acute angle entry. Subsequently the hand to be readjusted such that the ultrasound rays are perpendicular to the external anal sphincter fibers

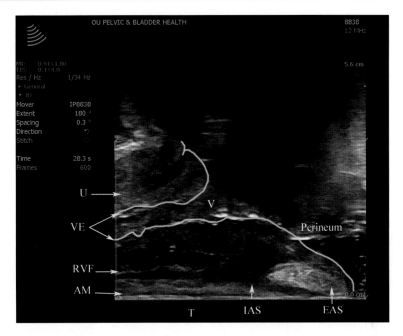

Fig. 2.45 8838 view of the perineal area upon anal entry. The external anal sphincter (EAS), internal anal sphincter (IAS), probe in the anorectum (T), anal mucosa (AM), rectovaginal fascia (RVF), vaginal epithelium (VE), urethra (U), and the vagina are marked (V) © SHOBEIRI 2013

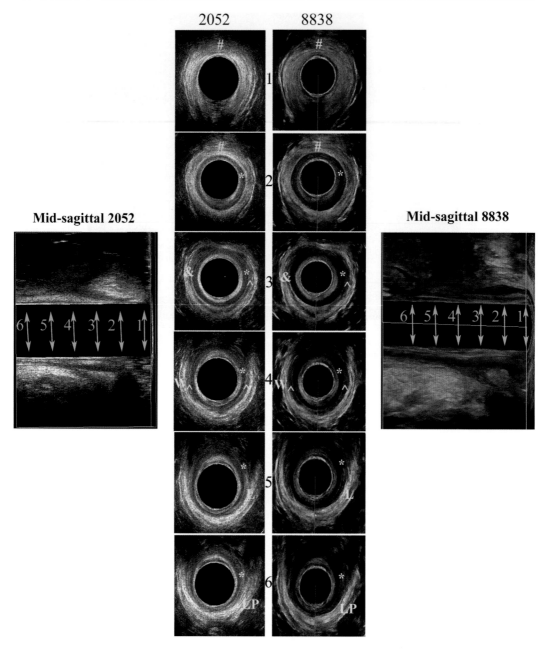

Fig. 2.46 Endoanal views of the levator plate and anal complex at different levels. The images to the *right* are from 8838 and the ones to the *left* from 2052. The axial images are placed side by side at levels 1–6 for comparison. 1. The subcutaneous part of the EAS is visualized with # mark. 2. The first hyperechoic layer, from inner to outer, corresponds to the interface of the probe with the anal mucosal surface; the second hyperechoic layer adjacent to the probe is the subepithelial tissue. Immediately adjacent to it is the internal anal sphincter (IAS) marked with *. The IAS merges with the circular muscle of the rectum, extending from the anorectal junction to approximately 1 cm below the dentate line. 3. The fourth main part of EAS is marked with &. 4. The winged portion of the EAS is marked with W. The longitudinal muscle (LM) has mixed echogenicity and is marked with ^. 5. The puborectalis fibers are seen winging out marked with L. 6. The levator plate fibers are seen winging out marked with LP © SHOBEIRI 2013

References

1. Haylen BT, De Ridder D, Freeman RM, Swift SE, Berghmans B, Lee JH, et al. An international urogynecological association (IUGA)/international continence society (ICS) joint report on the terminology for female pelvic floor dysfunction. Int Urogynecol J Pelvic Floor Dysfunct. 2010;21:5–26.

2. Stankiewicz A, Wieczorek AP, Wozniak MM, Bogusiewicz M, Futyma K, Santoro GA, et al. Comparison of accuracy of functional measurements of the urethra in transperineal vs. endovaginal ultrasound in incontinent women. Pelviperineology. 2008;27:145–7.

3. Santoro GA, Wieczorek AP, Shobeiri SA, Mueller ER, Pilat J, Stankiewicz A, et al. Interobserver and interdisciplinary reproducibility of 3D endovaginal ultrasound assessment of pelvic floor anatomy. Int Urogynecol J Pelvic Floor Dysfunct. 2011;22:53–9.

4. Shobeiri SA, LeClaire E, Nihira MA, Quiroz LH, O'Donoghue D. Appearance of the levator ani muscle subdivisions in endovaginal 3-dimensional ultrasonography. Obstet Gynecol. 2009;114:66–72.

5. Wieczorek AP, Wozniak MM, Stankiewicz A, Bogusiewicz M, Santoro GA, Rechberger T, et al. Assessment of normal female urethral vascularity with color doppler endovaginal ultrasonography. Pelviperineology. 2009;28:59–61.

6. Wieczorek AP, Wozniak MM, Stankiewicz A, Santoro GA, Bogusiewicz M, Rechberger T. 3-D high-frequency endovaginal ultrasound of female urethral complex and assessment of inter-observer reliability. Eur J Radiol. 2012;81(1):e7–12. PubMed PMID: 20970275. Epub 2010/10/26. eng.

7. Santoro GA, Wieczorek AP, Shobeiri SA, Stankiewicz A. Endovaginal ultrasonography: methodology and normal pelvic floor anatomy. In: Santoro GA, Wieczorek AP, Bartram CI, editors. Pelvic floor disorders: imaging and multidisciplinary approach to management. Dordrecht: Springer; 2010. p. 61–78.

8. Dal Corso HM, D'Elia A, De Nardi P, Cavallari F, Favetta U, Pulvirenti D'Urso A, et al. Anal endosonography: a survey of equipment, technique and diagnostic criteria adopted in nine Italian centers. Tech Coloproctol. 2007;11(1):26–33. PubMed PMID: 17357863. English.

9. Santoro GA, Wieczorek AP, Bartram C. Pelvic floor disorders: imaging and multidisciplinary approach to management. 1st ed. Italia: Springer; 2010. p. 729.

Instrumentation and Techniques for Translabial and Transperineal Pelvic Floor Ultrasound

3

Milena Weinstein and S. Abbas Shobeiri

Learning Objectives

1. To describe 2D and 3D sonographic anatomy of the pelvic floor structures
2. To understand the transperineal and translabial ultrasound technique with transducer position and image orientation and optimization
3. To provide overview of angles and measurements in transperineal and translabial pelvic floor US
4. To appreciate role of transperineal and translabial pelvic floor US in pelvic floor disorders

3.1 Introduction

Pelvic floor disorders include pelvic organ prolapse (POP) urinary and anal incontinence (UI and AI). Pelvic floor disorders have high prevalence in women of all ages [1]. Pelvic floor disorders may also manifest with myriad of urinary, defecatory, and pain symptoms. At times the symptoms of pelvic floor disorders and clinically observed findings do not correlate [2]. Imaging techniques have increased our understanding of pelvic floor disorders by providing more insight into pathophysiology of these conditions and enhancing clinical assessment. Imaging studies that are used to further understand pelvic floor disorders are defecography or dynamic fast-field magnetic resonance imaging (MRI) [3].

Defecography can demonstrate interaction of rectal evacuation with the other pelvic viscera and presumed relationship of pelvic musculature, but it requires multi-organ opacification and exposure to radiation [4]. Dynamic MRI imaging obtains high-resolution pelvic structures images; however MRI is an expensive and not widely available technique requiring radiology expertise. Furthermore provocative maneuvers for dynamic MRI are usually performed in non-physiologic positioning [3].

For the purposes of this chapter the ultrasound performed by placing an abdominal 2D/3D/4D probe between the labia to obtain pelvic floor volumes is referred to as Trans Labial Ultrasound (TLUS). The ultrasound performed by placing a 2D/3D/4D endovaginal ultrasound probe on the perineal area will be called Transperineal Ultrasound (TPUS). There is quite an overlap in terminology where TPUS and TLUS are used interchangeably. Transperineal ultrasound (TPUS) has been used for the past 25 years to assess the

M. Weinstein, M.D.
Department of Obstetrics and Gynecology, Massachusetts General Hospital, Boston, MA, USA

S.A. Shobeiri, M.D. (✉)
Female Pelvic Medicine and Reconstructive Surgery, The University of Oklahoma Health Sciences Center, WP 2410, 920 Stanton L. Young Blvd., Oklahoma City, OK 73104, USA
e-mail: Abbas-shobeiri@ouhsc.edu

S.A. Shobeiri (ed.), *Practical Pelvic Floor Ultrasonography: A Multicompartmental Approach to 2D/3D/4D Ultrasonography of Pelvic Floor*, DOI 10.1007/978-1-4614-8426-4_3,
© Springer Science+Business Media New York 2014

anatomy and physiology of the genitourinary tract [5–7]. TPUS provides noninvasive static and dynamic visualization of pelvic anatomy with use of easily accessible ultrasound platforms [8]. Despite the ease of use and long history pelvic floor ultrasound still remains mostly experimental technique with many possible applications in clinical practice. Large body of TPUS literature has emerged in the last decade making progress in developing the TPUS technique in investigation of pelvic floor disorders; however still much work is needed to standardize imaging terminology and outcome measures [9]. TPUS can investigate pelvic floor anatomy and function in variety of pelvic floor disorders, including UI, POP, and AI and can be used as an adjunct to pelvic muscle training. This chapter will focus on practical aspects of transperineal ultrasound techniques, pelvic floor biometry, and application of ultrasound in investigating different pelvic floor conditions.

3.2   Translabial Ultrasonography

3.2.1   2D Translabial Ultrasonography

Regardless of the intention to perform 3D Translabial Ultrasound (TLUS), Transperineal Ultrasound (TPUS) vs. a 3D Endovaginal Ultrasound (3D EVUS) or a 3D Endoanal Ultrasound (3D EAUS), the imaging should always start with a 2D overview of the pelvic floor in midsagittal view. In the case of a TLUS or TPUS, regardless of the machine used, the probe will be capable of obtaining a 2D view of the pelvic floor. The orientation on the screen will vary depending on the machine and the setting. In case of multicompartmental imaging with BK Ultraview or Flexfocus, an 8802 probe is used (Fig. 3.1). The transducer is placed between the labia majora with the on screen view that includes the pubic symphysis to the right of the screen and the anorectal angle to the left. In resting position you can see location of mesh and synthetic slings, but if you cannot see them, you may investigate further with 3D or 4D imaging. You may also notice the patient's resting prolapse. Although the 2D imaging can

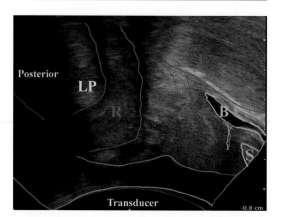

Fig. 3.1 This view demonstrates CORRECT positioning as the starting 2D field of view includes the pubic symphysis (S) anteriorly and the levator plate (LP) posteriorly. Also noted are the bladder (B), uterus (U), vagina (V), anorectum (R) © SHOBEIRI 2013

be done with stage 3 or 4 POP-Q defects, it will necessitate pushing the prolapse back in and the utility of imaging for indication of advanced prolapse alone is questionable. Imaging of the pelvic floor structures may be easier with endovaginal imaging precisely because the prolapse can be pushed in to look at the muscles. The patient is asked to perform the following maneuvers: (1) the patient is asked to squeeze her muscles. Observing a pelvic floor muscle contraction on ultrasound provides visual biofeedback to the patient and can be used for pelvic floor muscle training and for quantification of pelvic floor muscle activity. In the midsagittal plane, a cranioventral shift of the pelvic organs is observed as well as a narrowing of the levator hiatus and changes in bladder neck position.

Many patients may not know what you mean or what to do. So, you have to be specific finding phrases that are familiar to the patient such as please do a kegal or pretend you are holding your urine. This maneuver shows if the patient is discoordinated. Generally, a normal patient has a strong resting tone and the levator lifts slightly vs. a patient who has weak pelvic floor can move the levator plate to a longer distance but cannot reach normal woman's resting position (Fig. 3.2). (2) The patient is asked to perform Valsalva. You can say "bear down as if you are trying to have a bowel movement." It is important that this is the

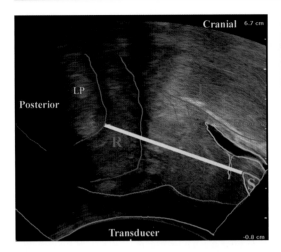

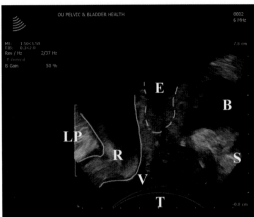

Fig. 3.2 The distance between the pubic symphysis and the levator plate (the *yellow line*) can be measured in resting, squeeze, and Valsalva position. In 2D images a pelvic floor muscle contraction can be quantified using displacement of the bladder neck, as well as a reduction of the midsagittal diameter (antero—posterior, AP) of the levator hiatus at the level of minimal hiatal dimensions © SHOBEIRI 2013

Fig. 3.3 Translabial imaging with Valsalva in this patient demonstrates a low rectocele (R). The bladder (B) does not demonstrate prolapse, however the shadow of an apical enterocele (E) is seen. Also noted are: the levator plate (LP), vagina (V), the transducer (T), and the pubic symphysis (S) © SHOBEIRI 2013

last thing you would ask the patient to do since if she has gas in the upper rectum, it may move down and obscure the 3D images you mean to obtain. If this happens you can ask the patient to perform Valsalva again and the gas and prolapse may move up cephalic. Much important information may be obtained with Valsalva. Rectocele (Fig. 3.3), enterocele or most commonly sigmoidocele (Fig. 3.4), cystocele (Fig. 3.5) or multicompartmental defects may come to view with Valsalva maneuver. Dynamic imaging with Valsalva shows the movement of slings and meshes and may show the point of defects above, below or lateral to the mesh (Figs. 3.6 and 3.7). More about this is discussed in chapter about imaging of meshes.

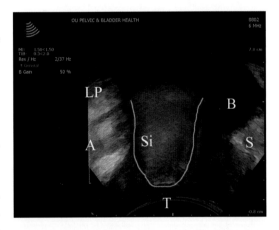

Fig. 3.4 Translabial imaging with Valsalva in this patient demonstrates a sigmoidocele (Si). Also noted are: the levator plate (LP), anus (A), bladder (B), vagina (V), the transducer (T), and the pubic symphysis (S) © SHOBEIRI 2013

3.2.2   3D/4D Translabial Ultrasonography (TLUS)

Three- and four-dimensional ultrasound has increased public interest in pelvic floor tremendously. The superficial axial plane faces the puborectalis portion of the levator ani, and all the levator subdivisions are better imaged by endocavitary transducers such as BK 2052 or BK 8838. However, endocavitary transducers impede Valsalva maneuver. Although the quality of translabial 3D/4D US are reasonable, the endocavitary transducers used transperineally have much higher resolution and may give better images.

If you have a BK ultrasound machine, the 8802 transducer is capable of free hand acquisition of 3D volumes (Figs. 3.8 and 3.9). However, freehand acquisition with 8802 is only advisable if you do not possess a 2052 or 8838. Performing freehand acquisition of a Translabial 3D volume (1) takes considerable skill to move the transducer at a constant speed as it sweeps radially from the patient's right to left. (2) The acquired 3D volume is not repeatable or reliable for measurement purposes and most importantly (3) if you have endocavitary 16 MHz transducers at your disposal which obtains automatic high-

resolution views of the levator ani muscles, it obviates the need for freehand translabial acquisition.

The most commonly published data comes from GE machines. Phillips, Hitachi, and others make similar or superior machines. However, GE's 4D View is available for offline analysis

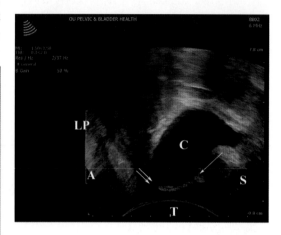

Fig. 3.7 Translabial imaging of a patient with anterior vaginal mesh. The image is with Valsalva. With Valsalva the patient demonstrates a cystocele (C) and detachment of the apical part of the mesh. The *double arrows* point to the cephalad end of the mesh, and the *single arrow* points to the caudad end of the mesh. Also noted are: the levator plate (LP), bladder (B), the transducer (T), and the pubic symphysis (S) © SHOBEIRI 2013

Fig. 3.5 Translabial imaging with Valsalva in this patient demonstrates a concomitant cystocele (C) and a rectocele (R). Also noted are: vagina (V), the transducer (T), and the pubic symphysis (S) © SHOBEIRI 2013

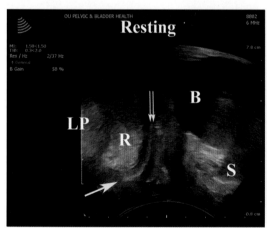

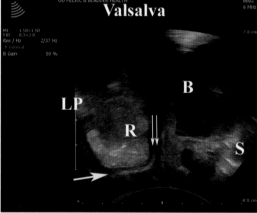

Fig. 3.6 Translabial imaging of a patient with anterior and posterior vaginal mesh. The anterior mesh cannot be seen as clearly. The image to the *left* is at rest. The *double arrows* point to the cephalad end of the mesh, and the *single arrow* points to the caudad end of the mesh. A resting rectocele (R) is seen behind the mesh. The image to the *right* is with

Valsalva. With Valsalva the patient demonstrates worsening of the rectocele and detachment of the apical part of the mesh. Also noted are: the levator plate (LP), bladder (B), the transducer (T), and the pubic symphysis (S) © SHOBEIRI 2013

and use with 4D ultrasound volumes obtained using GE's Voluson series systems. The cheapest and most easily available system is Voluson e or i (Fig. 3.10). Despite its compact size the system is very capable when used with a RAB4-8-RS transducer (Fig. 3.11). The systems where developed and designed to visualize fetus' surface structures and adapted for pelvic floor imaging.

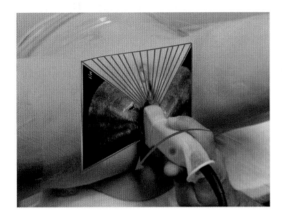

Fig. 3.8 The use of BK 8802 transducer for freehand acquisition of 3D volumes. The transducer is placed between the labia majora and swept at a constant rate from the patient's *left* to *right*. The time during which imaging is obtained can be set. However slower acquisition will result in higher quality 3d volumes © SHOBEIRI 2013

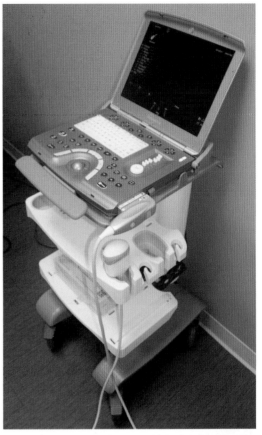

Fig. 3.10 A GE Voluson e ultrasound machine © SHOBEIRI 2013

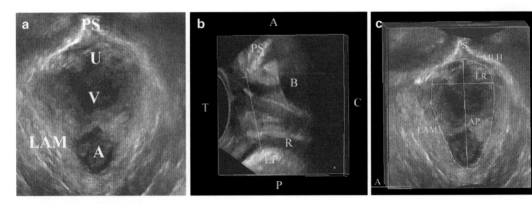

Fig. 3.9 (**a**) A 3D volume obtained using BK 8802 transducer. The 3D volume can be rotated to look at different areas. (**b**) Demonstrated is the right sagittal view of the pelvic floor. The anterior-posterior (AP) distance defined as the shortest distance between the pubic symphysis and the levator plate is drawn in a *yellow line*.

The AP line forms the AP line of the minimal levator hiatus (MLH) in (**c**). Also noted are: the levator plate (LP), bladder (B), the transducer (T), anorectum (R), anterior (A), posterior (P), caudad (C), the left-right line (LR) of the MLH, the levator ani muscle (LAM), and the pubic symphysis (PS or S) © SHOBEIRI 2013

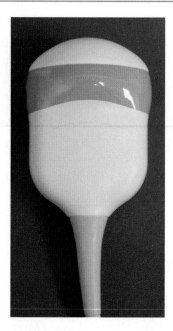

Fig. 3.11 A GE RAB4-8-RS transducer © SHOBEIRI 2013

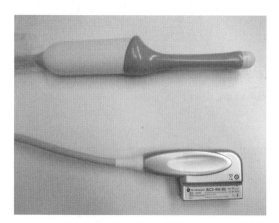

Fig. 3.12 A GE RIC5-9W-RS transducer

GE Kretz 4D view allows manipulation of image characteristics and output of stills, cine loops and rotational volumes in bitmap and AVI format. Slightly higher resolutions can be obtained if the endocavitary RIC5-9W-RS is used on the perineum (Fig. 3.12). The characteristics of these transducers are shown in Table 3.1.

The GE transducer is placed between labia majora and the 2D image as outlined above is displayed on the screen. Depending on the setting of your machine the image orientation may be dif-

ferent. We place the ultrasound machine to the patient's left and operate the probe with the left hand (Fig. 3.13) which leaves the right hand available for running the console (Fig. 3.14). Once you have the appropriate 2D view, maximize the angle of acquisition to 75°–85° and proceed with 3D imaging (Fig. 3.15). During or after acquisition of volumes it is possible to process imaging information into slices of predetermined number and spacing, reminiscent of computer tomography. This technique has been termed Tomographic Ultrasound Imaging (TUI) by manufacturers. The combination of true 4D (volume cine loop) capability and TUI allows simultaneous observation of the effect of maneuvers. Using this methodology, the minimal levator hiatus (MLH), defined in the midsagittal plane as the shortest line between the posterior surface of the symphysis pubis and the levator plate as the plane of reference, with 2.5 mm steps recorded from 5 mm below this plane to 12.5 mm above.

3.3   GE 4D View Software

The software is available on the GE machines and also through "Voluson club" for Voluson Ultrasound machine purchaser. Separate licenses for the software are expensive and not available to those who do not have a machine.

3.4   2D/3D/4D Transerineal Ultrasonography (TPUS)

3.4.1   Basic Procedure and Equipment

Ultrasonography has become a common place in Obstetrics, Gynecology, and Urology. Most ultrasound platforms are equipped with curved array and/or endovaginal transducers which are suitable for transperineal ultrasound imaging.

Positioning
As with gynecologic ultrasound most TPUS exams are performed with the woman in either lithotomy in a standard gynecologic examination

Table 3.1 Characteristics of GE RAB4-8-RS used for translabial ultrasound, and RIC5-9W-RS used for transperineal ultrasound

; RAB4-8-RS	Real time 4D convex transducer	63.6×37.8 mm	2–8 MHz	70°, V 85°×70°	Voluson *i*
	Real time 4D endocavity				
; RIC5-9W-RS	Next generation real time 4D micro-convex endocavitary transducer, with wide FOV	22.4×22.6 mm	4–9 MHz	146°, V 146°×120°	Voluson *i*

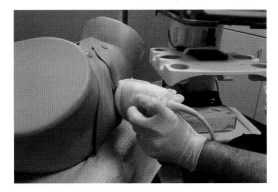

Fig. 3.13 Left-handed application of the transducer during Translabial ultrasonography © SHOBEIRI 2013

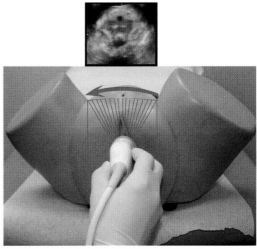

Fig. 3.15 3D pelvic floor volume acquisition with GE RAB4-8-RS transducer. The internalized mechanism in the probe moves the crystals obviating the need for hand movement. The hand and the elbow should be rested in a steady position for good quality imaging. The volume obtained is displayed on the screen © SHOBEIRI 2013

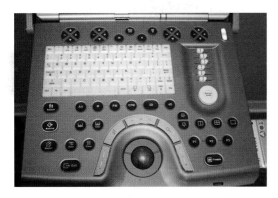

Fig. 3.14 The dominant hand generally operated the console. Unlike BK console, the GE Voluson e buttons on the console are multifunctional, and their function corresponds to the menu at the bottom of the screen © SHOBEIRI 2013

table or in a modified lithotomy position with cushion placed under buttocks and lower extremities in frog-legged position. For 3-dimensional imaging the examiner may also need to prop their arm or elbow as the imaging capture time can be as long as 15–20 s and the absolute stillness is critical for the optimal image quality. It is certainly

possible to do the TPUS with a patient standing, which could be especially useful in patients who are not as successful with dynamic maneuver in supine position.

Transducers and Probes

Transperineal ultrasound refers to ultrasound performed with the transducer position on the perineum. There are techniques described in literature that use translabial ultrasound, i.e., transducer is placed on the labia majora. Term introital ultrasound [10] is also used where transducer is placed at the vaginal introitus or posterior fourchette. The common denominator for all those techniques is placement of transducers externally on the patient's vulva rather than introduction of the transducer into vagina or anal canal. For the

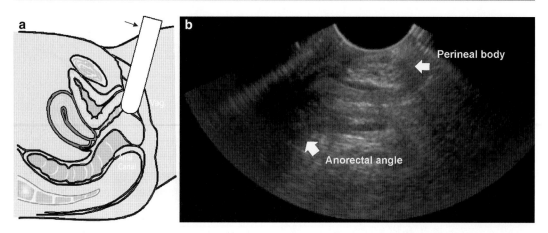

Fig. 3.16 Transperineal ultrasound of the anorectal structures: (**a**) schematic of endovaginal transducer positioned on the perineum and oriented caudally to visualize anorectum; (**b**) 2D transperineal sagittal image of the anorectum with perianal body easily visualized as an ovoid structure and anorectal angle marked

purposes of this chapter we will focus on transperineal ultrasound and mention other types of ultrasound where appropriate for specific studies. TPUS imaging can be performed with use of either trans-abdominal curvilinear transducers or with endovaginal transducer that is typically used for endovaginal gynecologic ultrasound. Curved array transducer is typically 4–8 MHz, whereas endovaginal transducers have frequencies up to 9.0 MHz. It is important to keep in mind that higher frequency transducers provide superior resolution, but have less tissue penetration. This trade-off is important for achieving images of diagnostic quality. For the purposes of this chapter, ultrasound performed with curved array transducers will be referred to as translabial ultrasound (TLUS) as the transducer is placed over the labia majora to visualize anatomic structures. With use of endovaginal transducer the transducer is mostly placed on the perineum or at the posterior fourchette and thus we will refer to it as transperineal ultrasound (TPUS). There is no agreement in nomenclature for these techniques.

Preparation

For transperineal ultrasound as with any ultrasound imaging use of coupling gel is a critical step as ultrasound waves do not pass through air. Whether trans-abdominal or endovaginal transducers are used the gel should be placed between the transducer and covering. For endovaginal transducers a disposable cover (e.g., male condom) and for curved trans-abdominal transducer glove or plastic wrap can be used. Additionally gel should be applied to the perineum to allow for better coupling. Warming the gel in a commercial warming device improves patient comfort. After each use, transducers should be cleaned and disinfected according to manufacturer recommendations.

3.4.2 Transperineal Ultrasound Orientation and Optimization

2D: Technique—Orientation

Different techniques have been described for transperineal and translabial pelvic floor imaging. Some investigators use a curved array transducer (4–8 MHz abdominal probe) [11–13]. The transducer oriented vertically with a mark (i. e., a groove or ridge on one side of the ultrasound transducer) facing up and placed firmly against symphysis pubis. The transducer can be placed on the labia or with labia parted. With the transperineal technique an endovaginal transducer is placed on the perineum with a mark facing up. In this chapter all the TPUS images are captured with endovaginal transducer. The image optimization depends on the goal of desired visualization. With imaging of the pelvic floor muscles and levator hiatus the transducer is directed cranially (Fig. 3.16a, b) with imaging of

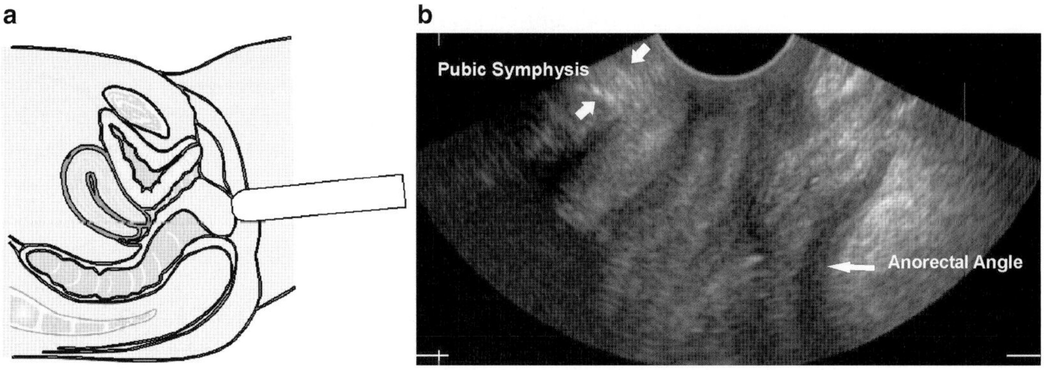

a

b

Fig. 3.17 Transperineal ultrasound of the pelvic floor hiatus: (**a**) schematic of endovaginal transducer positioned on the perineum and oriented cranially to visualize the pelvic floor hiatus; (**b**) 2D transperineal sagittal image of the pelvic floor hiatus with pubic symphysis and anorectal angle shown

the anorectum the transducer is usually oriented posteriorly towards the anal canal [14] (Fig. 3.17a, b). Care should be taken to avoid excessive pressure applied to the perineal structures. Most investigators advise to assure tissue contact enough to visualize anorectal structures avoiding any excessive pressure on the perineum. Compression of perineum may distort perineal anatomy and limit mobility of the pelvic floor during dynamic maneuvers.

In transperineal pelvic floor imaging the transducer is most commonly oriented with the mark facing up (12 o'clock position) with midsagittal orientation. The produced 2D image will represent anterior structures (pubic symphysis and urethra) at the left portion of the screen and the posterior structures (anorectum) at the right side of the screen (Fig. 3.17b). The 2D image produced by TPUS imaging allows for visualization of the urethrovesical junction (UVJ), anorectal angle, structures of the anal sphincter complex. This view can be used to observe pelvic floor mobility during pelvic floor maneuvers, like pelvic floor contraction (Kegel's exercise) and during straining.

In the midsagittal view the structures seen from left to right: pubic symphysis, urethra and bladder, vagina and anorectum. On the midsagittal view the pubic symphysis cross-section is usually oblong and bony structures of the pubic rami are not visible. Next, anterior and posterior urethral walls are delineated against periurethral tissues. Usually urethral mucosa and submucosa are imaged as a universally hypoechoic structure that appears as an open lumen. Vagina is usually seen as a collapsed structure, where vaginal walls are not clearly separated by ultrasound. Anorectum is seen as outline of hypoechoic internal anal sphincter (IAS) against the midline anal mucosa, which is usually echogenic with variable echogenicity due to fold of anal mucosa. Hyperechoic external sphincter surrounds the hypoechoic internal sphincter. The anorectal angle is normally easily visualized and changes with dynamic maneuvers of the pelvic floor muscles. Cross-section of the puborectalis muscle (PRM) is seen posterior to the anorectal angle.

3D TPUS: Technique

Three-dimensional (3D) ultrasound refers to two-dimensional static display of three-dimensional data. For acquiring and rendering 3D ultrasound dataspecial transducers and software are needed. The 3D ultrasound dataset is referred to as "volume." To obtain 3D ultrasound the transducer is held in the stationary position at the perineum during acquisition of the volume. The scanning angle is usually set to the widest available—depending on equipment this could be between 120° and 180°. The acquisition time depends on set image quality and varies between 2 and 15 s. The patients are usually instructed to hold her breath (or use shallow breathing) through the volume acquisition phase as any motion can introduce a motion artifact. For the static 3D volume acquisition the quality of acquisition (acquisition time) should be maximized for best quality images. The faster scanning modes usually compromise quality of image but can be useful during dynamic maneuvers. When 3D volumes of dynamic maneuvers are obtained the image quality could be sacrificed for faster acquisition since the subject has to sustain the dynamic state for the length of the acquisition. The dynamic conditions most commonly used for the imaging included pelvic floor contraction and the Valsalva maneuver. When acquiring volumes during the dynamic imaging the position of the transducer at rest may need to be adjusted to allow for the capturing of the dynamic state. The best imaging is achieved by assuring that patients maintain the dynamic state without movement. Any movement from operator or the subject can introduce motion artifact.

3D TPUS: Pelvic floor hiatus— Orientation, Optimization, and Rotation

To capture transperineal 3D US volume of the pelvic floor hiatus and the surround levator ani muscles the transducer placed on the perineum and the ultrasound beam is directed in the cranial direction (Fig. 3.17). The field of view is optimized by identifying the symphysis pubis on the left of the screen and the anal canal on the right side of the screen [15]. The operator should also maximize the midline alignment with assuring that the urethra is also visible in this view. After capturing the volume images can be stored on a compact disk or drive and assessed offline. The offline post possessing is done with equipment-specific software—this is usually proprietary software that allows rotation of the volume, thick and thin slicing of the volume, and multiple measurements. During the post-processing of volumes the 3D static images are rotated to be displayed in a symmetric orientation in the three orthogonal planes: coronal sagittal and transverse planes. A cursor dot is located in corresponding positions in all three orthogonal planes. A cursor dot allows for the exact position of an anatomical structure to be identified simultaneously in the three orthogonal planes (Fig. 3.18). One of the standardized rotation techniques described is demonstrated in the serial figures [15] (Fig. 3.19a–e).

1. The transverse (axial) 3D volume is rotated approximately 90° clockwise in the plane of the PRM for an appropriate anterior-posterior (AP) orientation of the image. (The plane is defined as a line joining the inferior border of the pubic symphysis and the apex of the anorectal angle.)
2. The cursor dot is placed in the area of the pubic bone that allows the symphysis pubis to come into view on the coronal view.
3. The coronal image is then analyzed millimeter-by-millimeter to identify and mark the location where the 2 pubic rami meet to form the inferior border of the symphysis pubis.
4. The sagittal plane is then rotated to align the inferior border of the symphysis pubis with the apex of the anorectal angle, noting that this allows the PRM to come into the full view on the transverse (axial) plane.

After post-processing rotation the pelvic floor hiatus is visualized in the transverse (or axial) plane. The visualization of the hiatal structures can be further optimized by tomographic function where the volume is sliced with predetermined thickness to visualized structures at different levels. The rendering function can also further assist in visualization of the specific anatomy. This "thick slice" technique is usually set at the thinnest slice ~1 cm. The normal appearance includes pubic rami and symphysis and the midline positioned urethral cross-section. The cross-section of the vagina normally has "butterfly" or H-appearance, which is due to lateral vaginal attachments of the vagina to the endopelvic connective tissues—to the arcus tendentious anteriorly and the posterior arcus posteriorly. The cross-section of the anal canal is also seen. The PRM surrounds the pelvic floor forms the most distal portion of the levator hiatus (Fig. 3.19e).

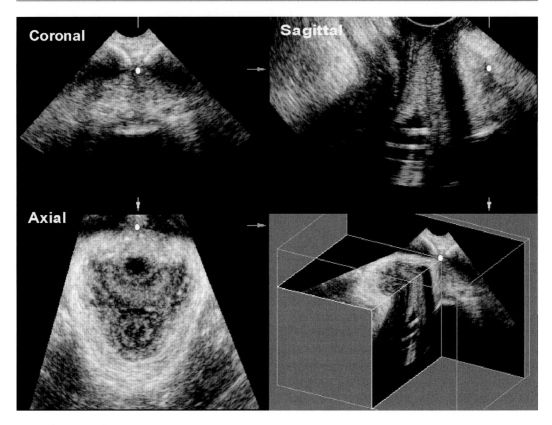

Fig. 3.18 Transperineal static 3D volume processed to demonstrate the relationship of the three orthogonal planes—coronal, sagittal, and axial. The cursor dot seen in each plane represents the exact same spot in each plane

3.5 Transperineal Ultrasound and Pelvic Floor Disorders

3.5.1 Pelvic Floor Biometry with TLUS/TPUS

Multiple TLUS/TPUS pelvic floor biometry measurements are described in the literature. The lower edge of the pubic symphysis, UVJ, and the anorectal angle are the most common used reference points in transperineal imaging. The biometry can be performed at rest and during dynamic maneuvers.

For assessment of bladder neck position and mobility in the sagittal plane variety of measurements have been described with use of 2D TPUS. In 1995 Schaer et al. [7] described a coordinate system for bladder neck and urethral mobility ultrasound appearance. X-axis determined by a straight line through the central portion of the pubic symphysis. The Y-axis is perpendicular to the x-axis at the lower border of the symphysis. The urethrovesical angle or the UVJ is measured by creating a perpendicular line from the X-axis on the image, and following this line to the margin of the bladder base when the patient is at rest [7]. The most common index in assessment of bladder neck position and urethral mobility are the urethral height (H), which is defined as the distance between the lower edge of the pubic symphysis and the bladder neck [10] (Fig. 3.20). The location of the symphysis is defined as an imaginary line drawn through the lower edge of the pubic symphysis. In addition, posterior urethrovesical angle can be measured. This is the angle between the urethral axis and the bladder floor. These indices can be measured at rest

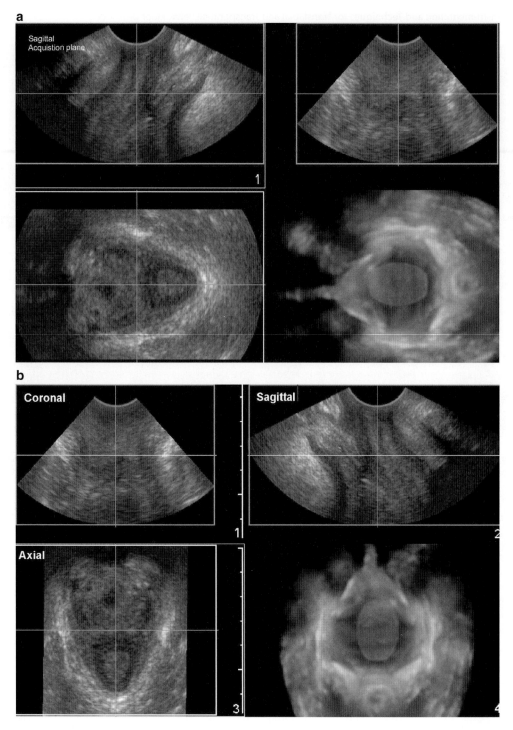

Fig. 3.19 3D TPUS—volume post-processing step-by-step: (**a**) transperineal ultrasound of the pelvic floor hiatus with the sagittal acquisition plane—sagittal plane optimized by visualizing the pubic symphysis and the anorectal angle; (**b**) volume is rotated to orient the axial plane upright. The multiplanar of the 3D transperineal volume shown with coronal, sagittal, and axial (transverse) planes identified; (**c**) the cursor dot is moved in the axial (transverse) plane in the area of the pubic symphysis. The pubic rami and pubic symphysis are visible in the coronal plane. The dot-marker is positioned on the pubic symphysis; (**d**) in the sagittal plane the volume is rotated to align the pubic symphysis with the anorectal angle—the represents the puborectalis muscle (PRM) plane. The PRM is seen encircling the pelvic floor hiatus in the transverse image; (**e**) the transperineal view of the pelvic floor hiatus after completion of the volume rotation. The rendered thick slice (10 mm) allows for more detailed assessment of the hiatal structures. The pelvic floor hiatus anatomy includes cross-section of the urethra, vagina, and the anorectum. The hiatus is encircled by the PRM

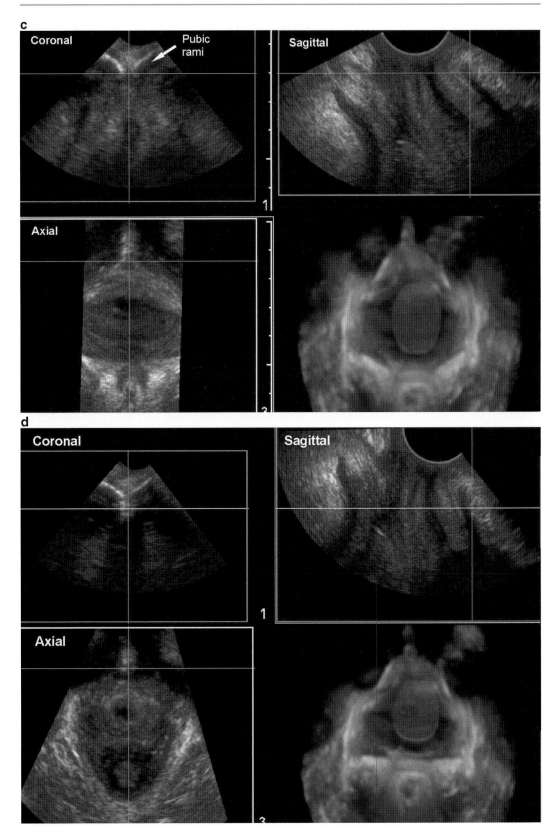

Fig. 3.19 (continued)

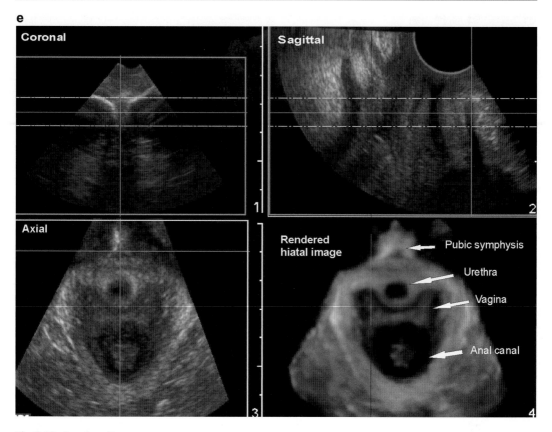

Fig. 3.19 (continued)

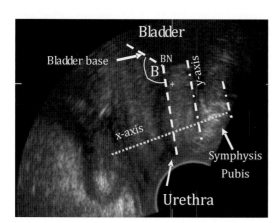

Fig. 3.20 The posterior urethrovesical angle measurement method with perineal ultrasound described by Schaer et al. [7]. The rectangular coordinate system was constructed with *y*-axis is at the inferior symphysis pubis and *x*-axis is perpendicular through the mid-symphysis pubis. The posterior urethrovesical angle (B) was measured with a line through the urethral axis and the other line through the at least one-third of the bladder base

and during dynamic maneuvers—pelvic floor contraction (squeeze), coughing and straining (Valsalva). In continent women normal values measured for urethrovesical angle is 96.8° at rest and 108.1° with Valsalva maneuver, and for height are 20.6 and 14.0 mm, respectively [10]. During Valsalva maneuver deviation of the indices of bladder neck mobility and concomitant funneling of the proximal urethra can be observed in incontinent women (Fig. 3.21). Correlation between ultrasound findings of bladder neck descent measurements and urodynamic testing has been inconsistent [16, 17] and largely do not help distinguish continent and incontinent women [18]. Transperineal ultrasound has also been used in the assessment of patients with urinary incontinence by imaging the urethral support and morphology and by measuring the urethra and its sphincter. A recent study showed that translabial 3D US is reliable in calculated

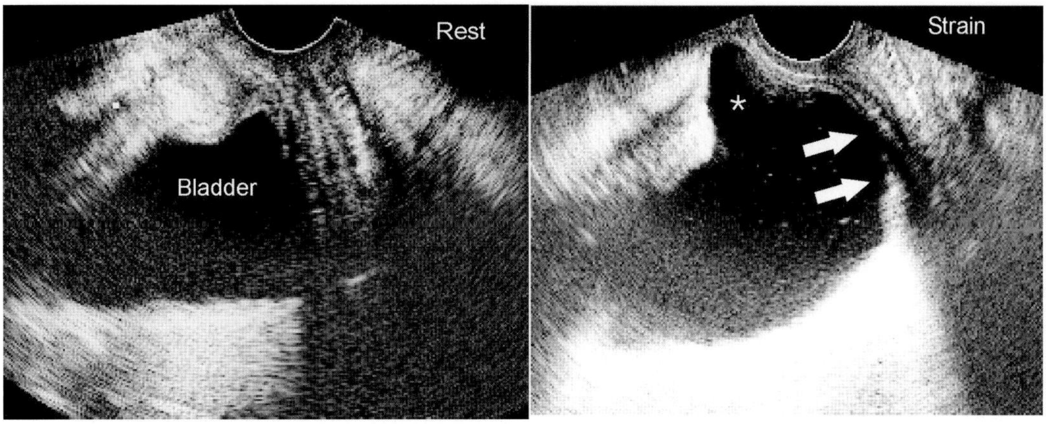

Fig. 3.21 Transperineal ultrasound of the sagittal bladder neck with the outline of the bladder easily seen on the rest image. The strain image shows descent of the bladder wall (*arrows*) and funneling (marked with *asterisk*)

volumes of the urethral sphincter in nulliparous women [19]. One ultrasound study showed that women with stress urinary incontinence have urethral sphincters that are shorter, thinner, and smaller in volume [20].

There are many measurements described to characterize the dimensions of the pelvic floor (or levator) hiatus. These measurements are usually done using 3D TPUS in the plane of minimal hiatus which is the shortest distance between the lower edge of the pubic symphysis and the edge of the levator plate posteriorly. The majority of the MLH border is lined with pubovisceralis muscle [21, 22]. It has been referred to as the puborectalis, pubovisceralis or pubococcygeus by multiple authors as the borders of these muscles cannot be delineated by transperineal imaging. In this chapter we will refer to the muscle that borders levator hiatus as the pubovisceralis muscle. The levator hiatus plane has defined reference points of inferior edge of the pubic symphysis and the anorectal angle. This plane is also referred to as "plane of minimal hiatal dimensions" [23]. Multiple biometric indices are described for this plane that can be obtained on the multiplanar image in axial (transverse) plane or on a rendered image. These measurements can be performed on volumes obtained at rest, pelvic floor contraction or during a Valsalva maneuver. In addition to measurements, PRM integrity can be assessed.

The measurements include linear measurements of the anterior-posterior hiatal diameter, lateral hiatal diameter, levator ani (PRM) thickness and angle. The most common biometric measurement used is anteroposterior hiatal diameter, which is measured in the plane of minimal dimensions and defined as the distance between lower edge of the pubic symphysis and the anorectal angle [15]. This measurement has been shown to consistently decrease with pelvic floor contraction. The levator hiatus measurements are reliable [15, 24] and can be easily learned [24]. The pelvic floor contraction is shown to decrease the hiatal area dimensions. The PRM inner perimeter is defined by a curvilinear measurement along the inner border of the pubovisceralis muscle to its insertion site on the pubic ramus. The pelvic floor hiatus inner area is defined as the area within the pubovisceralis muscle inner perimeter enclosed anteriorly by two straight lines, connecting the pubovisceralis insertion point on the pubic rami to the inferior edge of the symphysis pubis. The pelvic floor hiatus outer area is contained within the outer border of the puborectalis; it has the same borders as the pelvic floor hiatus inner area anteriorly. The puborectalis area has been calculated. The measurement is obtained by subtracting the pelvic floor hiatus from the outer area. This measurement represents the cross-sectional area of the puborectalis [15].

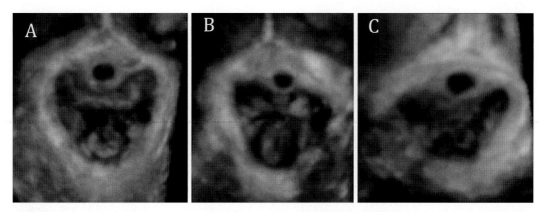

Fig. 3.22 3D TPUS of the axial 10 mm thick slice rendered hiatal image showing of normal hiatal structures (**a**) and example of the PRM injury (**b, c**). Note how urethra and vagina shift away from the midline to the side where the PRM injury is greater

Using 3D TPUS and vaginal manometry Jung et al. [25] characterized high-pressure zone of the vagina. They demonstrated that using vaginal fluid-filled bag the progressive distention initially increased lateral and only then anteroposterior dimensions of the pelvic floor hiatus and that anterior-posterior and not lateral dimensions decreased with pelvic floor contraction. This provides evidence that the PRM is responsible for creating high-pressure zone in the vagina.

3.5.2 TLUS/TPUS: Pelvic Floor (Levator) Hiatus and Pelvic Floor Musculature

Series of studies by MRI and 3D ultrasound have identified defects in the levator ani muscles in parous women. These morphological defects vary from minor abnormalities to major muscle damage. There is no agreement on classification of these defects [26, 27]. MRI studies have shown that the most common injury related to childbirth is an avulsion injury of the insertion of the pubovisceralis muscle on the pubic ramus [28] (Fig. 3.22).

There are series of studies that assess pelvic floor morphologic changes related to vaginal delivery. Many studies report that vaginal delivery is associated with levator muscles injury. Dietz and Lanzarone [29] showed that in a third of women delivering vaginally, the avulsions were associated with stress urinary incontinence at 3 months postpartum. Further data from the same group [30] suggests that levator trauma is associated with prolapse of anterior and apical compartment and not with bladder dysfunction or urinary incontinence. They also demonstrated that larger levator hiatus was correlated with POP. Further studies analyzing large retrospective cohort suggested that levator ani avulsions are associated with prolapse in women with previous pelvic surgery [31].

3.5.3 Anal Sphincter Complex and Anal Canal TPUS

When assessing anal canal the transducer can be oriented in either sagittal or axial orientation. Using endovaginal transducer positioned on the perineum and oriented caudally the sagittal image usually visualizes the anal canal and the anorectal angle (Fig. 3.17). Using 2D ultrasound the anorectal angle can easily be seen and measured. The dynamic changes in the displacement of the anorectal angle can provide visual biofeedback for levator ani activity and are easily understood and readily accepted by women [32].

When capturing 3D TPUS the sagittal orientation of the anal canal is optimal. The image is further optimized by assuring that the anorectal

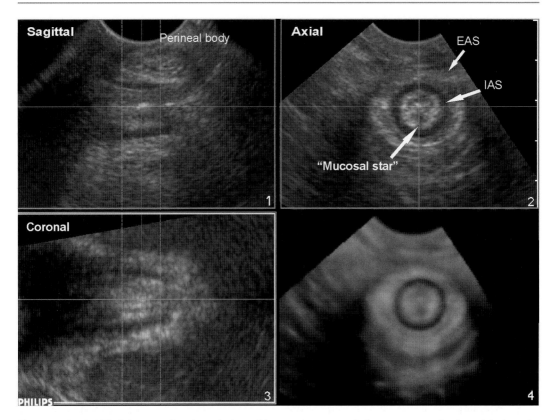

Fig. 3.23 3D TPUS of the normal anal canal: the multiplanar image with three orthogonal planes shown: sagittal, coronal, and axial identified. The rendered thick slice (10 mm) allows for integrated evaluation of the mid-anal sphincter portion. In the sagittal plane the perineal body is seen as an oval-shape structure. On the axial plane the mucosal fold—"mucosal star" and the classic representation of the mid-anal canal with hypoechoic internal anal sphincter (IAS) and hyperechoic external anal sphincter (EAS)

angle is visible. Alternatively anorectum can be visualized with 2D or 3D in the axial plane with when the transducer marker is oriented to 3 or 9 o'clock. Images can be captured at rest and during sustained anal sphincter and pelvic floor contraction. The offline assessment of 3D TPUS static images allows for volume rotation with symmetrical viewing of anal sphincter structures in standard coronal, sagittal and transverse (axial) planes. Additionally the sphincter structures can be further characterized using thick slice or multi-slice assessments tools. The inner portion of the axial sphincter image has been called "mucosal star" [14] (Fig. 3.23). The visualization of the mucosal folds of the anal canal differentiates TPUS from endoanal technique, where inserted transducer flattens folds of the anal mucosa. The appearance of the sphincter is different depending on the level of capturing. In the middle of the anal canal, the classical "target" sphincter appears. The echolucent IAS encircles the anal mucosal layer. IAS is encircled by the echogenic external anal sphincter (EAS). As with other structures use of tomographic sonography with 3D volume processing can enhance visualization (Fig. 3.24).

Contractions of the PRM are thought to decrease the anorectal angle and increased pressure in the proximal part of the anal canal, and when the EAS contracts, there is increased pressure in the distal part of the canal [33]. On 3-dimensional ultrasound, these contractions and associated measurements are well captured [34].

Use of TPUS also allows visualization of the sphincter defects. Limited data is available on clinical diagnostic utility of TPUS for imaging of

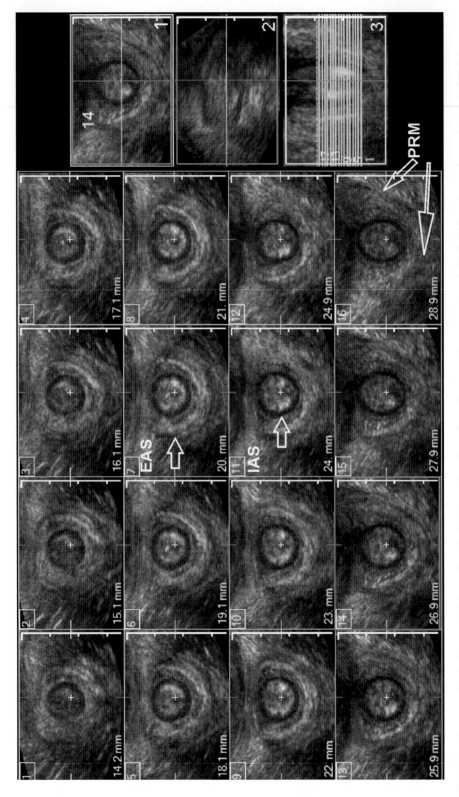

Fig. 3.24 3D transperineal ultrasound of the anal canal with 1 mm slices from the anal verge to the anorectal angle. IAS, EAS, and posterior portion of the PRM shown

anal sphincter. Endoanal ultrasound is the gold standard of assessing anal sphincter defects. A recent study compared transperineal and endovaginal ultrasounds to the endoanal ultrasound technique in evaluating women with postpartum anal sphincter injuries. The study found while TPUS was useful in identifying normal anatomy, the sensitivity for assessing anal sphincter defects was inferior to the gold standard—the endoanal approach [35].

3.5.4 3D US and MRI

MRI has gained in importance as a diagnostic and research tool for assessment of pelvic floor disorders. It certainly has capability of high-resolution superb imaging of the soft tissues of the pelvic floor and has been one of the modalities of choice for evaluation of the pelvic floor. However, the major technical limitation of MR imaging is its poor ability to fully capture present-time pictures as its spatial resolution is often spared as imaging time becomes faster. Other clinical limitation includes its high cost, time and space constrains, and limited availability. The utility of 3-dimensional ultrasound has been studied and compared to MR imaging [15, 25, 27, 36]. Some studies have shown poor correlation between MR imaging and ultrasound, but some authors believe that this is because previous studies did not use the same plane on ultrasound as was used on MRI [36]. Another study showed that the two modalities correlate at rest, but there is no correlation during maximum Valsalva. This is likely because of the physical limitations of MR imaging. When using MRI, it is difficult to predict the end point during Valsalva and because MRI is not done under real time, the true plane needed to adequately evaluate pelvic floor function is not as available to the degree that it is in ultrasound [36]. In more recent studies, transperineal 3D US has shown to be as effective, if not better, than MRI in imaging the pelvic floor [36]. With 3D US cine loop capabilities the functional pelvic floor anatomy assessment has superior spatial and temporal resolution, where multiple volumes of imaging obtained per second [37].

Dynamic 3D ultrasound, also known as 4D ultrasound, acquires volume datasets that can be used to produce single slices in any arbitrarily defined plane [38].

3.5.5 TLUS/TPUS in the Evaluation and Treatment of Urinary Incontinence

Transperineal or introital ultrasound has been used in assessment of bladder neck position before and after incontinence procedures and in assessment of implanted materials in treatment of stress urinary incontinence.

Bernstein showed that pelvic floor muscles thickness and function could be visualized by perineal ultrasound. He also demonstrated that pelvic floor muscle were thinner in women older than 60 years old and in women with SUI compared with continence controls. After pelvic floor muscle training all groups showed increase in muscle thickness and 60 % of SUI women showed subjective and objective improvement with UI. Dietz et al. [32] used translabial ultrasound as biofeedback in teaching women to perform a proper pelvic floor muscle contraction. They proved that translabial ultrasound is a useful adjunct in pelvic floor muscle training.

Prolene mesh, that is used for minimally invasive slings is highly echogenic and can easily be visualized with TPUS (Fig. 3.25). Schuettoff et al. [39] compared use of MRI and introital US and suggested that ultrasound is most suited for assessment for suburethral and periurethral mesh portion, whereas MRI is more suitable for retropubic mesh evaluation. Ultrasound can also show the spatial relationship between a suburethral sling, the urethra, and the symphysis pubis. Yalcin et al. published a pilot study in a group of women with SUI after Tension-free vaginal tape (TVT) operation [40]. It showed that bladder neck mobility measured on x-y coordinate system could discriminate successful and failed slings; however these measurements had large overlap. It has been shown to move variably as an arc around the posterior symphysis pubis. Movement closes the gap between the mesh and the bony

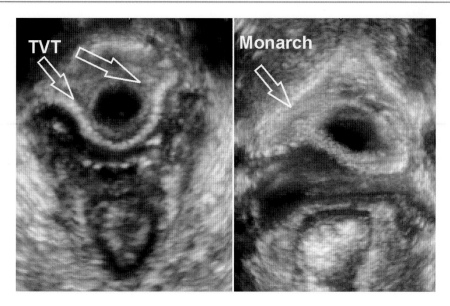

Fig. 3.25 3D transperineal ultrasound of the hiatus—axial image with 10 mm rendered thick slice—the mesh sling (TVT and Monrach) are shown

structure of the pelvic, thereby, compressing the urethra during increases in intra-abdominal pressure. The ability to visualize the variability in the location and the movement of the sling allows clinicians to understand why there is variability in the actual efficacy of the sling and to help determine if the sling needs to be adjusted [41]. Using 3D TPUS investigators showed that mid-urethral position is not necessary for minimally invasive slings success in treatment of SUI [42, 43].

Urethral bulking agents are used to improve continence by enhancing urethral coaptation. Periurethral collagen has been imaged by perineal ultrasound. Using perineal (introital) ultrasoundElia and Bergman found that optimal location of collagen implant was less than 7 mm from the bladder neck [44]. With use of 3D ultrasound, Defreitas et al. suggest that optimal periurethral collagen location is a circumferential distribution around the urethra, while an asymmetric distribution is associated with a significantly smaller improvement in incontinence symptoms [45]. Poon and Zimmern describe the use of 3D ultrasound as part of their standard algorithm in managing incontinence in patients who undergo periurethral collagen injection. If a patient has no or minimal improvement after collagen injection therapy and ultrasound shows low volume retention of collagen or an asymmetric distribution, the patient is offered a repeat injection in the area of deficiency. If there is no improvement but a circumferential pattern is seen on ultrasound, the injection is considered optimal and the patient is offered an alternative treatment [46].

3.5.6 TLUS/TPUS and Pelvic Organ Prolapse

TLUS/TPUS has been increasingly used as an adjunct in diagnostic evaluation of POP. There are many studies reporting use of TPUS to assess POP. In a pilot study, Beer-Gabel et al. [12] used dynamic transperineal ultrasound to identify pelvic floor descent. The assessment of anorectal angle was comparable to defecography. Rectoceles were also easily identified. Dietz and Steensma [47] showed that rectovaginal septal defects could be easily identified on translabial ultrasound, but a third of women with rectocele showed no sonographic abnormalities. Grasso et al. [48] reported a good to excellent correlation of introital ultrasound finding and defecography in evaluation of anorectal angle, presence of intussusception and rectocele. Recently Weemhoff et al. [49] reported that TPUS finding of intussusception was predictive of abnormal evacuation proctography, however prediction of enterocele findings was poor compared with evacuation proctography.

Some studies attempted to correlate clinical findings by Pelvic Organ Prolapse Quantification system (POP-Q) to the ultrasound findings. The reference for measurement in the ultrasound findings is different from the reference that is used in POP-Q, i.e., hymen. For ultrasound measurements of the prolapse the reference line is usually drawn parallel to the infero-posterior margin of pubic symphysis [50].

In a study by Lone et al. [51], the authors assessed the relationship between validated POP-Q measures and assessment made by dynamic 2D-TPUS. In this study only women with prolapse at or above the hymen were included for analysis. They also adjusted for reference points to minimize difference between the reference lines used with POP-Q and TPUS. They found that proportion of correctly assessed prolapse was around 60 % for anterior and posterior compartment (using points Ba and Bp) and only 33 % for the apical compartment (using point C).

3.6 Summary

2D and 3D Transperineal and Translabial pelvic floor ultrasound allows evaluating many aspects of pelvic floor anatomy and function and can compliment a careful physical examination. It shows promise in investigation of pelvic floor disorders. However no universal standard for its use exists to date. Some of the promising applications of the TLUS/TPUS include assessment of pelvic floor muscles integrity and biometry. TLUS/TPUS can be a useful adjunct to the pelvic floor muscle training and biofeedback. Some other potentially useful applications of TLUS/TPUS include investigation of posterior vaginal wall prolapse and assessment of implanted materials. Lack of standardized terminology and objective parameters and validation of diagnosis and assessment of pelvic floor disorders dampen the broader clinical application of TLUS/TPUS. In 2011, an international panel aimed to perform a meta-analysis to analyze pelvic floor ultrasound literature. They deemed the production of a systematic review impossible based on the type and quality of published literature [9]. They identified research priorities and advised on more coordinated and structured research effort into internal and external validity of pelvic floor ultrasound in assessment of pelvic floor disorders.

References

1. Lawrence JM, Lukacz ES, Nager CW, Hsu JW, Luber KM. Prevalence and co-occurrence of pelvic floor disorders in community-dwelling women. Obstet Gynecol. 2008;111(3):678–85.
2. Maglinte DD, Kelvin FM, Fitzgerald K, Hale DS, Benson JT. Association of compartment defects in pelvic floor dysfunction. AJR Am J Roentgenol. 1999;172(2):439–44.
3. Fielding JR, Griffiths DJ, Versi E, Mulkern RV, Lee ML, Jolesz FA. MR imaging of pelvic floor continence mechanisms in the supine and sitting positions. AJR Am J Roentgenol. 1998;171(6):1607–10.
4. Goei R, Kemerink G. Radiation dose in defecography. Radiology. 1990;176(1):137–9.
5. Kohorn EI, Scioscia AL, Jeanty P, Hobbins JC. Ultrasound cystourethrography by perineal scanning for the assessment of female stress urinary incontinence. Obstet Gynecol. 1986;68(2):269–72.
6. Creighton SM, Pearce JM, Stanton SL. Perineal video-ultrasonography in the assessment of vaginal prolapse: early observations. Br J Obstet Gynaecol. 1992;99(4):310–3.
7. Schaer GN, Koechli OR, Schuessler B, Haller U. Perineal ultrasound for evaluating the bladder neck in urinary stress incontinence. Obstet Gynecol. 1995; 85(2):220–4.
8. Kleinubing Jr H, Jannini JF, Malafaia O, Brenner S, Pinho TM. Transperineal ultrasonography: new method to image the anorectal region. Dis Colon Rectum. 2000;43(11):1572–4.
9. Tubaro A, Koelbl H, Laterza R, Khullar V, de Nunzio C. Ultrasound imaging of the pelvic floor: where are we going? Neurourol Urodyn. 2011;30(5):729–34.
10. Tunn R, Petri E. Introital and transvaginal ultrasound as the main tool in the assessment of urogenital and pelvic floor dysfunction: an imaging panel and practical approach. Ultrasound Obstet Gynecol. 2003;22(2):205–13.
11. Yagel S, Valsky DV. Three-dimensional transperineal ultrasonography for evaluation of the anal sphincter complex: another dimension in understanding peripartum sphincter trauma. Ultrasound Obstet Gynecol. 2006;27(2):119–23. Epub 2006/01/26.

12. Beer-Gabel M, Teshler M, Barzilai N, Lurie Y, Malnick S, Bass D, et al. Dynamic transperineal ultrasound in the diagnosis of pelvic floor disorders: pilot study. Dis Colon Rectum. 2002;45(2):239–45. discussion 45–8.

13. Dietz HP. Ultrasound imaging of the pelvic floor. Part II: three-dimensional or volume imaging. Ultrasound Obstet Gynecol. 2004;23(6):615–25.

14. Timor-Tritsch IE, Monteagudo A, Smilen SW, Porges RF, Avizova E. Simple ultrasound evaluation of the anal sphincter in female patients using a transvaginal transducer. Ultrasound Obstet Gynecol. 2005; 25(2):177–83.

15. Weinstein MM, Jung SA, Pretorius DH, Nager CW, den Boer DJ, Mittal RK. The reliability of puborectalis muscle measurements with 3-dimensional ultrasound imaging. Am J Obstet Gynecol. 2007; 197(1):68.e1–6.

16. Robinson D, Anders K, Cardozo L, Bidmead J, Toozs-Hobson P, Khullar V. Can ultrasound replace ambulatory urodynamics when investigating women with irritative urinary symptoms? BJOG. 2002;109:145–8.

17. Bai SW, Lee JW, Shin JS, Park JH, Kim SK, Park KH. The predictive values of various parameters in the diagnosis of stress urinary incontinence. Yonsei Med J. 2004;45(2):287–92.

18. Lukanovic A, Patrelli TS. Validation of ultrasound scan in the diagnosis of female stress urinary incontinence. Clin Exp Obstet Gynecol. 2011;38(4):373–8.

19. Digesu GA, Calandrini N, Derpapas A, Gallo P, Ahmed S, Khullar V. Intraobserver and interobserver reliability of the three-dimensional ultrasound imaging of female urethral sphincter using a translabial technique. Int Urogynecol J. 2012;23(8): 1063–8.

20. Athanasiou S, Khullar V, Boos K, Salvatore S, Cardozo L. Imaging the urethral sphincter with three-dimensional ultrasound. Obstet Gynecol. 1999;94(2):295–301.

21. Shobeiri SA, Rostaminia G, White DE, Quiroz LH. The determinants of minimal levator hiatus and their relationship to the puborectalis muscle and the levator plate. BJOG. 2012. doi:10.1111/1471-0528.12055

22. Kim J, Ramanah R, DeLancey JOL, Ashton-miller JA. On the anatomy and histology of the pubovisceral muscle enthesis in women. Neurourol Urodyn. 2011;30:1366–70.

23. Kruger JA, Heap SW, Murphy BA, Dietz HP. How best to measure the levator hiatus: evidence for the non-Euclidean nature of the 'plane of minimal dimensions'. Ultrasound Obstet Gynecol. 2010;36(6):755–8.

24. Siafarikas F, Staer-Jensen J, Braekken I, Bo K, Engh ME. Learning process for performing and analysing 3/4D transperineal ultrasound imaging and inter-rater reliability study. Ultrasound Obstet Gynecol. 2013;41:312–7.

25. Jung SA, Pretorius DH, Padda BS, Weinstein MM, Nager CW, den Boer DJ, et al. Vaginal high-pressure zone assessed by dynamic 3-dimensional ultrasound images of the pelvic floor. Am J Obstet Gynecol. 2007;197(1):52.e1–7.

26. Dietz HP. Quantification of major morphological abnormalities of the levator ani. Ultrasound Obstet Gynecol. 2007;29(3):329–34.

27. Weinstein MM, Pretorius DH, Jung SA, Nager CW, Mittal RK. Transperineal three-dimensional ultrasound imaging for detection of anatomic defects in the anal sphincter complex muscles. Clin Gastroenterol Hepatol. 2009;7(2):205–11.

28. DeLancey JO, Kearney R, Chou Q, Speights S, Binno S. The appearance of levator ani muscle abnormalities in magnetic resonance images after vaginal delivery. Obstet Gynecol. 2003;101(1):46–53. Epub 2003/01/09.

29. Dietz HP, Lanzarone V. Levator trauma after vaginal delivery. Obstet Gynecol. 2005;106(4):707–12.

30. Dietz HP, Steensma AB. The prevalence of major abnormalities of the levator ani in urogynaecological patients. BJOG. 2006;113(2):225–30.

31. Model AN, Shek KL, Dietz HP. Levator defects are associated with prolapse after pelvic floor surgery. Eur J Obstet Gynecol Reprod Biol. 2010;153(2): 220–3.

32. Dietz HP, Wilson PD, Clarke B. The use of perineal ultrasound to quantify levator activity and teach pelvic floor muscle exercises. Int Urogynecol J Pelvic Floor Dysfunct. 2001;12(3):166–8. discussion 8–9.

33. Choi JS, Wexner SD, Nam YS, Mavrantonis C, Salum MR, Yamaguchi T, et al. Intraobserver and interobserver measurements of the anorectal angle and perineal descent in defecography. Dis Colon Rectum. 2000;43(8):1121–6.

34. Padda BS, Jung SA, Pretorius D, Nager CW, Den-Boer D, Mittal RK. Effects of pelvic floor muscle contraction on anal canal pressure. Am J Physiol Gastrointest Liver Physiol. 2007;292(2):G565–71.

35. Roos AM, Abdool Z, Sultan AH, Thakar R. The diagnostic accuracy of endovaginal and transperineal ultrasound for detecting anal sphincter defects: the PREDICT study. Clin Radiol. 2011;66(7):597–604. Epub 2011/03/29.

36. Kruger JA, Heap SW, Murphy BA, Dietz HP. Pelvic floor function in nulliparous women using three-dimensional ultrasound and magnetic resonance imaging. Obstet Gynecol. 2008;111(3):631–8.

37. Dietz HP, Shek C, Clarke B. Biometry of the pubovisceral muscle and levator hiatus by three-dimensional pelvic floor ultrasound. Ultrasound Obstet Gynecol. 2005;25(6):580–5.

38. Jackson SL, Weber AM, Hull TL, Mitchinson AR, Walters MD. Fecal incontinence in women with urinary incontinence and pelvic organ prolapse. Obstet Gynecol. 1997;89(3):423–7.

39. Schuettoff S, Beyersdorff D, Gauruder-Burmester A, Tunn R. Visibility of the polypropylene tape after tension-free vaginal tape (TVT) procedure in women with stress urinary incontinence: comparison of introital ultrasound and magnetic resonance imaging in vitro and in vivo. Ultrasound Obstet Gynecol. 2006;27(6):687–92.

40. Yalcin OT, Hassa H, Tanir M. A new ultrasonographic method for evaluation of the results of anti-incontinence operations. Acta Obstet Gynecol Scand. 2002;81(2):151–6.

41. Dietz HP, Wilson PD. The 'iris effect': how two-dimensional and three-dimensional ultrasound can help us understand anti-incontinence procedures. Ultrasound Obstet Gynecol. 2004;23(3):267–71.

42. Dietz HP, Mouritsen L, Ellis G, Wilson PD. How important is TVT location? Acta Obstet Gynecol Scand. 2004;83(10):904–8.

43. Ng CC, Lee LC, Han WH. Use of three-dimensional ultrasound scan to assess the clinical importance of midurethral placement of the tension-free vaginal tape (TVT) for treatment of incontinence. Int Urogynecol J Pelvic Floor Dysfunct. 2005;16(3):220–5.

44. Elia G, Bergman A. Periurethral collagen implant: ultrasound assessment and prediction of outcome. Int Urogynecol J Pelvic Floor Dysfunct. 1996;7(6):335–8.

45. Defreitas GA, Wilson TS, Zimmern PE, Forte TB. Three-dimensional ultrasonography: an objective outcome tool to assess collagen distribution in women with stress urinary incontinence. Urology. 2003;62(2):232–6.

46. Poon CI, Zimmern PE. Role of three-dimensional ultrasound in assessment of women undergoing urethral bulking agent therapy. Curr Opin Obstet Gynecol. 2004;16(5):411–7.

47. Dietz HP, Steensma AB. Posterior compartment prolapse on two-dimensional and three-dimensional pelvic floor ultrasound: the distinction between true rectocele, perineal hypermobility and enterocele. Ultrasound Obstet Gynecol. 2005;26(1):73–7.

48. Grasso RF, Piciucchi S, Quattrocchi CC, Sammarra M, Ripetti V, Zobel BB. Posterior pelvic floor disorders: a prospective comparison using introital ultrasound and colpocystodefecography. Ultrasound Obstet Gynecol. 2007;30(1):86–94.

49. Weemhoff M, Kluivers KB, Govaert B, Evers JL, Kessels AG, Baeten CG. Transperineal ultrasound compared to evacuation proctography for diagnosing enteroceles and intussusceptions. Int J Colorectal Dis. 2013;28:359–63.

50. Broekhuis SR, Kluivers KB, Hendriks JC, Futterer JJ, Barentsz JO, Vierhout ME. POP-Q, dynamic MR imaging, and perineal ultrasonography: do they agree in the quantification of female pelvic organ prolapse? Int Urogynecol J Pelvic Floor Dysfunct. 2009;20(5):541–9.

51. Lone FW, Thakar R, Sultan AH, Stankiewicz A. Accuracy of assessing pelvic organ prolapse quantification points using dynamic 2D transperineal ultrasound in women with pelvic organ prolapse. Int Urogynecol J. 2012;23(11):1555–60.

3D Endovaginal Ultrasound Imaging of the Levator Ani Muscles

4

Lieschen H. Quiroz and S. Abbas Shobeiri

Learning Objectives

1. To describe 3D Endovaginal sono-graphic anatomy of the pelvic floor structures
2. To understand the 3D endovaginal ultrasound technique with transducer position and image orientation and optimization
3. To provide overview of angles and measurements in 3D Endovaginal pelvic floor US
4. To appreciate role of endovaginal US in pelvic floor disorders

4.1 Introduction

4.1.1 Imaging Modalities for Endovaginal Imaging

The pelvic floor is a complex three-dimensional structure, with a variety of functional and anatomical areas. It consists of a musculotendinous sheet that spans the pelvic outlet and consists of

paired levator ani muscle (LAM). It is broadly accepted that the LAM consists of subdivisions that have been characterized according to the origin and insertion points, consisting of the pubo-visceral, puborectal, and puboanal portions [1]. Although MRI descriptions of the pubovisceral subdivision included the puboperinealis, pubo-vaginalis, and puboanalis (Fig. 4.1), our more recent 3D endovaginal ultrasound literature groups iliococcygeus and pubococcygeus as part of the pubovisceralis [1]. Lateral to the pubovis-ceral division of the LAM is the puborectal division, which forms a sling around and behind the rectum, just cephalad to the external anal sphincter. Lastly, the iliococcygeus division forms a flat, horizontal shelf, spanning both pelvic side walls (Fig. 4.2) [2]. The validity of 3D EVUS to visualize LAM subdivisions has been established by meticulous anatomic studies [3]. These subdivisions were localized in cadaveric dissections (Fig. 4.3), then correlated with images seen in nulliparous women, based on origin and insertion points and were shown to have excellent interobserver reliability.

The pelvic floor muscles have the unique role of supporting the urogenital organs and the ano-rectum. Unlike most other skeletal muscles, the LAM maintains constant tone, except during voiding, defecation and a Valsalva maneuver [4]. At rest, the LAM keeps the urogenital hiatus closed, by compressing the vagina, urethra, and rectum against the pubic bone, and maintains the pelvic floor and pelvic organs in a cephalic

L.H. Quiroz, M.D., • S.A. Shobeiri, M.D. (✉)
Department of Obstetrics and Gynecology,
Female Pelvic Medicine and Reconstructive Surgery,
The University of Oklahoma Health Sciences Center,
WP 2410, 920 Stanton L. Young Blvd., Oklahoma
City, OK 73104, USA
e-mail: Abbas-shobeiri@ouhsc.edu

S.A. Shobeiri (ed.), *Practical Pelvic Floor Ultrasonography: A Multicompartmental Approach to 2D/3D/4D Ultrasonography of Pelvic Floor*, DOI 10.1007/978-1-4614-8426-4_4,
© Springer Science+Business Media New York 2014

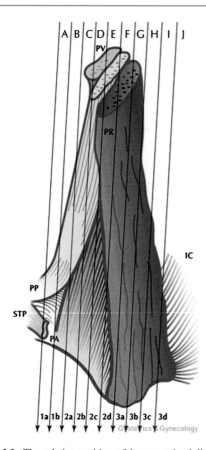

Fig. 4.1 The relative position of levator ani subdivisions during ultrasound imaging. Levels 1–3 are identified below the figure. The A–J markings on *top* of the figure correspond to the ultrasound images shown in Fig. 4.4. *IC* iliococcygeus, *PP* puboperinealis, *STP* superficial transverse perinea, *PA* puboanalis. Illustration: John Yanson. © Shobeiri. Ultrasonography Validation. Obstet Gynecol 2009

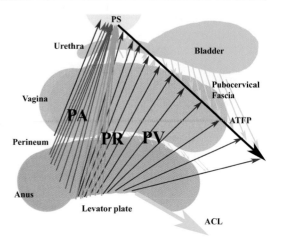

Fig. 4.2 Subgrouping of the pubovisceralis (PV), puborectalis (PR), and the puboanalis muscle groups. The lines of actions of these muscle groups and their relative contributions to the levator plate are shown. Anococcygeal ligaments (ACL), Arcus tendineus Fascia Pelvis (ATFP) are shown. © Shobeiri

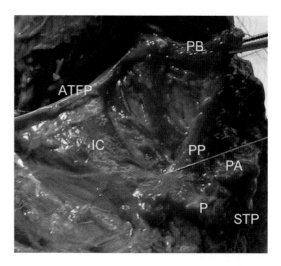

Fig. 4.3 Gross cadaveric dissection. A needle is seen inserted into the puboperinealis. *PB* pubic bone on pubic bone insertion, *ATFP* arcus tendineus fascia pelvis, *IC* iliococcygeus, *PP* puboperinealis, *PA* puboanalis, *P* perineum, *STP* superficial transverse perinei. Shobeiri. Ultrasonography Validation. Obstet Gynecol 2009

direction (Fig. 4.2) [2]. Pelvic floor muscles are integral to pelvic organ support, and while functioning properly, provide support to the pelvic organs, keeping the ligament and fascial attachments tension-free.

During parturition, the LAM stretches beyond its limits [5, 6] in order to allow passage of a term infant (Fig. 4.4). Studies have shown that LAM injury occur in 13–36 % of women who deliver vaginally [7–9]. There are various definitions of levator ani injury, according to mode of assessment and imaging modality. Most authors have used avulsion of the muscles as the end point of the study. However, more recent in publication studies using 3D endovaginal ultrasonography have found that up to 50 % of women may have hematoma formation after first delivery (Fig. 4.5). Assessment of the levator muscles is essential for a complete understanding of pelvic floor

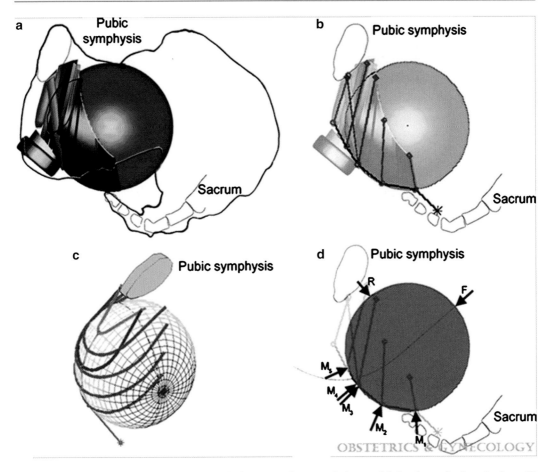

Fig. 4.4 (**a**) Initial geometry of the female pelvic floor at the beginning of the second stage of labor in a left lateral view. (**b**) Left lateral view of the pelvic floor model. (**c**) Left three-quarter view of the model. (**d**) A free body diagram of the model is shown in lateral view. (© Biomechanics Research Laboratory, University of Michigan). Lien. Efficacy of Maternal Effort. Obstet Gynecol 2009

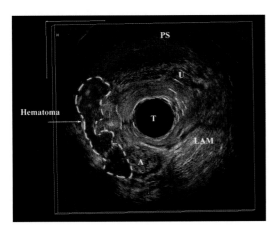

Fig. 4.5 Hematoma formation in the right levator ani muscle territory is outlined. Anus (A), transducer (T), urethra (U), pubic symphysis (PS). © Shobeiri

anatomy abnormalities, as well as of pelvic floor dysfunction.

4.1.2   3-D EVUS Technique for Levator Ani Imaging

All the endovaginal and endoanal images in this chapter are obtained from a Flex Focus (Fig. 4.6) or ProFocus Ultraview (Fig. 4.7) BK Medical scanner (BK Medical, Peabody, MA) as discussed in previous chapter on Instrumentations and techniques. For optimal images to be obtained, we recommend for the operator to have a clear understanding of the technique, as well as

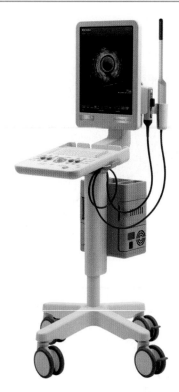

Fig. 4.6 BK flex focus ultrasound machine with a 2052 probe

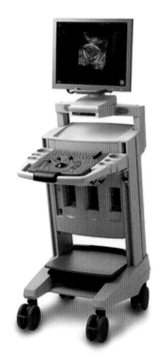

Pro Focus UltraView scanner

Fig. 4.7 BK ultrafocus ultrasound machine

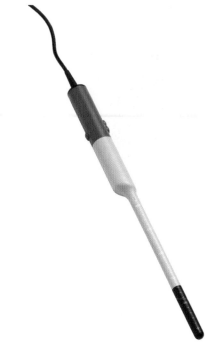

Fig. 4.8 BK 2052 transducer

familiarity with the controls of the machine. Most importantly, improper settings of the equipment can lead to artifact.

Two 360° probes can be used for endovaginal levator ani imaging. The 2052 transducer (Fig. 4.8) is its built-in 3D automatic motorized system (proximal-distal actuation mechanism is enclosed within the shield of the probe). This equipment allows for the acquisition of 300 images in 60 s for a distance of 60 mm. The 8838 probe is a 60 mm 360° rotational transducer and obtains an image every 0.55° for a total of 720 images (Fig. 4.9). The images are acquired automatically with the touch of the 3D button on the equipment console. The data from the closely spaced 2D images are combined as a 3D volume displayed as a data volume which can then be stored and analyzed separately.

No special patient preparation is required and no vaginal or rectal contrast is necessary. The patient is asked to keep a comfortable amount of urine in the bladder. The patient is placed on the dorsal lithotomy position and the probe is inserted in a neutral position, with care

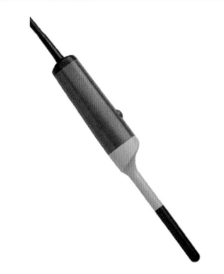

Fig. 4.9 BK 8838 transducer

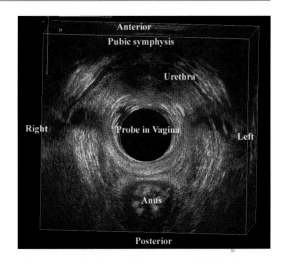

Fig. 4.10 An endovaginal 3D volume. © Shobeiri

not to press on the upper or lower vaginal areas so as not to distort anatomy. The probe should create a horizontal line with the body's axis. When placing the ultrasound gel in the probe cover, we recommend for air bubbles to be gently squeezed out of the probe cover, so as to minimize the potential for artifact.

Once the 3D endovaginal imaging is selected on the console, the rotating crystal will begin to rotate, signaling that the probe is ready for insertion. The probe is inserted as described in endovaginal instrumentations and techniques chapter. Based on our anatomic studies, we recommend placing the probe 6 cm inside the vagina, just 2 cm above the level of the urethrovesical junction. If using the 2052 probe, the two buttons that move the crystal cephalad and caudad should be facing the 12 o'clock position. Once the acquisition is started, it is important that the operator minimize movement by stabilizing the probe during the full length of the scan. This will help optimize image quality in obtaining the 3D cube (Fig. 4.10). We have characterized 3 levels for assessment of the axial plane [3] (Fig. 4.1).

Level 1: Contains all the muscles that insert into the perineal body, namely the superficial transverse perinei (STP), puboperinealis, and puboanalis. The STP serves as the reference point.

Level 2: Contains the attachment of the pubovaginalis, puboperinealis, puboanalis, puborectalis, and iliococcygeus to the pubic bone.

Level 3: Contains the subdivisions cephalad to the inferior pubic ramus, namely the pubococcygeus and iliococcygeus, which wing out towards the ischial spine.

Functionally and based on the levator ani volume measurements, we divide the muscles into: (1) Puboanalis (Puboperinealis + Puboanalis), (2) Puborectalis, and (3) Pubovisceralis (Pubococcygeus + Iliococcygeus) (Fig. 4.2). By 3D endovaginal ultrasound reconstruction of nulliparous subjects, puboanalis, puborectalis, and pubovisceralis groups had the volume of 4.4 cm^3 (Range 2.1–6.7 cm^3), 4.2 cm^3 (Range 1.9–6.5 cm^3), 4.5 (Range 2.2–6.8 cm^3) respectively. Although they have a wide range in volumes, the proportions remain constant within the individual [10].

When analyzing a 3D volume caudad to cephalad, the first structure to visualize as a landmark is the STP muscle (Fig. 4.11). Visualization of this structure will consistently point to the most caudad structure seen by the probe in the vaginal canal. In normal nulliparous individuals, the external anal sphincter may be visualized just below the STP. If using the 2052 probe, there are two buttons used to move the rotating crystal caudally or cephalad located on the dorsal portion of the probe handle. By pressing the cephalad button the rotating crystal can be slowly moved cephalad and the perineal body and puboperinealis muscle come to view (Fig. 4.12a, b). The puboperinealis is hard to find consistently for the untrained eyes because it perhaps has less than 30 muscle fibers and lies very close to the vaginal epithelium. At the same level but more

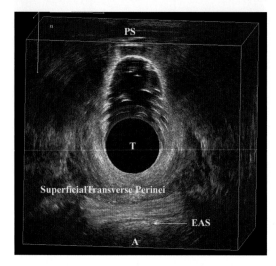

Fig. 4.11 The most caudad muscles seen by 3D endovaginal ultrasound imaging is the superficial transverse perinei muscle which is highlighted. External anal sphincter (EAS), anus (A), transducer (T), pubic symphysis (PS). © Shobeiri

laterally are the fibers of the puboanalis that travel at a 45° to surround the anal canal and insert into longitudinal fibers of the anus at the level of the external anal sphincter (Fig. 4.13). Continuing to move the crystal cephalad will show the puborectalis forming a sling around the rectum and it can be followed to its insertion into the inferior margin of the pubic symphysis and the perineal membrane. Moving further cephalad will show the medial relationship of the iliococcygeus muscle in its medial relationship to the puborectalis (Fig. 4.14).

The reliability of visualization of levator ani subdivisions have been reported in nulliparous patients. The levator ani subdivisions in these scans were examined at levels 1, 2, and 3 (Fig. 4.1). The visibility was scored by two blinded observers. Interrater reliability was calculated by taking the number of agreements and dividing by the number of observations in the total number of subjects. There was 98 %, 96 %, and 92 % agreement for level 1, 2, and 3 muscles respectively. Cohen's kappa index/standard error were calculated for individual muscles as below: STP and puborectalis were seen by both raters 100 %, puboperinealis 0.645/0.2, pubovaginalis, and puboanalis 0.645/0.2 (95 % confidence interval 0.1–1), iliococcygeous 0.9/0.2 (95 % confidence interval 0.6–1).

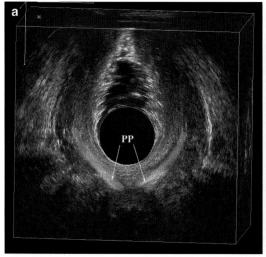

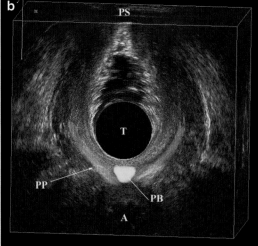

Fig. 4.12 (a) The scant fibers of the puboperinealis muscles (PP) are highlighted. (b) The perineal body (PB) is highlighted in the same axial view as 3a. Pubic symphysis (PS), transducer (T), puboperinealis (PP), perineal body (PB), anus (A). © Shobeiri

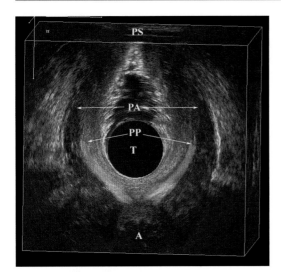

Fig. 4.13 The puboanalis (PA) is shown at the same level as the Fig. 4.12. PA lies just lateral to the puboperinealis (PP) and they are part of the same functional groups. Anus (A), transducer (T), pubic symphysis (PS). © Shobeiri

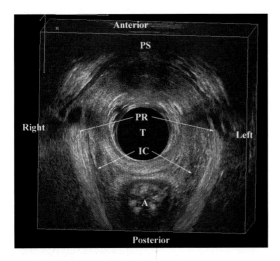

Fig. 4.14 The puborectalis (PR) is shown at its cephalad insertion point to the pubic symphysis (PS). Note that PR has a wide insertion area which includes the PS, and the perineal membrane which is more caudad. The iliococcygeus muscle (IC) fibers are seen medial to the puborectalis fibers. Anus (A), transducer (T). © Shobeiri

In addition to the visualization of the muscle subdivisions, the interobserver and the interdisciplinary repeatability of (1) Levator hiatus length; (2) Levator hiatus width; (3) Levator hiatus area; (4) LAM attachment to the pubic rami, on both sides; (5) Anorectal angle (ARA); (6) Urethral thickness measurements using 3D

endovaginal ultrasound have been established [11]. A team of six investigators of three different specialties (urogynecology—UGN, radiology—RAD, colorectal surgery—CRS) was formed. Each discipline included two investigators: UGN #1, UGN #2; RAD #1, RAD #2; CRS #1, CRS #2. Prior study initiation, a dedicated training session was completed and preliminary trial measurements were performed. For the training session, an expert 3D reader demonstrated to each of the readers the technique for measurements, including bony and soft tissue landmarks to be utilized. Readers discussed and refined the measurement technique for each parameter until all readers were in agreement regarding measurement methodology. In order to minimize the effect of imaging variations on the final measurements, a standardized protocol for review of the study datasets was strictly defined and jointly approved by all investigators.

Each ultrasound volume was displayed in a symmetrical orientation in the coronal, sagittal, and transverse planes and assessed in standardized sequences. The overall interobserver repeatability for levator hiatus dimensions was good to excellent (ICC, 0.655–0.889), for urethral thickness was good (ICC, 0.624), and for ARA was moderate (ICC, 0472) (Table 4.1). The interdisciplinary repeatability for levator hiatus indices was good to excellent (ICC, 0.639–0.915), for urethral thickness was moderate to good (ICC, 0.565–0.671), and for ARA was fair to moderate (ICC, 0.204–0.434) (Table 4.2) [11].

4.1.3   Clinical Applications

Pelvic floor disorders are common, costly, and distressing conditions for women resulting in greater than 300,000 operations per year, leading to considerable suffering from conditions not readily cured by surgery [12]. Fifty-five percent of women with pelvic organ prolapse (POP) have visible major LAM damage compared to 15 % of women with normal support making it the strongest known factor to be associated with both vaginal birth and POP [13]. The ability to diagnose injury to the LA muscle relies on advancements

Table 4.1 Overall means and standard deviations (SD) of various measurements of individual readers

Observer	LH length (mm)	LH width (mm)	LH area (cm²)	Urethral thickness (mm)	ARA (degrees)
UGN #1	50.42 (SD: 4.18)	35.03 (SD: 3.50)	10.48 (SD: 1.51)	12.82 (SD: 1.6)	133.1 (SD: 12.3)
UGN #2	48.62 (SD: 4.87)	34.21 (SD: 3.30)	10.60 (SD: 1.31)	13.06 (SD: 1.41)	144.2 (SD: 7.03)
RAD #1	48.71 (SD: 4.84)	33.76 (SD: 3.50)	10.72 (SD: 1.70)	12.86 (SD: 1.73)	143.04 (SD: 12.5)
RAD #2	47.55 (SD: 5.62)	33.54 (SD: 3.32)	11.76 (SD: 1.35)	12.61 (SD: 1.32)	141.1 (SD: 7.99)
CRS #1	47.95 (SD: 4.20)	34.52 (SD: 3.38)	10.82 (SD: 1.60)	12.23 (SD: 1.77)	143.8 (SD: 9.97)
CRS #2	47.20 (SD: 4.05)	34.06 (SD: 2.96)	10.14 (SD: 1.60)	12.30 (SD: 1.44)	136.1 (SD: 5.94)

UGN urogynecologist, *RAD* radiologist, *CRS* colorectal surgeon, *LH* levator hiatus, *ARA* anorectal angle
From Santoro: Interobserver and interdisciplinary reproducibility. IUGJ 2011

in imaging. Levator ani avulsion as imaged by transperineal ultrasound appears to double the risk of any significant anterior and central compartment prolapse [14].

4.2 Levaror Ani Injury

Recent literature has identified the distal subdivisions of the levator ani, classifying them based on attachment points, using magnetic resonance imaging. By MRI the LAM has been divided to pubovisceralis (to include pubovaginalis, puboanalis, puboperinealis, pubococcygeus and iliococcygeus) and puborectalis [1]. Morgan et al. have described levator ani defects and scored unilateral muscle defects separately [15]. The terminology for EVUS is different and in order to better functionally describe these LAM subdivisions, we group them as the puboanalis, puborectalis, and pubovisceralis (Fig. 4.2). Our technique and the anatomical descriptions were first authenticated in female cadavers and then in live human female volunteers, documenting superior, dynamic imaging, and visualization of these structures [3]. LAM injury has been described on MRI studies as a "defect" or "avulsion," attributed to causes such as obstetric factors, aging or hormonal changes. 3D endovaginal ultrasonography has been used for visualization of the levator ani avulsion before and after bridging repair using fascia lata graft [16] (Fig. 4.15). This repair was done remote from delivery due to the patients' symptoms. The goal of pelvic floor reconstruction is to restore the anatomy and hope that will translate into restoration of physiology

and ultimately improve the patient's symptoms. To restore the normal anatomy, if we repair the LAMs, normal functioning of the muscles may resume as long as the innervations is intact. Current "routine" surgical practice does not address these defects, but the sequalea of pelvic floor injury appears years after its occurrence. There is still the question of whether the identification and repair of these muscles early on will spare the patient from future POP and incontinence. Since identification of the muscle fibers is difficult without a localization technique, attempts at repairing these muscles without intraoperative visualization may have questionable results. In the absence of symptoms prompting LAM repair, it will require a large cohort and long term follow-up to determine if preemptive repair of the LAMs will translate into reduction of incontinence or POP [17]. In a case of bilateral levator ani injury (Fig. 4.16) after vaginal delivery, a patient underwent 3D endovaginal ultrasound and under ultrasound guidance (Fig. 4.17), the detached levator muscles were tagged with J-hook needles (MPM Medical, Elmwood Park, NJ) bilaterally. The needle could be manipulated to identify the torn ends of muscles. A vertical incision was made on the lateral wall of the vagina cephalad to the puboperinealis muscle which is the muscle traversing between the pubic symphysis and the perineal body. The dissection was made laterally to reach the area of needle. The tissue was grasped and then, with a finger in the rectum to ascertain rectal elevation, 2.0 vicryl sutures were passed (Fig. 4.3), 1 cm apart, and these were brought anteriorly to the level of the arcus tendineous insertion into the pubic bone

Table 4.2 Interobserver, intra- and interdisciplinary repeatability of three-dimensional endovaginal ultrasound parameters

Repeatability	LH length		LH width		LH area		Urethral thickness		ARA	
	ICC	95%CI	ICC	95%CI	ICC	95%CI	ICC	95%CI	ICC	95%CI
Overall	0.655	0.509–0.794	0.889	0.822–0.940	0.810	0.707–0.894	0.624	0.472–0.772	0.331	0.179–0.528
Intradisciplinary										
UGN #1 vs. UGN #2	0.643	0.359–0.819	0.889	0.773–0.948	0.857	0.713–0.932	0.660	0.385–0.829	0.035	−0.339–0.402
RAD #1 vs. RAD #2	0.717	0.473–0.860	0.981	0.958–0.991	0.893	0.781–0.950	0.601	0.298–0.795	0.569	0.252–0.777
CRS #1 vs. CRS #2	0.883	0.761–0.945	0.910	0.815–0.958	0.887	0.770–0.947	0.735	0.501–0.869	0.216	−0.167–0.544
Interdisciplinary										
RADs vs. CRSs	0.677	0.514–0.815	0.915	0.855–0.956	0.831	0.724–0.909	0.651	0.482–0.798	0.434	0.241–0.639
RADs vs. UGNs	0.639	0.467–0.790	0.897	0.826–0.946	0.851	0.755–0.921	0.565	0.380–0.739	0.327	0.139–0.549
UGNs vs. CRSs	0.694	0.536–0.826	0.874	0.790–0.934	0.783	0.656–0.882	0.671	0.506–0.811	0.204	0.032–0.431

ARA anorectal angle, *CI* confidence interval, *CRS* colorectal surgeon, *ICC* interclass correlation coefficient, *LH* levator hiatus, *RAD* radiologist, *UGN* urogynecologist
From Santoro: Interobserver and interdisciplinary reproducibility. IUGJ 2011

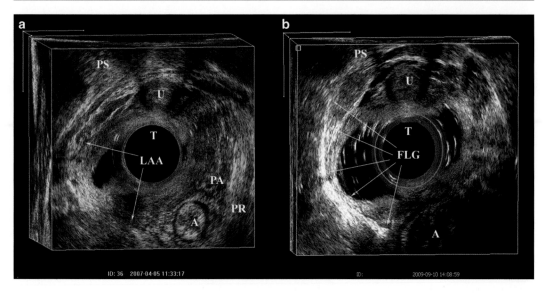

Fig. 4.15 (**a**) 3D EVUS of the patient with right levator ani avulsion (LAA). The *arrows* point to the extent of the defect. (**b**) 3D EVUS of the same patient almost 2.5 years after repairs point to the fascia lata graft (FLG) in correct position. © Shobeiri

Fig. 4.16 Bilateral puborectalis avulsion in endovaginal 360° 3D volume. The lines demonstrate the measurements of the urethra-levator gap. LAM: levator ani, anus (A), transducer (T), urethra (U), pubic symphysis (PS). © Shobeiri

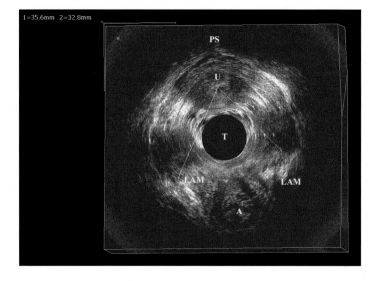

under direct visualization and tied sequentially. The procedure was repeated on the contralateral side with palpable lift of ARA.

Besides the dramatic presentation of the levator ani detachment from the pubic bone, there are ultrasound images which show muscles with scant fibers or muscles that are lax. Although no comparative studies have been published, these findings on 3D EVUS are perhaps analogous to transperineal 4D ultrasonog-raphy findings of what has been called microtrauma or ballooning. The absence of the LAM in MRI and ultrasound studies has been denoted as a defect or an avulsion attributed to many different causes such as labor and delivery, aging, or hormonal changes. Hudson referred to these changes collectively as "pelvic floor defi-ciency" [18]. We will denote the degree of leva-tor ani defects seen by ultrasound as "levator ani deficiency, or LAD."

4.2.1 LAD: Levator Ani Deficiency Score

Unlike the terms "defect" and "avulsion" which may imply an all or none phenomenon, the term "LAD" implies a measurable gradient. While documenting the presence or absence of injury is important, LA muscle damage after childbirth leading to symptomatic pelvic floor disorders, or a decrement in muscle strength, may depend on the location and severity of the injury. Identifying specific location and severity of defects in LA muscle subdivisions may help us correlate specific defects to corresponding clinical findings, providing further insight into the form and function of this complex muscle group. Recent imaging has pointed to the pubovisceral insertion (PVM) of the levator ani as the most often injured portion of the LAM group (Fig. 4.4) [19].

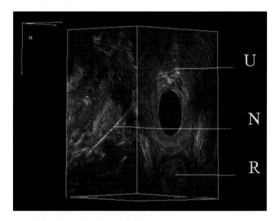

Fig. 4.17 J-hook needle in puborectalis muscle by endovaginal 360° ultrasound. Urethra (U), needle (N), rectum (R). © Shobeiri. Surgical repair of bilateral levator ani muscles. IUGJ 2012

4.2.2 Scoring System

A LAD scoring system to grade levator injury has been developed according to the morphology and clarity of the each subdivision's origin-insertion points, scored unilaterally. This is analogous to the scoring system used in the MR imaging [15]. Subgroups were evaluated and were scored (0 = no defect, 1 = minimal defect with ≤50 % muscle loss, 2 = major defect with >50 % muscle loss, 3 = total absence of the muscle) on each side based on thickness and detachment from the pubic bone (Table 4.3). Each muscle pair score ranged from 0, indicating no defects, to maximum score of 6, indicating total muscle absence. For the entire LAM group, a cumulative LAD score that ranged between 0 and 18 was possible. Scores were categorized as 0–6 = mild (Fig. 4.18) 7–12 = moderate (Fig. 4.19) and >13 = severe deficiency (Fig. 4.20) [20].

In a study to evaluate if there is a LAD threshold above which prolapse occurs, 220 patients were analyzed. Table 4.4 shows the distribution of stages of prolapse and associated LAD scores. Kruskal-Wallis test demonstrated that the distribution of scores significantly differed by stage of prolapse ($p < 0.0001$). The distribution of LAD status (mild, moderate, severe) was also significantly different between stages of prolapse (Table 4.5). A moderate positive correlation was demonstrated between LAD score and stage of prolapse ($r_s = 0.44$, $p < 0.0001$). When trying to find a threshold of LAD above which vaginal prolapse developed, no subjects with stage 3 prolapse had a score lower than 6, no subjects with stage 4 prolapse had a LAD score lower than 9 (Fig. 4.21). While all patients with stage 3 and 4 prolapse had moderate

Table 4.3 EVUS validated scoring system for levator ani muscle deficiency (LAD)

Score	0 (No muscle damage)	1 (Mild abnormality)	2 (Moderate abnormality)	3 (Complete muscle loss)	Subtotal 0–3	Total 0–18
(L) Puboanalis (PA + PP)						
(R) Puboanalis (PA + PP)						
(L) Puborectalis						
(R) Puborectalis						
(L) Pubovisceralis (IC + PC)						
(R) Pubovisceralis (IC + PC)						

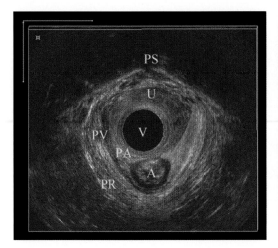

Fig. 4.18 3D ultrasound volume of a normal nulliparous woman with LAD score of 0. Anus (A), vagina (V), urethra (U), pubic symphysis (PS), puboanalis (PA), puboviceralis (PV), puborectalis (PR). © Shobeiri, Levator Ani Deficiency and Pelvic Organ Prolapse severity, Obstet Gynecol 2013

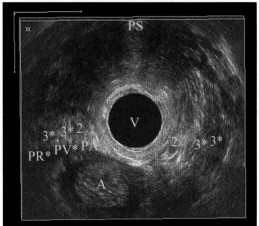

Fig. 4.20 The axial view of pelvic floor muscles with severe LA muscle deficiency. *Asterisks* denotes a missing muscle and numbers are muscle scores. Anus (A), vagina (V), pubic symphysis (PS), puboanalis (PA), pubovisceralis (PV), puborectalis (PR). © Shobeiri, Levator Ani Deficiency and Pelvic Organ Prolapse severity, Obstet Gynecol 2013

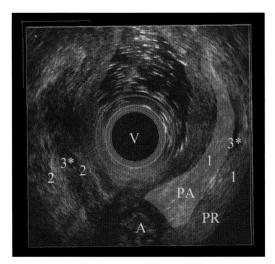

Fig. 4.19 The axial view of pelvic floor muscles with moderate LA muscle deficiency. *Asterisks* denotes a missing muscle and numbers are muscle scores. Anus (A), vagina (V), puboanalis (PA), puborectalis (PR). © Shobeiri, Levator Ani Deficiency and Pelvic Organ Prolapse severity, Obstet Gynecol 2013

Table 4.4 Distribution of stages of prolapse and associated total LA scores.

	n (%)	LA score (median, range)	p-value[a]
Stage 0	50 (22.7)	6 (0, 18)	<0.0001
Stage 1	57 (25.9)	8 (0, 18)	
Stage 2	60 (27.3)	10 (0, 18)	
Stage 3	43 (19.6)	14 (6, 18)	
Stage 4	10 (4.6)	13 (9, 18)	

Shobeiri, Levator ani deficiency, Obstet Gynecol 2013
[a]Based on Kruskall-Wallis test results

Table 4.5 Severity of LA deficiency by compartment and stage of prolapse

	Minimal LAD	Moderate LAD	Severe LAD	
	n, (%)	n, (%)	n, (%)	p-value
Stage 0	32, (42.1)	12, (15.2)	6, (9.2)	<0.0001[a]
Stage 1	22, (29.0)	24, (30.4)	11, (16.9)	
Stage 2	16, (21.1)	27, (34.2)	17, (26.2)	
Stage 3	6, (7.9)	11, (13.9)	26, (40.0)	
Stage 4	0, (0.0)	5, (6.3)	5, (7.7)	

Shobeiri, Levator ani deficiency, Obstet Gynecol 2013
[a]Based on chi-square test

to severe LAD, in the group of patients with no prolapse there were 15.2 % with moderate, and 9.2 % with severe LAM deficiency. The frequency of severe LAD increased progressively with increasing stage of POPQ (Fig. 4.22). Final adjusted logistic regression demonstrated a significant rela-

tionship between LAD score and the presence of clinically significant POP (Table 4.6). Likelihood ratio, c-statistics, and Hosmer-Lemeshow goodness of fit tests each indicated excellent model fit

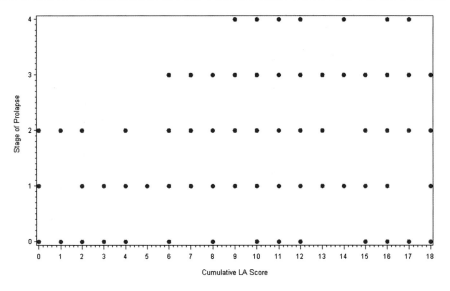

Fig. 4.21 Scatter plot of stage of prolapse and cumulative LA score. © Shobeiri

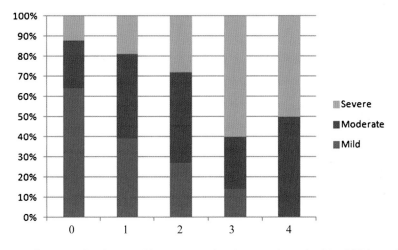

Fig. 4.22 Bar chart for stage of prolapse and LA score frequency. *Y* axis denotes the percentile of patients with mild, moderate, or severe LAD. *X* axis denotes the stage of prolapse as determined by POPQ staging system. © Shobeiri, Levator Ani Deficiency and Pelvic Organ Prolapse severity, Obstet Gynecol 2013

Table 4.6 Severity of LA deficiency by clinically significant prolapse

	Minimal defect	Moderate defect	Severe defect	
	(*n*, %)	(*n*, %)	(*n*, %)	*p*-value[a]
Stage 0–1	54 (71.1)	36 (45.6)	17 (26.2)	<0.0001
Stage 2–4	22 (29.0)	43 (54.4)	48 (73.9)	

[a]Based on chi-square test

(Table 4.6, Fig. 4.23). After controlling for age, parity, and menopausal status, patients with a moderate LAD have 3.2 times the odds of significant POP than those with only minimal deficiency; those with severe LAD have 6.44 times the odds of significant POP than those with minimal deficiency. Thus, worsening LAD scores as identified by 3D EVUS is a predictor of clinically significant POP [20]. From a biomechanical perspective, this data is important, since pelvic floor support provided by these muscles will be weak, and the load will shift from the deficient muscles to the supportive connective tissues and cause their failure [21]. However, two women with identical levator ani defects may present with different POP presentations. Finite element modeling have demonstrated that, in addition to LAM deficiency, development of prolapse, such as a cystocele, also requires an increase in abdominal pressure and apical and paravaginal support defect [22].

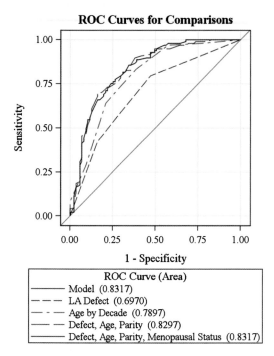

Fig. 4.23 ROC curve for comparison. © Shobeiri, Levator Ani Deficiency and Pelvic Organ Prolapse severity, Obstet Gynecol 2013

4.3　Changes of Levator Ani with Aging

Injuries to the LA after a vaginal delivery are associated with difficult vaginal birth, and with older age [23]. Age is commonly cited as a risk factor for developing prolapse, however few studies have examined the effect of aging on pelvic floor structures and function in the absence of childbirth trauma [24]. The role of age as a factor impacting possible age-related abnormalities in nulliparous women is understudied.

It is not known whether atrophic changes related to age will affect the visualization of the LA muscles, or mimic defects. This is important because the thickness of normal muscles varies among nulliparous women [25]. We performed a study to evaluate the visibility of LA muscles in 80 community dwelling nulliparous women LAD scoring system. Unilateral and bilateral levator ani subdivisions were scored according the LAD score system described above. Two observers read all the ultrasound cubes, with a resulting exact agreement for bilateral scoring of each levator ani subdivision ranged from 82 to 84 % [26]. There was no correlation between increasing age and total LA muscle scores

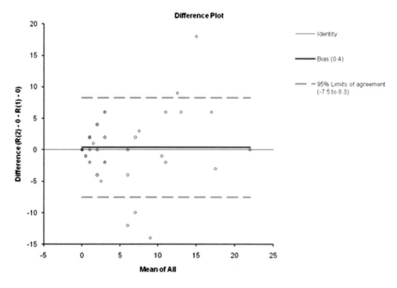

Fig. 4.24 Bland Altman plot showing mean difference of measurements between readers. © Quiroz, *Does age affect visualization of the levator ani in nulliparous women*? Int Urogynecol J. 2013

($r=0.20$, $p=0.072$). We found high levels of agreement among observers in assessing 3D EVUS scans of LAM subdivisions of nulliparous women of different ages, suggesting that age alone does not significantly impact reliable visualization of the LA muscle on 3-D EVUS (Fig. 4.24).

4.3.1 Levator Plate Descent Angle and Minimal Levator Hiatus

It is known that the normal shape of LAMs become distorted with different degrees of prolapse. Despite the association between prolapse and levator damage, there are women with prolapse who do not have levator defects and women with normal support who do have levator defects [27]. The minimal levator hiatus (MLH) dimensions, levator plate angle (LPA), iliococcygeal angle, and ARA have been used for assessing the impact of levator damage on static and dynamic imaging features [28, 29]. The puborectalis muscle is recognized as one of the components of the levator ani that forms the vaginal high pressure zone.

The puborectalis muscle is commonly thought to undergo injury during vaginal childbirth, in the form of avulsion from its insertion on the pubic ramus [23, 30, 31]. There had been no argument on what constitutes an avulsion mainly because it was thought that the puborectalis is the muscle injured. Avulsion of muscles from the pubic bone is known to have a marked effect on levator dimensions [32]. The MLH, which is the smallest fibromuscular dimension of the pelvic floor outlet, is thought to be made of levator fibers.

Due to variations in terminology, the borders of the MLH had not been consistently defined in the literature. The borders of the MLH have been recently described in detail using 3D EVUS [33]. 3D ultrasounds in this study were first performed in fresh frozen cadavers and structures were then confirmed in cadaveric dissections. Excellent interobserver and interdisciplinary reproducibility of 3D endovaginal ultrasound in measuring levator hiatus dimensions has been previously reported [11].

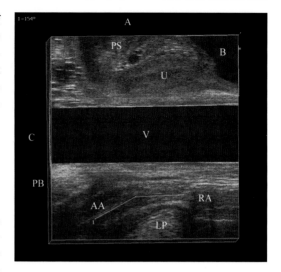

Fig. 4.25 Anorectal angle in midsagittal view by transvaginal 360° ultrasound. *A* anterior, *AA* anal axis, *B* bladder, *C* caudad, *LP* levator plate, *PB* perineal body, *PS* pubic symphysis, *RA* rectal axis, *U* urethra, *V* vagina. © Shobeiri. The determinants of minimal levator hiatus. BJOG 2012

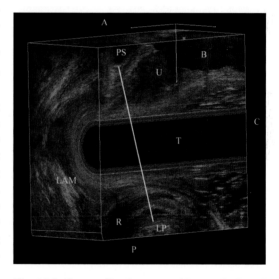

Fig. 4.26 Shortest line between pubic symphysis and levator plate in right midsagittal view by 3D EVUS; *A* anterior, *B* bladder, *C* cephalad, *LAM* levator ani muscle, *LP* levator plate, *P* posterior, *PS* pubic symphysis, *R* rectum, *T* transducer, *U* urethra. © Shobeiri

We measured the MLH area, puborectalis area, ARA, and levator plate descent angle (LPDA). We used the midsagittal view to measure the ARA, defined as the angle between the rectal and anal canal axis (Fig. 4.25). The ARA can be measured in the midsagittal plane as the

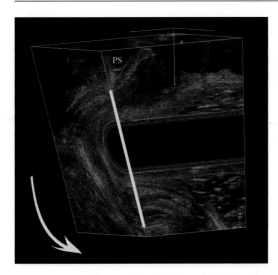

Fig. 4.27 The axial plane is rotated posteriorly and was advanced cephalad parallel to the shortest line between pubic symphysis and levator plate. *PS* pubic symphysis. © Shobeiri

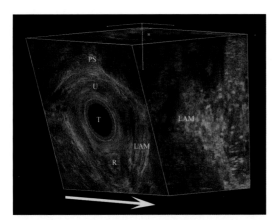

Fig. 4.28 The midsagittal plane was expanded to make the whole volume visible. *LAM* levator ani muscle, *PS* pubic symphysis, *R* rectum, *T* transducer, *U*: urethra. © Shobeiri

angle formed by the longitudinal posterior border of the anal canal and the posterior rectal wall. The posterior walls may be obscured at times due to presence of gas in the rectum. We located the shortest distance between pubic symphysis and the levator plate which formed the anterior-posterior (AP) diameter of the MLH. To obtain MLH we first draw a line between the pubic symphysis and the most anterior point on the levator plate (Fig. 4.26). The MLH is not in the axial plane. This is the strength of the BK software as it can

easily tilt the plane to become parallel to the MLH (Fig. 4.27) and once the 3D volume is expanded, the full MLH comes to view (Fig. 4.28). To obtain correct measurements, the observers should recognize the pubic symphysis and the anal canal for an appropriate anterior-posterior orientation of the image. In this plane, the levator ani was visualized as a multilayer hyperechoic sling coursing lateral to the vagina and posteriorly to the anal canal and attaching to the inferior pubic rami. The plane of minimal hiatal dimensions can be identified as the minimal distance between the inferior edge of the pubic symphysis and the anterior border of the levator ani at the ARA. In order to ensure that the minimal hiatal dimensions are found, the axial and sagittal planes should be carefully observed. The area of the levator hiatus can be calculated as the area within the levator ani inner perimeter enclosed by the inferior pubic rami and the inferior edge of the pubic symphysis. The length (anterior-posterior diameter) of the levator hiatus (LH) should be measured from the inferior border of the pubic symphysis to the 6 o'clock inner margin of the levator ani. The width (latero-lateral, or Left-Right diameter) of the levator hiatus should be taken on the widest part, perpendicular to levator hiatus anterior-posterior diameter [11].

The AP line of the MLH corresponds to the H line in MRI imaging [34]. We created the Pubic Levator Ultrasound Reference Assessment Line or in short the PLURAL plane which is a line drawn through the anterior-posterior axis of the mid-pubic symphysis and extended posteriorly. The data volume was then rotated such that the PLURAL plane was vertical. The relative position of the MLH to the PLURAL plane was measured using an angle which we termed the Levator Plate Descent Angle, or LPDA (Fig. 4.29). The MLH was measured along the puboanalis muscle medially, pubic bone anteriorly, and the levator plate posteriorly (Fig. 4.30). In order to measure the area created by the puborectalis muscle (puborectalis muscle hiatus), the puborectalis muscle borders were determined in the semi-axial view in a plane that had the puborectalis laterally, pubic symphysis anteriorly, and the levator plate posterior (Fig. 4.31). When the puborectalis muscle hiatus was approached from the sagittal

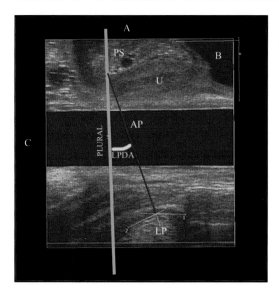

Fig. 4.29 Levator plate descent angle in midsagittal view by transvaginal 360° ultrasound. *A* anterior, *AP* antero-posterior line of minimal levator hiatus (*blue line*), *B* bladder, *C* caudad, *LP* levator plate, *LPDA* levator plate descent angle, *PLURAL* pubic levator ultrasound reference assessment line (*green line*), *PS* pubic symphysis, *U* urethra. © Shobeiri. The determinants of minimal levator hiatus. BJOG 2012

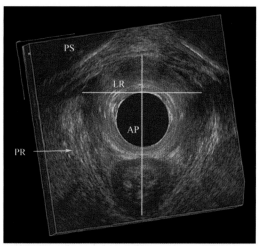

Fig. 4.31 Puborectalis hiatus in the same patient in axial view by transvaginal 360° ultrasound. *AP* antero-posterior line of minimal levator hiatus, *LP* levator plate, *PR* puborectalis, *PS* pubic symphysis. © Shobeiri. The determinants of minimal levator hiatus. BJOG 2012

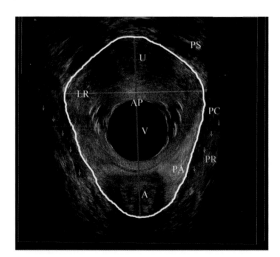

Fig. 4.30 Minimal levator hiatus area in axial plane by transvaginal 360° ultrasound. AP line is in blue. Puborectalis-pubococcygeus border is delineated with *small arrows*. *A* anus, *AP* antero-posterior line of minimal levator hiatus (*blue line*), *LR* left-right axis of minimal levator hiatus, *PC* pubococcygeus, *PR* puborectalis, *PS* pubic symphysis, *U* urethra, *V* vagina. © Shobeiri. The determinants of minimal levator hiatus. BJOG 2012

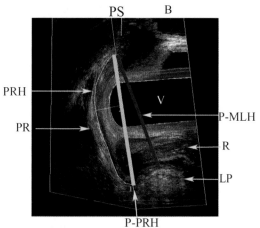

Fig. 4.32 Ultrasound showing plane of MLH and PRH in right sagittal view. *AP* antero-posterior line of minimal levator hiatus (*blue line*), *B* bladder, *LP* levator plate, *LPDA* levator plate descent angle, *P-MLH* plane of minimal levator hiatus (*blue line*), *P-PRH* plane of puborectalis hiatus (*purple line*), *PR* puborectalis, *PRH puborectalis hiatus*, *PS* pubic symphysis, *R* rectum, *V* vagina. © Shobeiri. The determinants of minimal levator hiatus. BJOG 2012

plane, its position relative to the MLH was clarified (Fig. 4.32).

In order to determine the normality, we used 80 nulliparous women and measured MLH area,

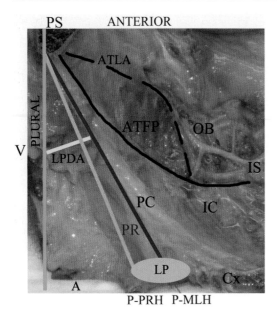

Fig. 4.33 Cadaver dissection of the right hemipelvis with the pelvic floor muscles visible. The plane of MLH and PRH are outlined. *A* anus, *AP* antero-posterior line of minimal levator hiatus (*blue line*), *CX* coccyx, *IC* iliococcygeus, *IS* ischial spine, *LP* levator plate, *LPDA* levator plate descent angle, *OB* obturator vessels, *PLURAL* pubic levator ultrasound reference assessment line (*green line*), *P-MLH* plane of minimal levator hiatus (*blue line*), *P-PRH* plane of puborectalis hiatus (*purple line*), *PB* perineal body, *PC* pubococcygeus, *PR* puborectalis, *PS* pubic symphysis, *V* vagina. © Shobeiri. The determinants of minimal levator hiatus. BJOG 2012

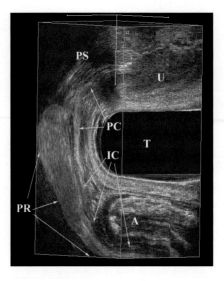

Fig. 4.34 The right sagittal view of a 3D EVUS showing the MLH muscles and their contribution to the levator plate. *A* anus, *PC* pubococcygeus, *PR* puborectalis, *PS* pubic symphysis, *IC* iliococcygeus, *T* transducer, *U* urethra. © Shobeiri

puborectalis hiatus area, ARA, and the LPDA. Having normal ranges of measurements helps investigators to define abnormality and perform further research on how to restore normalcy. In summary, the pubococcygeus forms the inner lateral border and anterior attachment of the MLH to the pubic bone (Fig. 4.33). The puboanalis fibers are immediately lateral to pubococcygeus attachments at the level of the pubic bone. There are variable contributions of the puborectalis fibers lateral to the puboanalis attachment. The posterior border of the MLH is formed by the levator plate. Eighty community dwelling nulliparous women underwent 3D endovaginal ultrasound (Fig. 4.34). The median age was 47 (range 22–70). The mean of MLH and puborectalis hiatus areas were 13.4 cm^2 ($\pm$1.89 SD) and 14.8 cm^2 ($\pm$2.16 SD). The mean anorectal and LPDAs were 156 ($\pm$10.04 SD) and 15.9 ($\pm$8.28 SD) degrees [33].

Our cadaveric dissections demonstrated the anterior border of the MLH is comprised of pubococcygeus and puboanalis fibers. Kim and colleagues named this area the "pubovisceralis entheses" [35]. Lateral to these fibers is a variable number of puborectalis fibers. Therefore, levator ani injury at childbirth at this location would most certainly involve the pubococcygeus as shown by 3D modeling by Lien et al. [5], and cephalad edge of the puborectalis attachment if the injury extends beyond the puboanalis fibers. In our opinion total unilateral or bilateral disruption of all the muscles involved in the anterior attachment of the MLH would constitute what has been called levator avulsion in the literature. A levator avulsion which is a total detachment of the levator entheses at the level of the pubic bone would result in widening of the levators and the ARA. To our knowledge, the contribution of the puboanalis muscle to this area has not been documented previously. The injury to the puboanalis fibers alone can potentially result in perineal and anal protrusion. The current repair methods for perineal and anal protrusion do not involve the investigation or the repair of the puboanalis muscle. The inner border of the MLH is mostly pubococcygeus, and the posterior border is the levator plate which forms the ARA.

The LPA as studied by the investigators measured the anterior-posterior movement of the levator plate relative to the horizontal reference line. Berglas and Rubin used levator myography to demonstrate that with straining, women with prolapse have greater inclination of the levator plate [36]. Goodrich quantified the difference in the LPA of 10 normal volunteers and five prolapse patients before and after surgery [37]. Interestingly, they found that women who had surgical repair of prolapse had a 10° more cephalad oriented LPA as well as a larger levator hiatus during straining even without recurrence of prolapse. Ozasa and colleagues compared the levator plate of 14 women with prolapse and 19 women without prolapse [38]. They found that a best fit line through the levator plate always crossed the pubic bone in women with normal support but never crossed the pubic bone in those with prolapse. DeLancey and colleagues showed that in women with normal support, the levator plate has a mean angle of 44.3° relative to a horizontal reference line during Valsalva, and women with prolapse have a 9.1° more vertically oriented LPA, which was statistically different [39]. In our study, we measured the LPDA which is the position of the levator plate along the caudad-cephalad plane relative to the PLURAL plane. This angle quantifies the levator plate position in reference to pubic bone and perineal body at rest. LPDA is potentially useful as a separate marker of levator function.

4.4 Conclusions and Future Research

Advances in technology have allowed a better appreciation of the functional anatomy of the pelvic floor. Initially, various modalities have documented the radiographic visualization of what can be observed during a physical examination. With more refined understanding of the unitary and global interaction of the pelvic floor and its contents, it has become possible to image what could only previously be determined on physical examination in the upright position. 3D imaging of the pelvic floor has provided an enrichment of knowledge about the complex dimensions of the pelvic floor, and allowed for clinicians to have an in vivo view of pelvic floor structures, observe dynamic changes on prompting, all during a bedside assessment.

Technology offers a driving progress. The wealth of knowledge that is rapidly being gained by recognizing what is visible, yet unseen. This raises the question of the clinical management relevance of the technologic advances of imaging. Technologic progress should be paralleled by clinical progress and understanding of all the extraordinary data afforded by recent new and exciting research. Clinical management should continue to rely on historical and clinical evaluation, and we must recognize that an adjunct imaging study may provide further insight into complex pelvic floor disorders. The true role of radiologic imaging in pelvic floor dysfunction clinical management is yet to be defined.

References

1. Kearney R, Sawhney R, DeLancey JO. Levator ani muscle anatomy evaluated by origin-insertion pairs. Obstet Gynecol. 2004;104(1):168–73.
2. Leigh DR, Baker AR, Mesiha M, Rodriguez ER, Tan CD, Walker E, et al. Effect of implantation site and injury condition on host response to human-derived fascia lata ECM in a rat model. J Orthop Res. 2012;30(3):461–7. PubMed PMID: 21858856. Pubmed Central PMCID: 3264843. Epub 2011/08/23. eng.
3. Shobeiri SA, Leclaire E, Nihira MA, Quiroz LH, O'Donoghue D. Appearance of the levator ani muscle subdivisions in endovaginal three-dimensional ultrasonography. Obstet Gynecol. 2009;114:66–72. PubMed PMID: 19546760.
4. Lercker G, Rodriguez-Estrada MT. Chromatographic analysis of unsaponifiable compounds of olive oils and fat-containing foods. J Chromatogr A. 2000;881(1–2):105–29. PubMed PMID: 10905697. Epub 2000/07/25. eng.
5. Lien KC, Mooney B, DeLancey JO, Ashton-Miller JA. Levator ani muscle stretch induced by simulated vaginal birth. Obstet Gynecol. 2004;103(1):31–40. PubMed PMID: 14704241. Pubmed Central PMCID: 1226707. Epub 2004/01/06. eng.
6. Richter HG, Tome MM, Yulis CR, Vio KJ, Jimenez AJ, Perez-Figares JM, et al. Transcription of SCO-spondin in the subcommissural organ: evidence for down-regulation mediated by serotonin. Brain Res

Mol Brain Res. 2004;129(1–2):151–62. PubMed PMID: 15469891. Epub 2004/10/08. eng.

7. Valsky DV, Lipschuetz M, Bord A, Eldar I, Messing B, Hochner-Celnikier D, et al. Fetal head circumference and length of second stage of labor are risk factors for levator ani muscle injury, diagnosed by 3-dimensional transperineal ultrasound in primiparous women. Am J Obstet Gynecol. 2009;201(1):91.e1–7. PubMed PMID: 19481726. Epub 2009/06/02. eng.

8. Model AN, Shek KL, Dietz HP. Levator defects are associated with prolapse after pelvic floor surgery. Eur J Obstet Gynecol Reprod Biol. 2010;153(2):220–3. PubMed PMID: 20832929.

9. Martin JF, Trowbridge EA. Theoretical requirements for the density separation of platelets with comparison of continuous and discontinuous gradients. Thromb Res. 1982;27(5):513–22. PubMed PMID: 7179205. Epub 1982/09/01. eng.

10. Shobeiri SA, Rostaminia G. Relative contributions of the levator ani subdivisions to levator ani movement. International urogynecology journal. 2013;24 (Suppl 1): S1–152. Epub 2013/07/03. eng.

11. Santoro GA, Wieczorek AP, Shobeiri SA, Mueller ER, Pilat J, Stankiewicz A, et al. Interobserver and interdisciplinary reproducibility of 3D endovaginal ultrasound assessment of pelvic floor anatomy. Int Urogynecol J. 2011;22(1):53–9. PubMed PMID: 20700728.

12. Boyles SH, Weber AM, Meyn L. Procedures for pelvic organ prolapse in the United States, 1979–1997. Am J Obstet Gynecol. 2003;188(1):108–15. PubMed PMID: 12548203. Epub 2003/01/28. eng.

13. DeLancey JO, Morgan DM, Fenner DE, Kearney R, Guire K, Miller JM, et al. Comparison of levator ani muscle defects and function in women with and without pelvic organ prolapse. Obstet Gynecol. 2007;109 (2 Pt 1):295–302. PubMed PMID: 17267827. Epub 2007/02/03. eng.

14. Dietz HP, Simpson JM. Levator trauma is associated with pelvic organ prolapse. BJOG. 2008;115(8):979–84. PubMed PMID: 18503571.

15. Morgan DM, Umek W, Stein T, Hsu Y, Guire K, DeLancey JO. Interrater reliability of assessing levator ani muscle defects with magnetic resonance images. Int Urogynecol J Pelvic Floor Dysfunct. 2007;18(7):773–8. PubMed PMID: 17043740. Pubmed Central PMCID: 2289432. Epub 2006/10/18. eng.

16. Shobeiri SA, Chimpiri AR, Allen A, Nihira MA, Quiroz LH. Surgical reconstitution of a unilaterally avulsed symptomatic puborectalis muscle using autologous fascia lata. Obstet Gynecol. 2009;114(2 Pt 2):480–2. PubMed PMID: 19622969.

17. Rostaminia G, Shobeiri SA. Surgical repair of bilateral levator ani muscles with ultrasound guidance: reply. Int Urogynecol J. 2012. doi:10.1007/s00192-012-1986-6

18. Hudson CN. Female genital prolapse and pelvic floor deficiency. Int J Colorectal Dis. 1988;3(3):181–5. PubMed PMID: 3053945.

19. DeLancey JO, Kearney R, Chou Q, Speights S, Binno S. The appearance of levator ani muscle abnormalities in magnetic resonance images after vaginal delivery. Obstet Gynecol. 2003;101(1):46–53.

20. Rostaminia G, White D, Hegde A, Quiroz LH, Davila GW, Shobeiri SA. Levator ani deficiency and pelvic organ prolapse severity. Obstet Gynecol. 2013;121(5): 1017–24. DOI: 10.1097/AOG.0b013e31828ce97d.

21. Ashton-Miller JA, Delancey JO. On the biomechanics of vaginal birth and common sequelae. Annu Rev Biomed Eng. 2009;11:163–76. PubMed PMID: 19591614. Pubmed Central PMCID: 2897058.

22. Chen L, Ashton-Miller JA, DeLancey JO. A 3D finite element model of anterior vaginal wall support to evaluate mechanisms underlying cystocele formation. J Biomech. 2009;42(10):1371–7. PubMed PMID: 19481208. Pubmed Central PMCID: 2744359.

23. Kearney R, Miller JM, Ashton-Miller JA, DeLancey JO. Obstetric factors associated with levator ani muscle injury after vaginal birth. Obstet Gynecol. 2006; 107(1):144–9.

24. Jundt K, Kiening M, Fischer P, Bergauer F, Rauch E, Janni W, et al. Is the histomorphological concept of the female pelvic floor and its changes due to age and vaginal delivery correct? Neurourol Urodyn. 2005;24(1):44–50.

25. Tunn R, Delancey JO, Howard D, Ashton-Miller JA, Quint LE. Anatomic variations in the levator ani muscle, endopelvic fascia, and urethra in nulliparas evaluated by magnetic resonance imaging. Am J Obstet Gynecol. 2003;188(1):116–21. PubMed PMID: 12548204. Epub 2003/01/28. eng.

26. Quiroz LH, White D, Shobeiri SA, Wild RA. Does age affect visualization of the levator ani in nulliparous women? Int Urogynecol J. 2013 Feb 15. [Epub ahead of print] PMID: 23411510

27. Hoyte JJM, Warfield SK, et al. Levator ani thickness variations in symptomatic and asymptomatic women using magnetic resonance-based 3-dimensional color mapping. Am J Obstet Gynecol. 2004;191: 856–61.

28. Lone FW, Thakar R, Sultan AH, Stankiewicz A. Accuracy of assessing pelvic organ prolapse quantification points using dynamic 2D transperineal ultrasound in women with pelvic organ prolapse. Int Urogynecol J. 2012;23:1555–60. PubMed PMID: 22543548. Epub 2012/05/01. Eng.

29. Hsu Y, Chen L, Huebner M, Ashton-Miller JA, DeLancey JO. Quantification of levator ani cross-sectional area differences between women with and those without prolapse. Obstet Gynecol. 2006;108(4):879–83. PubMed PMID: 17012449. eng.

30. Dietz HP, Lanzarone V. Levator trauma after vaginal delivery. Obstet Gynecol. 2005;106(4):707–12. PubMed PMID: 16199625.

31. Shek KL, Dietz HP. Intrapartum risk factors for levator trauma. BJOG. 2010;117(12):1485–92. PubMed PMID: 20735379.

32. Otcenasek M, Krofta L, Baca V, Grill R, Kucera E, Herman H, et al. Bilateral avulsion of the puborectal muscle: magnetic resonance imaging-based three-dimensional reconstruction and comparison with a model of a healthy nulliparous woman. Ultrasound Obstet Gynecol. 2007;29(6):692–6. PubMed PMID: 17523155.

33. Shobeiri SA, Rostaminia G, White D, Quiroz LH. The determinants of minimal levator hiatus and their relationship to the puborectalis muscle and the levator plate. BJOG. 2013 Jan;120(2):205–11. doi: 10.1111/1471-0528.12055. Epub 2012 Nov 12. Erratum in: BJOG. 2013 Apr;120(5):655.

34. Lakeman MM, Zijta FM, Peringa J, Nederveen AJ, Stoker J, Roovers JP. Dynamic magnetic resonance imaging to quantify pelvic organ prolapse: reliability of assessment and correlation with clinical findings and pelvic floor symptoms. Int Urogynecol J. 2012;23:1547–54. PubMed PMID: 22531955. Eng.

35. Kim J, Ramanah R, DeLancey JOL, Ashton-miller JA. On the anatomy and histology of the pubovisceral muscle enthesis in women. Neurourol Urodyn. 2011;30:1366–70.

36. Berglas B, Rubin IC. Study of the supportive structures of the uterus by levator myography. Surg Gynecol Obstet. 1953;97:677–92.

37. Goodrich MA, Webb MJ, King BF, Bampton AE, Campeau NG, Riederer SJ. Magnetic resonance imaging of pelvic floor relaxation: dynamic analysis and evaluation of patients before and after surgical repair. Obstet Gynecol. 1993;82(6):883–91. PubMed PMID: 8233259. English.

38. Ozasa H, Mori T, Togashi K. Study of uterine prolapse by magnetic resonance imaging: topographical changes involving the levator ani muscle and the vagina. Gynecol Obstet Invest. 1992;34:43–8.

39. Hsu Y, Summers A, Hussain HK, Guire KE, Delancey JOL. Levator plate angle in women with pelvic organ prolapse compared to women with normal support using dynamic MR imaging. Am J Obstet Gynecol. 2006;194(5):1427–33. PubMed PMID: 16579940. Pubmed Central PMCID: Source: NLM. NIHMS10238. Source: NLM. PMC1479225.

Endovaginal Urethra and Bladder Imaging

5

Andrzej Pawel Wieczorek
and Magdalena Maria Wozniak

Learning Objectives

1. The review of available endovaginal 3D ultrasound techniques in the urethral and bladder imaging
2. The efficiency of each of the transducers in the assessment of the morphology of the urethra and bladder
3. The influence of technology used in various transducers for the quality of image and range of available information
4. The demonstration of techniques of examination with each transducer and practical tips (patient position, preparation, method of acquisition)

5.1 Introduction

Female urethra is anatomically and functionally a complex organ conditioning urinary continence. Normal anatomy, proper position, and relations of the urethra to the surrounding pelvic floor structures guarantee normal function of the organ [1–3]. Until recently most published studies focused on transperineal ultrasound (TPUS) assessment of the urethra, its hypermobility, and hyper-rotation recognized as factors in the pathogenesis of urinary incontinence (UI) in females. Transperineal 2D/3D/4D approach is however based on the low frequency transducers (3–8 MHz) and has number of other limitations resulting in the lack of the possibility of analytic assessment of urethral morphology.

Introduction to pelvic floor diagnostics rotational transducers with perpendicular ultrasound beam formation to examined organs, using high frequency (12–16 MHz), working in 2D/3D modes and with Doppler options opened the opportunity of very detailed assessment of pelvic organs complexity, including the urethra. The technical differences among the transducers, various crystals, and modes of acquisition allowed to obtain a variety of focuses in the detailed examinations of the urethra. This chapter describes the characteristics of the endovaginal transducers and optimal conditions in the examinations of the urethra.

5.2 Equipment, Technology, and Methodology

Endovaginal examinations of the urethra and bladder may be performed with the use of three various types of transducers, each of them involving different beam formation technology. These transducers include rotational mechanical transducer (type 2050 or its newer version type

A.P. Wieczorek • M.M. Wozniak, M.D., Ph.D. (✉)
Department of Pediatric Radiology, Medical University of Lublin, Al. Raclawickie 1, 20-059 Lublin, Poland
e-mail: mwozniak@hoga.pl

S.A. Shobeiri (ed.), *Practical Pelvic Floor Ultrasonography: A Multicompartmental Approach to 2D/3D/4D Ultrasonography of Pelvic Floor*, DOI 10.1007/978-1-4614-8426-4_5,
© Springer Science+Business Media New York 2014

2052), biplane electronic transducer (type 8848), and rotational electronic transducer (type 8838). Technical characteristics of each of the transducers have been described in the chapter on 3D/4D instrumentations and techniques but discussed here briefly.

5.2.1 Patient Position

Patients are placed in a dorsal lithotomy position on a flat couch or gynaecological chair while the endovaginal ultrasound (EVUS) is performed. In some patients, particularly those with pelvic organ prolapse (POP); when the scan obtained in the lying position is insufficient to make the final diagnosis examination in standing position may be helpful. Scanning on a gynaecological chair would be recommended for patients who are assessed with the transducer type 8848 and the use of the automatic mover because the dimensions of the mover do not allow performing the examination on a flat couch.

5.2.2 Patients Preparation

The patients are recommended to have a comfortable volume of urine in the bladder. No patient preparation is required and no rectal or vaginal contrast is used for the examination.

5.2.3 Methodology

The methodology of obtained image depends on the type of the transducer used. A silicon cover for all the transducer is required. The amount of the gel should be adjusted and equally distributed on the whole surface of the transducer, without air bubbles. Transducer is inserted into the vagina in a neutral position to avoid distortion of anatomy due to excessive pressure on surrounding structures. Proper 2D/3D assessment of the urethra with the use of endovaginal approach with each of the above-mentioned transducers is dependent on the proper acquisition in various sections based on different reference points.

Transducer Type 2050/2052

This rotational 360° mechanical transducer (See specifications in the chapter on instrumentations and techniques) has two arrays working in the range of frequencies from 9 to 16-MHz. It provides a good topographical overview of the pelvic floor anatomy on the maximal length of 60 mm, which can be obtained during 60 s of automatic acquisition if the best resolution—minimum spacing (0.2 mm) is chosen. Larger spacing (possible up to 3 mm) shortens the acquisition time and decreases the quality of the image. The transducer enables individual optimization of the image depending on the selected anatomical structure in focus e.g., urethra. The acquisition on the length of 60 mm enables visualization of the urethra in axial section from the bladder base (level I according to Santoro et al.) to distal orifice (defined as level IV). Ability of downward and upward movement of the crystal inside the transducer is manipulated by pressing the buttons on the transducer which minimizes moving artefacts coming from the operator. Holding the transducer in stable position during the acquisition ensures good quality of obtained 3D volume dataset. Even a small asymmetry during the insertion of the transducer into the vagina and lack of neutral position results in asymmetry and/or compression of the examined organs. The offline assessment of the 3D file requires 3D viewer and may be performed either in the scanner or in an external computer. The 3D viewer enables also performing the measurements of the examined structures from the recorded 3D file. The 3D file covers all pelvic floor organs both anterior, middle, and posterior compartment on all levels. Measurements of all pelvic floor structures may be performed in all sections, including very detailed measurements of the urethra [4, 5].

The reference points to maintain symmetry of the image in the axial section for transducer type 205/2052 are the rami of symphysis pubis and the urethra on the screen at 12 o'clock position. The image obtained at this particular section is named the "gothic arch" as previously reported [5] (Fig. 5.1). The review of 3D file allows good assessment of the urethra, including the differentiation for its three main parts being intramural part, mid-urethra, and distal urethra. Tiling of the acquired 3D image in certain section may be adjusted to the maximal cross-section and midsagittal axial and coronal section of the particular organ which allows for obtaining reliable anatomy (Fig. 5.2b) and reliable measurement. Using 3D volume dataset recorded during the

examination all required measurements of the urethra and its surrounding structures may be reliably performed.

The main advantage of the transducer is a large region covered during acquisition (360°, all compartments) which provides a very good overview of all pelvic floor organs making the transducer universal for many specialties and many purposes. An important prone is also a wide selection of scanning time and the quality of obtained image. The universal character of the 2050/2052 transducer makes it a gold standard diagnostic tool in proctology [6, 7] and for pelvic floor diagnostics, as described in 2009 by Santoro et al. [4, 5, 8].

The main limitation of this technology is the total length of the transducer of 54 cm which is not particularly handy, difficult for operation, hard to be kept in a stable position, and also often recognized by patients as extremely long which creates an extra anxiety for the patient. From the methodological point of view mechanical character of the transducer does not allow to obtain the same resolution in all sections, only the axial section (the section of acquisition) has the best quality and all other sections coming from postprocessing of the 3D volume dataset have lower resolution.

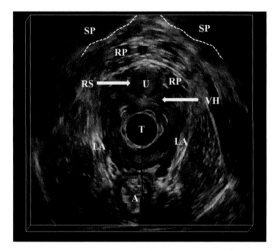

Fig. 5.1 Axial section gray-scale 3D image, transducer 8838. Symphysis pubis ("gothic arch")—reference points of symmetry in axial section for transducers 8848, 2050, and 2052 (B–K Medical). *SP* symphysis pubis, *RP* Retzius plexus, *U* urethra, *RS* rhabdosphincter, *T* transducer in vagina, *VH* vaginal hammock, *LA* levator ani, *A* anal canal

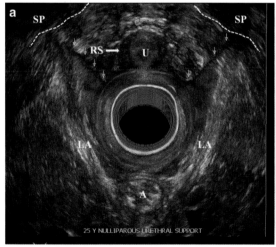

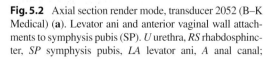

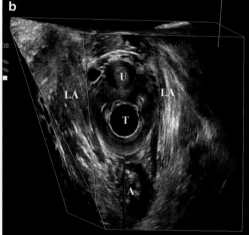

Fig. 5.2 Axial section render mode, transducer 2052 (B–K Medical) (**a**). Levator ani and anterior vaginal wall attachments to symphysis pubis (SP). *U* urethra, *RS* rhabdosphincter, *SP* symphysis pubis, *LA* levator ani, *A* anal canal;

Multisurface 3D reconstruction, transducer type 8838 (B–K Medical) (**b**). Attachments of levator ani fibers to symphysis pubis are well demonstrated on oblique sections. *U* urethra, *T* transducer in vagina, *LA* levator ani, *A* anal canal

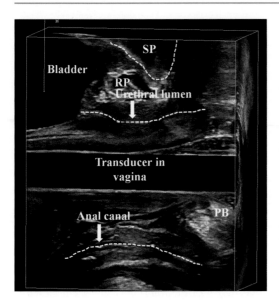

Fig. 5.3 Sagittal section 3D gray-scale image with a biplane 12-MHz transducer (type 8848, B–K Medical). Entire urethral lumen from the bladder neck to the external orifice as reference point of symmetry in sagittal section for transducers 8848, 8838, 2050, and 2052 (B–K Medical). *SP* symphysis pubis, *RP* Retzius plexus, *PB* perineal body

The 8848 Transducer

This is an electronic biplane, high frequency 5–12 MHz, multielement high-resolution transducer, working both in 2D and 3D modes with 6.5 cm linear and convex views transducer (See specifications in the chapter on instrumentations and techniques). The transducer has the focal range from 3 to 60 mm and contact surface in axial section of 127 mm^2, in sagittal section 357 mm^2. High frequency provides high resolution of examined organs allowing for very good assessment of urethral morphology. It gives the best broad view of anterior and posterior compartments for functional and anatomical studies. This transducer requires an external mover to obtain reliable 3D volumes. Obtained 3D volume dataset of the anterior compartment of pelvic floor may be analyzed in midsagittal, axial, coronal, and oblique sections.

Sagittal Section

The reference organ to maintain symmetry in the sagittal section is the visualization of the urethral lumen on the entire length from the bladder neck to the external orifice (Fig. 5.3). A longitudinal

array enables to obtain 2D and 3D volume dataset in a sagittal section as a free-hand acquisition, during maximum time of 13.4 s with minimal spacing of 0.2 mm. Free-hand acquisition may be connected to artefacts due to uneven move of the hand in time, which may distort the anatomy and create an artificial nonexisting asymmetrical position of urethra and the pelvic floor structures and their abnormal shape. Free-hand acquisition may be however performed on a normal flat couch. Reproducible 3D studies may be performed with external mover. The examination can be performed both in B-mode and in Color/Power Doppler modes.

To avoid artefacts connected to free-hand acquisition the examination may be performed with the use of automatic external mover (as described in the chapter on 3D/4D instrumentation and techniques). In order to safely use the mover the examination must be performed on a gynaecological chair. With the use of the mover the ultrasound acquisition may be performed in a maximum of 179°, during 46.5 s in B-mode and in 51.2 s in Color Doppler.

Axial Section

The reference points to maintain symmetry of the image in the axial section is the "gothic arch" the same as in 2050/2052 transducer (Fig. 5.1). Any asymmetrical insertion of the transducer to the vagina may cause bias in the obtained image, in the echostructure of the examined organs and their dimensions and measurements.

The length of acquisition may be selected by operator. In axial section choosing minimal spacing of 0.2 mm the acquisition time of 11.91 s covers 6 cm. The button placed on the transducer switches the image between the two arrays.

The 3D acquisition in axial section may be only free-hand, which may result in inappropriate urethral measurements due to distorted 3D anatomy. This section in 2D and the offline analysis of the 3D volume dataset allows for differentiation of various parts of the urethra such as intramural anatomical elements (layer structure of the trigone, trigonal ring), mid-urethra (differentiation for rhabdosphincter, longitudinal and circular smooth muscle, submucosal venous plexus) and the distal urethra (fibers of the compressor

Table 5.1 Endovaginal (EVUS) 2D/3D of the urethra—characteristics of the transducers and reference points

Transducer	Arrays	Sections of acquisition	Type	Frequency (MHz)	Doppler	3D acquisition	Reference points	Range of view
2050/2052	Two arrays (low and high frequency crystals)	Axial	Mechanical	9–16	No	Automatic built-in	Gothic arch (axial)	360°
8848	Two arrays (linear multielement, transverse multielement)	Axial / Sagittal	Electronic	5–12	Yes	Free-hand or external mover	Gothic arch (Axial) / Urethral lumen (sagittal)	180°
8838	Linear multielement array	Sagittal	Electronic	6–12	Yes	Automatic built-in	Urethral lumen (sagittal)	360° (tiny blank stitch)

urethra) and reliable assessment of the urethral relations to external anatomical structures such as vaginal wall or attachments of levator ani muscle fibers to the symphysis pubis.

Transducer Type 8838

This is an electronic transducer, for endovaginal and endoanal/endorectal imaging, with automatic high resolution 3D acquisition transducer (See specifications in the chapter on instrumentations and techniques). Built-in linear array rotates 360° inside the transducer with no need for additional accessories or external mover. It enables both dynamic 2D and 3D scanning at wide frequency range from 6 to 12 MHz. Its slim diameter (16 mm) is more comfortable for the patient, easy to hold and manipulate for the operator. Two-dimensional scanning plane is controlled remotely from the system keyboard. The image field of 65 mm is covering the entire urethra from the bladder base to the external orifice. Two-dimensional acquisition can be obtained only in longitudinal (sagittal) section. The reference section to obtain symmetry is the lumen of the urethra visualized on the entire length similarly as in the sagittal section with use of 8848 transducer (Fig. 5.3). The urethra may be assessed as a separate organ with a small region of interest (ROI) e.g., 45° or as a part of the entire overview examination of all pelvic floor in a 3D file of almost 360° (with a tiny blank stitch) with the time of acquisition at maximal length equaling 41.9 s with spacing of 0.4°. The spacing may be changed which influences the examination time.

Electronic character of the transducer allows assessing the vascularity and flow in Power and Color Doppler modes. The Doppler assessment may be performed either as a 2D examination and can be recorded as a video life file on a selected section or as a static 3D volume dataset.

The axial section may be obtained only in post-processing from the 3D volume dataset. Lack of axial acquisition limits the possibility to use the symphysis pubis ("gothic arch") as a reference point of symmetry. Inappropriate position of the transducer and B-mode obtained only in sagittal section may result in asymmetry of the organs in a 3D file (Table 5.1).

5.2.4 Vascular Render Mode and Maximum Intensity Projection

Volume render mode is a technique for the analysis of the information inside 3D-volume by digital enhancing of individual voxels (Fig. 5.2a, b). It is currently one of the most advanced and computer-intensive rendering algorithm available for computed tomography and can also be applied to high-resolution 3D-US data volume [9]. The typical ray/beam-tracing algorithm sends a ray/beam from each point (pixel) of the viewing screen through the 3D space rendered. The beam passing through the volume data, reaches the different elements (voxels) in the data set. Depending on the various render mode settings, the data from each voxel may be stored as a referral for the next voxel and further used in a filtering calculation, may be discarded or may modify the existing value of the beam. The final displayed pixel color is computed from the color, transparency, and reflectivity of all the volumes and surfaces encountered by the beam. The weighted summation of these images produces the volume-rendered view [9]. Vascular render mode refers to the application of render mode to 3D-data volume with Color Doppler acquisition to provide the visualization of the spatial distribution of the vascular networks.

Maximum intensity projection (MIP) is a 3D visualization modality involving a large amount of computation. It can be defined as the aggregate exposure at each point, which tries to find the brightest or most significant color or intensity along an ultrasound beam. Once the beam is projected through the entire volume, the value displayed on the screen is the maximum intensity value found (the highest value of gray or the highest value associated with a color). The application of MIP in a 3D color mode reduces the intensity of the gray-scale voxels so that they appear as a light fog over color information, which is in this way highlighted. In a color volume the colors are mapped to a given value in the volume.

Urinary Bladder

Specific features of each of the transducers parameters condition the range of obtained anatomical information. However, none of the described transducers is appropriate for the assessment of the entire urinary bladder due to endovaginal access and the beam formation perpendicular to the organ. The bladder may be visualized only partially, in the range depending on bladder filling. The assessment of the entire bladder has to be performed by transabdominal ultrasound or with the use of endovaginal end-fire transducers used widely in gynecology or urology.

5.3   Anatomy of Female Urethra and Bladder

5.3.1   Ultrasound Morphology

Endovaginal insertion of the transducer can influence the position of examined organs and may limit the reliability of the dynamic studies such

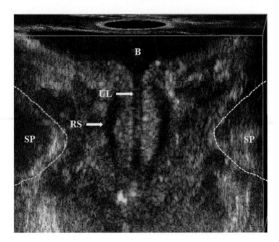

Fig. 5.4 Coronal 3D section showing bladder neck and urethral lumen with a transducer type 2050 (B–K Medical). *B* bladder, *UL* urethral lumen, *RS* rhabdosphincter, *SP* symphysis pubis

as Valsalva and squeeze maneuvers. Stankiewicz et al. proved that in incontinent women with no coexisting POP both ultrasound methods (TPUS and EVUS) have the same accuracy in the measurements of urethral complex and bladder-symphysis distance (BSD) at rest and during Valsalva maneuver. The study demonstrated that in females suffering from stress urinary incontinence (SUI) and coexisting POP, the endovaginal examination is not reliable in the assessment of the urethral mobility due to alterations of anatomical relations that result from introduction of the transducer into the vagina. Endovaginal approach is more appropriate for detailed assessment of urethral morphology (Fig. 5.4), while TPUS is the method of choice for dynamic assessment [8].

All described transducers used in EVUS allow proper assessment of ultrasound morphology of the pelvic floor organs including the urethra and the surrounding structures on different pelvic floor sections and levels as previously defined by Santoro et al. [5, 10]:

Level I: the highest level visualizing the bladder base on the screen at 12 o'clock position and the inferior third of the rectum at 6 o'clock position;

Level II: corresponds to the bladder neck, the intramural region of the urethra, and the anorectal junction;

Table 5.2 Measurements of the urethral structures obtained by 3D-EVUS taken by three observers

| | Observer 1 | Observer 2 | Observer 3 | |
	Mean (SD)	Mean (SD)	Mean (SD)	ICC (95 % CI)
BSD (mm)	34.01 (5.1)	33.9 (5.05)	33.9 (5.2)	0.964 (0.931–0.983)
Urethra length (mm)	41.2 (5.6)	40.9 (4.56)	40.7 (5.2)	0.975 (0.918–0.980)
Urethra width (mm)	13.1 (1.44)	13.24 (1.5)	13.1 (1.45)	0.892 (0.801–0.947)
Urethra thickness (mm)	11.6 (1.3)	11.02 (3.2)	11.4 (1.25)	0.848 (0.697–0.929)
Urethra volume (ml)	4.99 (1.3)	5.12 (1.38)	4.82 (1.32)	0.925 (0.86–0.964)
Intramural length (mm)	7.3 (1.7)	7.3 (1.25)	7.5 (1.5)	0.870 (0.764–0.936)
RS length (mm)	18.6 (2.9)	19.1 (2.6)	19.0 (2.6)	0.942 (0.889–0.972)
RS width (mm)	35.3 (4.07)	35.2 (4.1)	34.3 (3.9)	0.85 (0.728–0.926)
RS thickness (mm)	2.4 (0.21)	2.47 (0.23)	2.4 (0.24)	0.611 (0.390–0.789)
RS volume (ml)	1.27 (0.35)	1.28 (0.38)	1.24 (0.32)	0.909 (0.829–0.957)

Statistical analysis: intraclass coefficient correlation (ICC) [11]

Level III: corresponds to the mid-urethra and to the upper third of the anal canal. To facilitate the assessment of the position of these structures, a geometric reference point, termed as the "gothic arch," was defined at 12 o'clock position, specifically at the point where the inferior branches of the pubic bone join at the symphysis pubis (SP). At this level, the pubovisceral muscle (PVM) (synonymous with the term pubococcygeus/puborectalis muscle) can be completely visualized as a multilayer highly echoic sling lying posteriorly to the anal canal and attaching to the pubic bone;

Level IV: the outer level, the superficial perineal muscles, the perineal body, the distal urethra, and the middle and inferior third of the anal canal can be evaluated. To visualize these structures in their entirety, the reconstructed axial section should be tilted from the most protruding surface of the SP anteriorly to the ischiopubic rami laterally. In the same scan the urogenital hiatus (UGH) can be evaluated.

The following measurements of the urethra may be performed (Table 5.2) (Fig. 5.5):

In midsagittal plane
1. Urethral length (Ul) measured from the bladder neck to the external meatus along the urethral longitudinal axis.
2. BSD measured from bladder neck to the lowest margin of the symphysis pubis. According to Wieczorek et al. [11] frequency the mean value of the BSD varied from 33.9 to 34.01 mm for depending on the observer.
3. Rhabdosphincter length (RSl) measured in anterior part of the urethra.
4. The distance between bladder neck and rhabdosphincter corresponding to the intramural part of the urethra.

In axial plane of the mid-urethra
5. Urethral complex width (Uw).
6. Urethral complex thickness including Rhabdosphincter (Ut).
7. Width of the rhabdosphincter measured along its external border, where it is attached with the smooth muscle to the rhabdosphincter raphe—a tissue connection to the anterior vaginal wall (RSw); this is a summing value of the linear measurements performed by the use of tools available in B–K 3D Viewer. Rhabdosphincter appears in the axial section as a slightly hyperechoic (compared with urethral smooth muscle) structure surrounding ventral and lateral sides of the mid-urethra and forming a raphe connected to the anterior vaginal wall. Thus, rhabdosphincter has its typical omega shape [11].

According to integral theories described by Petros and Ulmsten between the mid-urethra and the vaginal anterior wall there are pubourethral ligaments and the suburethral vaginal hammock [1, 2]. This hammock is attached to the endopelvic fascia, and laterally the urethra is limited by periurethral space including Retzius vascular plexus, and by the elements of levator ani. On the section when levator hiatus is well visible also the paravaginal spaces can be determined, located

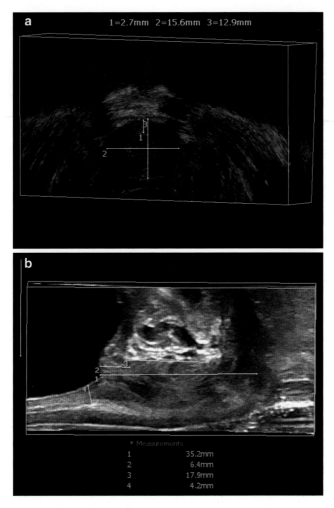

Fig. 5.5 Axial (**a**) and sagittal (**b**) section, 3D gray-scale mode with a transducer type 8848 (B–K Medical) demonstrating measurements of the urethra performed in the 3D viewer

between the lateral border of the vaginal wall and the medial border of the PVM. Shobeiri et al. demonstrated levator ani subdivisions visible on endovaginal three-dimensional ultrasonography at three levels, where level 2 contained the attachment of the pubovaginalis, puboperinealis, puboanalis, puborectalis, and iliococcygeus to the pubic bone [12]. It is possible to explain deterioration of continence with time in terms of age-related connective tissue laxity of the vaginal hammock. Improvement in continence after anticontinence surgery with time can be explained by tightening of the hammock via paraurethral scar contraction with time [13].

The review of the literature shows significant differences in the assessment of the anatomy of the urethra, its dimensions and volume [4, 5, 11, 14–17]. Santoro et al. in the study performed with high-resolution three-dimensional EVUS 2050 transducer demonstrated urethral length of 38.2 mm, urethral volume of 3.06 ml, and rhabdosphincter volume of 0.45 ml [5]. The results published by Wieczorek et al. [11] performed with the same type of transducer (2050) where urethral length was reported at 41.0 mm, urethral volume 4.9 ml, and rhabdosphincter volume 1.2 ml. The difference between rhabdosphincter volume between Santoro and Wieczorek results most probably from different mathematical algorithm used for calculating the volume and also unclear borders in sagittal section which may be interpreted differently by various operators. Similar results were presented also by Shobeiri et al. in the study on anterior and posterior compartment 3D EVUS with 8848 probe based on direct histologic comparison where urethral length was reported as 36.0 mm [18]. Additionally Shobeiri et al. obtained the following mean measurements of other pelvic floor structures: striated urogenital sphincter area 0.6 cm^2; longitudinal and circular smooth muscle area 1.1 cm^2; urethral complex width 14 mm; and urethral complex area 1.3 cm^2. The agreement for visualization of structures was as follows: vesical trigone 96 %, trigonal ring 94 %, trigonal plate 84 %; longitudinal and circular smooth muscle 100 %; compressor urethra 97 %; and striated urogenital sphincter 97 % [18].

The above results are concordant also with those obtained by Kondo et al., where morphology obtained in transvaginal ultrasonography was confirmed on cadaver specimens. The rhabdosphincter (peripheral zone) thickness was reported in various patients' groups: continent, patients with SUI and UUI as 2.78 mm, 2.14 mm, and 2.87 mm, respectively [19]. Above results are also accordant to those obtained by Macura et al. in the MR study on urethral morphology [20]. These results are slightly different to those obtained by Umek et al. who presented sagittal urethral diameter of 8.4 mm if measured in endovaginal access and 11.5 mm measured from endoanal access, urethral volume of 1.6 ml (both anatomical accesses) and rhabdosphincter volume of 0.7 and 0.8 ml accordingly [16]. In the study performed by Santoro et al. with 2050 transducer [4] involving the interobserver, intra and interdisciplinary reproducibility of pelvic floor measurements the sole urethral dimension measured was urethral thickness. The results were concordant with urethral dimensions obtained in all the above studies [4]. Moreover, as the study focused mainly on the reproducibility of the performed measurements in EVUS among various specialties (urogynecologists, colorectal surgeons, radiologists) and different experience

in ultrasound diagnostics of operators and the conclusions from the study were that 3D-EVUS yields reproducible measurements of levator hiatus dimensions and urethral thickness in asymptomatic nulliparous women. Agreement was best where landmark edges were well defined (LH dimensions) and acceptable where more reader judgment was needed (urethral thickness in the oblique axial plane). Using standardized criteria, the evaluation of these pelvic floor structures appeared to be independent from the different background training of the readers. The method appeared a reproducible technique for urethral measurements [4].

The rhabdosphincter may be also evaluated during intraurethral ultrasound as reported by Frausher et al. This technique provides excellent high-resolution images and allows for real-time visualization of the sphincter mechanism [21]. The rhabdosphincter thickness for patients with urge incontinence and for patients with combined stress and urge incontinence was reported as 3.2 mm.

However, the volumes of rhabdosphincter given generally in the literature seem to be significantly lower than reported by Digesu et al. [14] and Derpapas et al. [17]. The study by Digesu et al. demonstrated the rhabdosphincter volume of 3.79 ml in patients with successful surgical procedure due to SUI, while in patients with failures 1.09 ml. In the paper by Derpapas et al. the rhabdosphincter volume was 8.88 ml in black women and 5.97 ml in white females. Both studies were performed from transperineal (TPUS) access: the study by Digesu et al. with the use of sector, endovaginal transducer and the study by Derpapas et al. with 3D/4D curved array probe [14, 17].

The differences may result from the various nomenclature of urethral anatomy treated differently by different authors. There are many controversies in female urethral anatomy which have a significant impact for understanding urinary continence [22]. Variability of obtained results among authors may also result from various frequencies of the transducers used, different anatomical accesses, and various patient groups (age, race, BMI, parity, etc.). The differences in urethral morphology and physiology between black and white women have been already reported in the literature [17, 23]. Howard et al. reported that black women demonstrated difference in ultrasonically measured vesical neck mobility during a maximum Valsalva effort compared to white females (blacks = −17 mm vs. whites = −12 mm). Functional and morphologic differences exist in the urethral sphincteric and support system of nulliparous black and white women [23].

Moreover, the diagnostics of such a small organ as urethra may relatively easily result in variability of the measurements obtained in various techniques among the authors. Moreover, the review of the literature concerning 3D diagnostics of urethral complex shows that most researchers perform only one acquisition in axial plane to obtain 3D dataset, which also may potentially influence obtaining reliable measurements in all three planes.

5.3.2 Urethral Vascularity

Vascularity is one of the major factors contributing to maintaining the normal function of the urethra. The vascularity, and particularly the presence of cushioning blood vessels within the submucosa, conditions the normal tension of the urethral mucosal wall [24, 25]. Sphincteric closure of the urethra is normally provided by urethral striated muscles, the urethral smooth muscle, and the vascular elements within the submucosa. Each is believed to contribute equally to resting urethral closure pressure [24]. The submucosal vascular systems become engorged with blood, which causes swelling of the submucosa and decreasing the diameter of the urethral lumen [22]. Furthermore, the vascularity system is also responsible for the proper synthesis of factors that influence surface sealing of the urethral lumen.

Up to now, the assessment of urethral vascularity has mainly been based on selected Doppler parameters (velocity [V], resistive index [RI], pulsatility index [PI]), measured with transperineal ultrasound (TPUS) [26, 27]. Siracusano et al. [27] demonstrated the usefulness of color Doppler and spectral Doppler scans in the assessment of urethral vascularization in healthy young women,

defining the RI in urethral vessels at three parts of the urethra (proximal, middle, and distal), and reporting an increased RI in the intramural part of the urethra. Also the attempts of the assessment of vascularity after intravenous contrast agents administration were undertaken [27, 28] from transperineal approach. Siracusano et al. performed the examinations after intravenous application of ultrasound contrast in order to enhance Doppler signals from the urethral vessels, which seemed to generate good results. The application of invasive and relatively expensive diagnostic methods, such as intravenous contrast agent administration seems to be unnecessary considering the recent advances in ultrasound diagnostics, particularly in high frequency endoluminal ultrasonography (12 MHz) in urological practice, which can generate an ultrasound beam that is perpendicular to the urethra and in almost direct contact with the organ, thus enabling vascular assessment [29, 30].

The usefulness of Color Doppler in the quantitative assessment of the urethral vascularity has been already described [29]. The studies performed by Wieczorek et al. [29] demonstrated that high frequency transvaginal ultrasound with the use of Color Doppler mode is a very reliable method enabling visualization of urethral vessels distribution. The vascularity differs in different parts of the urethra with the mid-urethra being the most vascularized part of the organ. In the best oral poster by a fellow during ICS 2012, Lone et al. showed significant reduction in the vascularity parameters in all measured variables in urinary continent women when parity was accounted for [31].

Quantitative assessment of the urethral vascularity may be performed with the use of an independent external software package (Chameleon Software, Freiburg, Germany) which has been proved as a valuable tool for providing reproducible quantitative analysis of vascular parameters for the entire urethra [29, 30]. The analysis is based on video files recorded in Color Doppler mode. The video files may be recorded using transducers type 8848 or 8838. The vascular pattern may be obtained both in sagittal section at the level of urethral lumen and axial section at the

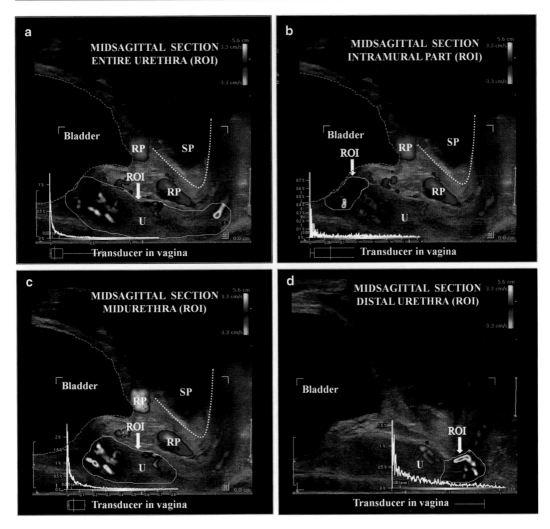

Fig. 5.6 Endovaginal ultrasound with a biplane 12-MHz transducer (type 8848, B–K Medical) using linear array. Analysis of the vascular parameters with the use of Pixel Flux software in the longitudinal (sagittal) section. Four regions of interest (ROIs) are defined: at the entire urethra from the bladder neck to the external orifice (**a**), the intramural part of the urethra (**b**), the mid urethra (**c**), and the distal urethra (**d**). *SP* symphysis pubis, *RP* Retzius plexus

level of mid-urethra with the use of the transducer type 8848 or in sagittal section at the level of urethral lumen with the use of the transducer type 8838. The data must be registered as video files in a stable position of the probe.

The vascular pattern may be analyzed within manually defined ROIs. The software automatically calibrates distances and color hues as flow velocities and calculates the color pixel area and flow velocity—encoded by each pixel—inside a ROI of a video sequence (20–90 images). Videos with movement artefacts are automatically or manually excluded from perfusion quantification.

In sagittal section regions of interest could be set at sequence at 3 levels (intramural, mid-urethra, and distal urethra) (Fig. 5.6a–d). In axial plane two regions of interest could be defined for each patient—one comprising the rhabdosphincter (the outer ring of urethra) and the second comprising the circular smooth muscle, the longitudinal smooth muscle, and the submucosa (the inner ring of the urethra) (Fig. 5.7a–c).

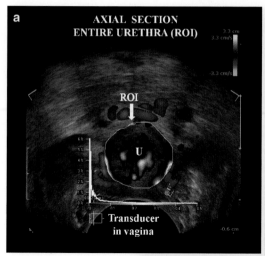 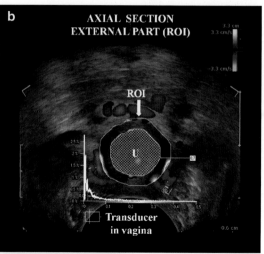

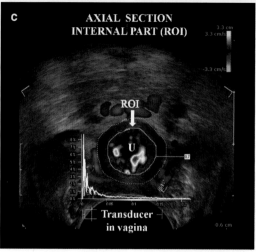

Fig. 5.7 Endovaginal ultrasound with a biplane 12-MHz transducer (type 8848, B–K Medical) using transverse array. Analysis of the vascular parameters with the use of the Pixel Flux software in the axial section at the level of mid-urethra. Three regions of interest (ROIs) are defined: entire urethra (**a**), the external part of the urethra (rhabdosphincter) (**b**), and at the internal part of the urethra (including the lisosphincter muscle that comprises the circular smooth muscle, the longitudinal smooth muscle, and the submucosa) (**c**)

The following parameters may be automatically computed for each single frame of the video within each ROI:

– The velocity (*V*), corresponding to the color hue of the pixels inside the ROI
– The perfused area (*A*), given by the number of perfused pixels inside the ROI
– The perfusion intensity (*I*), defined as the ratio $I = VA/AROI$, where AROI denotes the total area of the ROI

In this way, the perfusion intensity increases with the perfusion velocity, but decreases if less of the total area of the ROI is perfused. This parameter is calculated for every image in each video, in order to compute averages and pulsation indices of the parameters, always with respect to the duration of a full cardiac cycle. Inside the ROI, the whole area occupied by the colored pixels is calculated. This calculation is automatically repeated for the same ROI for all images of a digital video. The detection of one full heart cycle is also done automatically by the software.

The output is the measure of flow quantity inside the ROI, called "perfusion intensity,"

calculated in terms of the hue of the pixels in the ROI:
– The pulsatility index (PI)
– The resistance index (RI)

Each parameter is calculated including data from all imaged vessels in Color Doppler mode coded as red and blue reflecting the direction and velocity of blood particles movement. Results represent the sum of "red" and "blue" values named as "mix" value for each parameter (Vmix, Imix, Amix, PImix, and RImix.) [29, 30].

5.4   Clinical Applications of Urethral Ultrasound

According to Chaudhari et al. the introduction of high-resolution surface and intracavitary transducers in conjunction with three-dimensional acquisition has enhanced the role of US in the diagnostics of urethra [32]. From the clinical point of view recent advances in ultrasound allow more detailed evaluation of urethral and periurethral abnormalities enabling categorization the patients suffering from pelvic floor disorders for various groups, with or without existing anatomical abnormalities. It is very important to define prior the treatment if the cause of the abnormality has the anatomical background or is purely functional disturbance as it significantly influences the choice of treatment. Chaudhari et al. stated that in case of the presence of anatomical pathologies the distinctive imaging features and locations of the various diseases aid in narrowing the differential diagnosis. Real-time US has exciting potential as the tool for more comprehensive analysis of the pathophysiologic features of the complex disorders that affect the female urethra and periurethral tissues [32].

There are numerous risk factors for the development of pelvic floor dysfunction, including age, multiparity, and history of vaginal delivery, menopausal status, obesity, and history of hysterectomy. Patients present with signs and symptoms that often overlap with those of urethral diverticula and periurethral cystic lesions, including pelvic pain, incontinence, dyspareunia, incomplete emptying, and, at times, visible organ protrusion (Fig. 5.8) [32].

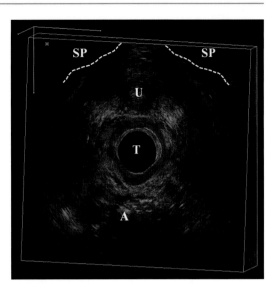

Fig. 5.8 Axial section 3D B-mode with a transducer type 2052 (B–K Medical). Urethra and symphysis pubis in pelvic organ prolapse (POP 3) and urinary incontinence (UI). Lack of differentiation of anatomical pelvic floor structures. Enlargement of urogenital hiatus. *U* urethra, *SP* symphysis pubis, *T* transducer in vagina, *A* anal canal

High frequency endovaginal 3D morphology of the urethra can significantly enrich our knowledge about abnormalities which are not clinically evident which may play role as causative factors of urinary incontinence. According to Wang et al. the urological anatomies can be generally categorized into three types: abnormal communication of urogenital tracts, malformation of bladder or ectopic ureter, and anomalies of urethral orifice. Ectopic ureters and ureteroceles are typically diagnosed in childhood and rarely present in adults. Nevertheless, ureteral ectopia should be included in the differential diagnosis of older patients who present with urinary tract infections or urinary incontinence (Fig. 5.9) [33]. Surgical corrections are helpful for most cases [34]. This has been confirmed by Tunn et al. [35] in updated recommendations on ultrasonography in urogynecology, where he concluded that ultrasonography is a supplementary, indispensable diagnostic procedure and that TPUS and ERUS are the most useful techniques. In patients undergoing diagnostic work-up for urge incontinence, US occasionally demonstrates urethral diverticula, leiomyomas, and cysts in the vaginal wall [35]. High frequency high-resolution EVUS allows

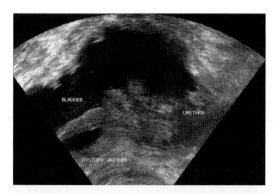

Fig. 5.9 Gray-scale axial section, transducer 8848 (B–K Medical). Dystopic urether entering the urethra

comprehensive evaluation of both congenital and acquired pathologies including diverticula, abnormal urethral insertion, dystopic/ectopic urethers, calcifications, ureterocele, fistulas, and other urethral and paraurethral lesions [36]. Among periurethral cystic lesions abnormalities such as Gartner duct cyst, Bartholin gland cyst, Skene duct cyst, müllerian cyst, epidermal inclusion cyst, perineal-vulvovaginal endometriomas, and injected collagen may be diagnosed. It is important for radiologists to be aware of the imaging characteristics of these entities, in particular their location, to differentiate them from urethral diverticula [32]. Although the exact mechanism of diverticular formation is unknown, the most commonly accepted theory implicates the periurethral glands. Obstruction of the periurethral gland duct is associated with infection which results in abscess formation, which subsequently ruptures into the urethral lumen forming the diverticulum. Yang et al. showed on two cases of paraurethral abnormalities such as urethral diverticulum and paraurethral abscess that transvaginal sonography, with its high-resolution visualization of the lower urinary tract, may aid in the diagnosis and treatment of such disorders. Using three-dimensional technology, the internal architecture of the paraurethral abnormalities and their spatial relationship to the urethra and bladder, important considerations at surgery, are clearly demonstrated on ultrasonography. Complete excision of complex paraurethral anomalies may be performed under transvaginal sonographic monitoring without

inadvertent injury to the bladder or urethra [36]. Urethral diverticulum has been reported in 1.4 % of women with stress urinary incontinence (Fig. 5.10) [37]. In total population of females the prevalence of this pathology is estimated for approximately 0.6–6 % [32]. EVUS enables reliable diagnostics of urethral diverticula, preoperative assessment and if necessary the diagnostics of postoperative complications. For preoperative planning, it is vital to evaluate the diverticula in terms of location, size, number, configuration, possible sac contents, mass effect, and position of the neck, resection of which is critical in preventing recurrence [32]. Complications of urethral diverticula include infection, calculus formation, and neoplasm development [32]. EVUS seems to play an important role in the diagnostics of periurethral abscesses. A case report by Huang et al. showed the usefulness of EVUS in the diagnostics of vaginal abscess mimicking a cystocele and causing voiding dysfunction after Burch colposuspension [38]. According to Chaudhari urethral fistulas are divided into urethrovaginal, rectourethral, and urethroperineal subtypes [32]. The study by Rostaminia et al. showed that visualization of periurethral structures by 3D endovaginal ultrasonography (EVUS) in midsagittal plane is not associated with SUI status. There were no differences in visualization of defects in the trigonal ring, vesical trigone, trigonal plate, longitudinal muscle, and striated muscle between groups. The authors found no meaningful statistical difference in the visualization of striated muscle by continence status, but the proportion of striated muscle defect visualized in incontinent women was 21 % more than in continent women [39].

EVUS is a very important modality in the algorithm of the diagnostics and monitoring of treatment of urethral tumors [40]. Urethral leiomyomas are extremely rare, benign smooth muscle tumors that may grow during pregnancy and result in dysuria. A well-defined homogeneous tumor with increased vascularity is the typical US manifestation. Urethral carcinoma is a rare neoplasm that accounts for less than 0.02 % of all malignancies in women. Squamous cell carcinoma (70 % of cases) classically involves the distal urethra and the external urethral meatus.

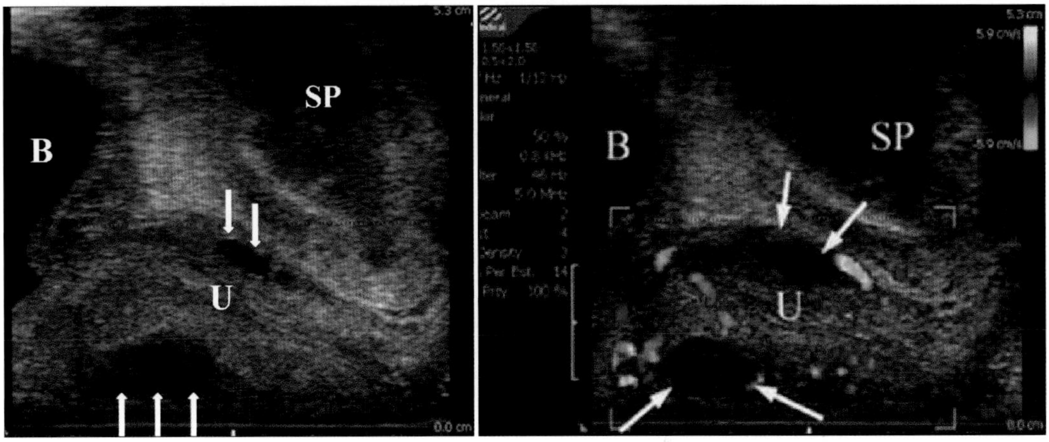

Fig. 5.10 Sagittal section gray-scale (**a**) and Color Doppler (**b**) mode with 8848 transducer (B–K Medical) demonstrating vaginal diverticula (*arrows*). The image performed in Color Doppler mode (**b**) presents hypervascularity due to the infection of the diverticula. *B* bladder, *U* urethra, *SP* symphysis pubis

Transitional cell carcinoma (20 %) and adenocarcinoma (10 %) typically involve the proximal urethra. Urethral malignancies exclusively involving the distal third of the urethra are known as anterior urethral tumors, with the remainder of malignancies being referred to as entire urethral tumors [32].

Secondary urethral carcinomas are rare tumors that extend contiguously from the urinary bladder, cervix, vagina, uterus, and anus, may occur during urethral instrumentation or by hematogenous tumor spread [32]. High frequency US may be a very important diagnostic tool in the assessment of these pathologies, their distribution, and relations to the surrounding tissues.

EVUS helps in demonstration of bladder diverticula, foreign bodies in the bladder, and bullous edema. Moreover, this diagnostic procedure allows documentation of functional and morphologic findings, such as position and mobility of the bladder neck.

Urethral mobility, urethral vascularity, funneling of the internal urethral meatus, bladder neck descent, and bladder wall thickness (Fig. 5.11) may be evaluated on TPUS and EVUS. In patients with stress incontinence, but also in asymptomatic women [41], urethral funneling (UF) may be observed on Valsalva maneuver and sometimes also at rest. Its morphologic basis is unknown and its incidence is reported to range from 18.6 to

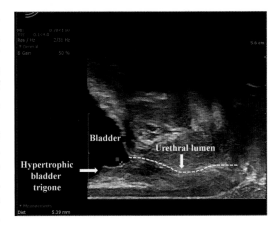

Fig. 5.11 Sagittal section 3D gray-scale image with a biplane 12-MHz transducer (type 8848, B–K Medical). Hypertrophy of the bladder trigone

97.4 %. Funneling is often associated with leakage, and occasionally weak grayscale echoes may be observed in the proximal urethra, suggesting urine flow and therefore incontinence during straining. However, funneling may also be observed in urge incontinence. Marked funneling has been shown to be associated with poor urethral closure pressures [42, 43]. Tunn et al. [44] performed introital US in stress urinary incontinence to distinguish patients with and without UF. The two groups were compared for clinical history, urodynamic results, and MRI findings. The results of this study, however, could not elucidate the pathogenesis of UF.

The demonstration of UF crucially depends on the examination technique employed [44].

EVUS is a relatively new technique showing the relations of bladder neck and the urethra. Up to date publications concerning these relationships were based mainly on TPUS, such as the paper published by Schaer et al. who evaluated the bladder neck in continent and stress incontinent women (5 MHz curved linear array transducer) with the help of US contrast medium (galactose suspension-Echovist-300). This method allowed quantification of the depth and diameter of bladder neck dilation, showing that both incontinent and continent women may have bladder neck dilation and that urinary continence can be established at different locations along the urethra [41]. Parity seemed to be a main prerequisite for a proximal urethral defect with bladder neck dilation. Dietz et al. reported that bladder neck mobility and maximum urethral closure pressure are strong predictors of the diagnosis of urinary stress incontinence, provided that major confounders such as previous incontinence or prolapse surgery, pelvic radiotherapy, or urethral kinking on ultrasound are excluded. Bladder neck descent explains 29 % and urethral closure pressure 12 % of overall variability. Bladder neck mobility appears to be the strongest predictor [45]. Petros et al. demonstrated that dynamic perineal ultrasound studies show that mid-urethral anchoring of vagina prevents bladder neck descent, funneling, and urine loss on effort. Appearances are consistent with continence control by a musculoelastic mechanism [46].

Hall et al. performed a comparison of periurethral blood flow resistive indices and maximum urethral closure pressure in women with stress urinary incontinence. They reported that translabial ultrasound (TLUS) and Doppler spectral waveform can confidently include assessment of morphology and urethral resistive indices [47].

Khullar et al. [48] described a technique of measuring bladder wall thickness using EVUS. Ultrasonographic measurements showed a good intra- and interobserver reproducibility. Women with urinary symptoms and detrusor instability were found to have significantly thicker bladder walls than women with urodynamically diagnosed stress incontinence. This result was confirmed in another study by the same authors, who reported that a mean bladder wall thickness greater than 5 mm at EVUS is a sensitive screening method for diagnosing detrusor instability in symptomatic women without outflow obstruction [49].

Assessment of the urethral sphincter using a 3D ultrasound scan predicts the outcome of continence surgery [14]. By performing 3D-TPUS with the use of a sector endovaginal probe, Digesu et al. found that the rhabdosphincter volume was a predictive factor for surgical outcome [14]. The study by Klauser et al. performed by dynamic intraurethral sonography with a 12.5-MHz transducer in the diagnostic evaluation of the function of the rhabdosphincter in female patients with urinary stress incontinence in relation to patient age an age-related decrease in rhabdosphincter function was found [50]. Perucchini et al. suggested that aging is connected to the loss of urethral muscle fibers which in ultrasonography is observed as increase in echogenicity of the urethra and particularly the rhabdosphincter and/or coexisting decrease in rhabdosphincter volume [51–54]. Post-inflammatory changes may include intra- and periurethral calcifications, fibrosis, and diverticula (Figs. 5.12 and 5.13).

Comparative studies have shown good correlation between TPUS and radiological methods in the assessment of urinary incontinence and voiding dysfunction [55, 56]. There are still no comparative studies between EVUS and radiological imaging as the method is still relatively new. In the prospective blinded comparative clinical study 125 women by Dietz videocystourethrography and cystometry as well as transperineal ultrasound as part of their diagnostic work-up for urinary incontinence or after incontinence-correcting surgery were compared. Mean bladder neck descent was significantly greater with ultrasound compared to VCU. Rotation of the proximal urethra was not always seen on X-ray, but when it was there was good correlation with US. There was also good agreement between both tests regarding visualization of funneling or opening of the proximal urethra, with both tests showing equivalent results in 95 out of 117 patients. Overall a good correlation between ultrasound and radiological findings was

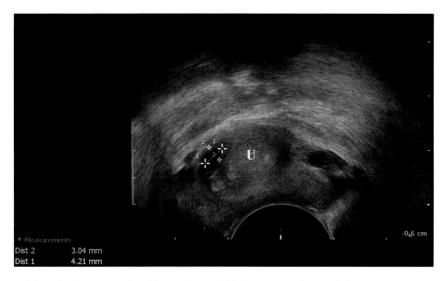

Fig. 5.12 Axial section 2D gray scale with transducer 8848 (B–K Medical). Post-inflammatory changes of the urethra—small diverticulum, calcifications, fibrosis, lack of differentiation of the rhabdosphincter

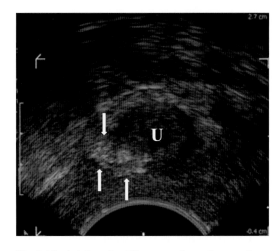

Fig. 5.13 Axial section 3D gray-scale mode, transducer 8848 (B–K Medical) image demonstrating urethral calcifications

observed. Both methods allowed anatomic assessment of the bladder neck and had different strengths and weaknesses. Ultrasound imaging may be preferable as it is cheaper, requires less technological back-up and avoids the risks of radiation exposure and allergic reactions to contrast medium [55]. Gordon et al. also found good correlation between perineal ultrasound scanning and radiologic scanning of the bladder neck [56].

Ultrasonography allows evaluation of anti-incontinence procedures and helps in understanding their failure [40]. The study performed by Kociszewski et al. performed with introital ultrasound (3.6–8.3-MHz vaginal probe, 160° ultrasound beam angle) revealed specific ultrasound findings that can be obtained if the tape is either too close to the urethra or too far away and that these findings were associated with a lower cure rate and higher rate of complications. Outcome was best in women in whom US demonstrated the elastic sling to lie parallel to the urethra at rest and assume a transient C-shape during straining. The authors assumed that this ultrasound finding suggests tension-free orthotopic positioning of the tape and that this position makes optimal use of the tape's elasticity reserve, thereby ensuring sufficient compression of the urethra during Valsalva maneuver. Published data also indicated that if ultrasound showed tape functionality at 6-month, the patient can expect mid-term cure and a low mid-term complication rate [57, 58].

Ultrasound is particularly useful in the assessment of postoperative voiding dysfunction. The minimum gap between implant and symphysis pubis on maximal Valsalva maneuver seems to be the single most useful parameter in the postoperative evaluation of suburethral tapes, as it is associated negatively with voiding dysfunction and positively with both SUI and UUI [59]. Occasionally, sonographic findings will suggest

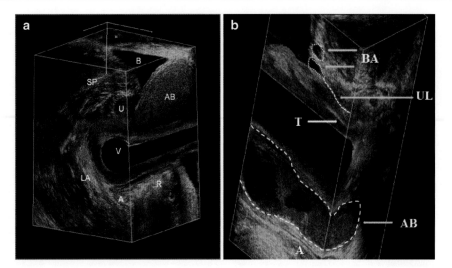

Fig. 5.14 (**a**) Multisurface 3D reconstruction, transducer type 2050 (B–K Medical) demonstrating postoperative hematoma. (**b**) Multisurface 3D reconstruction, transducer type 2050 (B–K Medical) demonstrating bulking agents protruding to the bladder lumen above the bladder neck, suburethral tape, and retrovaginal abscess. *B* bulking agents, *UL* urethral lumen, *T* tape, *AB* abscess, *A* anal canal

tape perforation (partial or complete), with the implant found within the rhabdosphincter muscle, or even crossing the urethral lumen. At times it is necessary to divide an obstructive tape, and ultrasound can help in locating the tape, as well as in confirming tape division postoperatively [60].

It is important to recognize postoperative changes in the urethra and periurethral tissues and to differentiate these changes from primary urethral disease. Periurethral injection of collagen for stress urinary incontinence can give rise to an echogenic lesion that may be mistaken for a neoplasm. Periurethral calcification can be seen in patients with suture granulomas and in patients who have undergone Durasphere injection which is an injectable agent for stress urinary incontinence. Suture granulomas that develop as a hypersensitivity reaction by the host to suture material may appear as discrete, echogenic foci [61]. Defreitas et al. used endocavitary 3D-US to examine the distribution of periurethral collagen and to incorporate this technology into a practical treatment decision algorithm for women with stress urinary incontinence requiring collagen injection [62]. Forty-six women who received periurethral collagen injection were assessed with 3D US 7.5-MHz transvaginal 3D probe placed beneath the urethral meatus to document the position and volume of collagen around the urethra. Patients with a good clinical response were observed with serial 3D US scans. Circumferential distribution of collagen around the urethra was associated with a higher likelihood of clinical success. The authors found that ultrasonographic evaluation of collagen volume and periurethral location was an affordable, noninvasive, and objective technique to predict improvement after periurethral collagen injection [62].

EVUS is also a very good method for the diagnostics of postoperative complications such as haematomas (Fig. 5.14a, b) or fistulas (Fig. 5.15a, b). It enables the visualization of the pathology and also very precise defining of its dimensions, distribution, and relations to surrounding structures being very helpful in clinical decision concerning the type of treatment of the complications. The advantage of the method is also the possibility of detailed assessment in patients who undergone multiple pelvic floor surgeries (Fig. 5.14b) as well as complications following vaginal deliveries and obstetrical trauma (Fig. 5.16).

Ultrasonographic imaging findings, however, do not always correlate with clinical findings

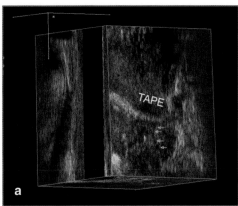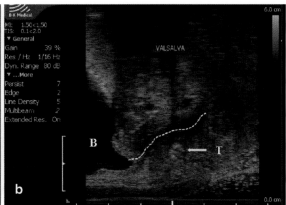

Fig. 5.15 (**a**) Multisurface 3D reconstruction, transducer type 2050 (B–K Medical) demonstrating tape, folded and elongated in the distal part, with coexisting postoperative fistula (*arrows*); (**b**) Sagittal section with the transducer type 8848 (B–K Medical) during Valsalva maneuver showing the tape protruding to the urethra due to too tight insertion and causing bladder outlet obstruction

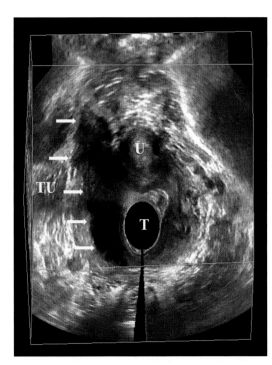

Fig. 5.16 Coronal section 3D gray scale with transducer 8838 (B–K Medical). Lack of symmetry, massive thickening of the vaginal wall on the right side due to the obstetrical trauma and episiotomy. *U* urethra, *SP* symphysis pubis, *V* vagina, *T* transducer in vagina

and patient symptoms, nor does anatomical correction always lead to functional correction. Nevertheless, the goal of pelvic surgery is to relieve patient symptoms and to restore anatomy and function whenever possible. There is no doubt that the additional knowledge gained from multicompartmental ultrasonography of the pelvic floor, with a systematic "integrated" approach, will improve our chances of actually reaching this goal. Imaging findings are already leading to either modification or a choice of specific operative procedures [60].

5.5 Conclusions and Future Research

5.5.1 3D Endovaginal (EVUS) Ultrasound

The 3D EVUS with use of all above-described transducers due to high frequencies of the probes and the possibility of 3D acquisition enable to get coronal, axial, and oblique sections of pelvic floor and deliver analytic insight into all pelvic floor structures including the urethral morphology and defining its normal anatomy or existing abnormalities, which may be responsible for pelvic floor disorders. Described transducers differ among themselves with type of data acquisition, different reference points to obtain optimal view and other details. The electronic character of the crystals, very high resolution of obtained images together with option for the assessment of the vascularity of examined organs decide about the unique imaging opportunities impossible before for all the pelvic floor structures, particularly the urethra and its detailed anatomical and dynamic assessment. The publications by Shobeiri et al. concerning the anatomy of anterior and posterior compartment confirmed with cadaveric studies are a real breakthrough in the attitude to future correlations of the ultrasound morphology, clinical methods, and additional examinations for the understanding of many elements influencing the continence/incontinence in women [12, 18]. It is important to remember that these techniques were described for the first time at the end of the year 2000 [5, 58]. The availability of these transducers is incomparably less than the transducers used for TPUS, but they have universal character and may be used by many specialties dealing with pelvic floor diseases. The main advantages apart from very analytic view of examined structures are wider accessibility of ultrasonography than other imaging techniques, simplicity of the performance, and easiness of understanding and interpretation together with clinical examination and additional tests.

5.5.2 3D EVUS in Interventional Treatment

The most important application of 3D EVUS of the urethra is the understanding and the attempt of explanation the causes of the high percentage of failures in surgical treatment of patients with urinary incontinence and POP. The influence of the tape and mesh position implemented in the restoration of anatomy continuous to be still unclear. The opportunity of static and dynamic three-dimensional examinations and their recording will bring new light into the explanation of the causes of surgical failures. The advantage of 3D EVUS is also the assessment of the tension of tapes and their mobility, particularly in patients with postoperation bladder outlet obstruction or voiding dysfunctions. Another advantage of 3D EVUS is the possibility of detailed assessment of the dimensions and the distribution of the postop-

erative fistulas in the pelvic floor. Important advantage of 3D EVUS is also the possibility of defining localization and dimensions of abnormal fluid collections such as hematomas or empyemas. It is also important to remember that among all available imaging modalities only ultrasound scanner with biopsy attachment may be used not only in diagnostics and monitoring of treatment but also for interventions in the operating theatre. Aspiration of abnormal fluid collections with subsequent lavage and sclerotization can reduce the number of surgical interventions.

5.5.3 Future Applications and Directions of Development

The knowledge of normal and abnormal anatomy of the pelvic floor conditions proper understanding of all these clinically complex processes. Most probably in future years there will be many publications about newly discovered previously unknown and not described anatomical elements and their relations, not only in urethra but also in all pelvic floor structures in various groups of clinical disturbances. One of the most important advantages of 2D/3D EVUS of the urethra is the possibility of assessment of vascularization. It is known that the pregnancy and the labor may deteriorate nerve, muscular, and vascular supply. Recent reports concerning the changes of urethral vascularity depending on parity is the example of hopes which can be fulfilled in the future in comparison to other methods such as urodynamic studies [31]. The possibility of delineating very small ROIs gives hope for creating the opportunity of defining vascularity of tiny organs and their parts for example rhabdosphincter or other parts of the urethra. 3D EVUS and quantification of vascularity together with detailed morphological image of urethra, its location, and relations to other organs may give many new information about the prediction for the effectiveness of surgery. The ultrasonography undergoes huge development; 2D techniques are developed into 3D; these techniques enable to get better resolution; they are enriched with dynamic studies for example motion tracking and color vector mapping which enable the assessment of biomechanical properties of tissues and organs. Computer-aided vector-based ultrasound appears to be a feasible and valuable tool for the assessment of bladder neck and urethral mobility and the evaluation of posterior compartment muscles displacement [63, 64]. More often the fusion of various techniques images is possible for example MR and US, which may bring new information about morphological and dynamic information about urinary incontinence (UI) and POP.

References

1. Petros PE, Ulmsten UI. An integral theory and its method for the diagnosis and management of female urinary incontinence. Scand J Urol Nephrol Suppl. 1993;153:1–93. PubMed PMID: 8108659.
2. Petros PE, Ulmsten UI. An integral theory of female urinary incontinence. Experimental and clinical considerations. Acta Obstet Gynecol Scand Suppl. 1990;153:7–31. PubMed PMID: 2093278.
3. Petros PE, Woodman PJ. The integral theory of continence. Int Urogynecol J Pelvic Floor Dysfunct. 2008;19(1):35–40. PubMed PMID: 17968480.
4. Santoro GA, Wieczorek AP, Shobeiri SA, Mueller ER, Pilat J, Stankiewicz A, et al. Interobserver and interdisciplinary reproducibility of 3D endovaginal ultrasound assessment of pelvic floor anatomy. Int Urogynecol J. 2011;22(1):53–9. PubMed PMID: 20700728.
5. Santoro GA, Wieczorek AP, Stankiewicz A, Wozniak MM, Bogusiewicz M, Rechberger T. High-resolution three-dimensional endovaginal ultrasonography in the assessment of pelvic floor anatomy: a preliminary study. Int Urogynecol J Pelvic Floor Dysfunct. 2009;20(10):1213–22. PubMed PMID: 19533007.
6. Haylen BT, de Ridder D, Freeman RM, Swift SE, Berghmans B, Lee J, et al. An International Urogynecological Association (IUGA)/International Continence Society (ICS) joint report on the terminology for female pelvic floor dysfunction. Neurourol Urodyn. 2010;29(1):4–20. PubMed PMID: 19941278.
7. Toozs-Hobson P, Freeman R, Barber M, Maher C, Haylen B, Athanasiou S, et al. An International Urogynecological Association (IUGA)/International Continence Society (ICS) joint report on the terminology for reporting outcomes of surgical procedures for pelvic organ prolapse. Neurourol Urodyn. 2012;31(4):415–21. PubMed PMID: 22517068.
8. Stankiewicz A, Wieczorek AP, Wozniak MM, Bogusiewicz M, Futyma K, Santoro GA, Rechberger T. Comparison of accuracy of functional measurements of the urethra in transperineal vs. endovaginal ultrasound in incontinent women. Pelviperineology. 2008;27:145–7.
9. Santoro GA, Fortling B. The advantages of volume rendering in three-dimensional endosonography of the anorectum. Dis Colon Rectum. 2007;50(3):359–68. PubMed PMID: 17237912.
10. Santoro GA, Wieczorek AP, Shobeiri SA, Stankiewicz A. Endovaginal ultrasonography: methodology and normal pelvic floor anatomy. In: Santoro GA, Wieczorek AP, Bartram CI, editors. Pelvic floor disorders: imaging and multidisciplinary approach to management. Dordrecht: Springer; 2010. p. 61–78.
11. Wieczorek AP, Wozniak MM, Stankiewicz A, Santoro GA, Bogusiewicz M, Rechberger T. 3-D high-frequency endovaginal ultrasound of female urethral complex and assessment of inter-observer reliability. Eur J Radiol. 2012;81(1):e7–12. PubMed PMID: 20970275.
12. Shobeiri SA, Leclaire E, Nihira MA, Quiroz LH, O'Donoghue D. Appearance of the levator ani muscle subdivisions in endovaginal three-dimensional ultrasonography. Obstet Gynecol. 2009;114(1):66–72. PubMed PMID: 19546760.
13. Petros PP. Medium-term follow-up of the intravaginal slingplasty operation indicates minimal deterioration of urinary continence with time. Aust N Z J Obstet Gynaecol. 1999;39(3):354–6. PubMed PMID: 10554951.
14. Digesu GA, Robinson D, Cardozo L, Khullar V. Three-dimensional ultrasound of the urethral sphincter predicts continence surgery outcome. Neurourol Urodyn. 2009;28(1):90–4. PubMed PMID: 18726938.
15. Umek WH, Laml T, Stutterecker D, Obermair A, Leodolter S, Hanzal E. The urethra during pelvic floor contraction: observations on three-dimensional ultrasound. Obstet Gynecol. 2002;100(4):796–800. PubMed PMID: 12383551.
16. Umek WH, Obermair A, Stutterecker D, Hausler G, Leodolter S, Hanzal E. Three-dimensional ultrasound of the female urethra: comparing transvaginal and transrectal scanning. Ultrasound Obstet Gynecol. 2001;17(5):425–30. PubMed PMID: 11380968.
17. Derpapas A, Ahmed S, Vijaya G, Digesu GA, Regan L, Fernando R, et al. Racial differences in female urethral morphology and levator hiatal dimensions: an ultrasound study. Neurourol Urodyn. 2012;31(4):502–7. PubMed PMID: 22190140.
18. Shobeiri SA, White D, Quiroz LH, Nihira MA. Anterior and posterior compartment 3D endovaginal ultrasound anatomy based on direct histologic comparison. Int Urogynecol J. 2012;23(8):1047–53. PubMed PMID: 22402641.
19. Kondo Y, Homma Y, Takahashi S, Kitamura T, Kawabe K. Transvaginal ultrasound of urethral sphincter at the mid urethra in continent and incontinent women. J Urol. 2001;165(1):149–52. PubMed PMID: 11125385.
20. Macura KJ, Genadry R, Borman TL, Mostwin JL, Lardo AC, Bluemke DA. Evaluation of the female urethra with intraurethral magnetic resonance imag-

ing. J Magn Reson Imaging. 2004;20(1):153–9. PubMed PMID: 15221821.

21. Frauscher F, Helweg G, Strasser H, Enna B, Klauser A, Knapp R, et al. Intraurethral ultrasound: diagnostic evaluation of the striated urethral sphincter in incontinent females. Eur Radiol. 1998;8(1):50–3. PubMed PMID: 9442128.

22. Haderer JM, Pannu HK, Genadry R, Hutchins GM. Controversies in female urethral anatomy and their significance for understanding urinary continence: observations and literature review. Int Urogynecol J Pelvic Floor Dysfunct. 2002;13(4):236–52. PubMed PMID: 12189429.

23. Howard D, Delancey JO, Tunn R, Ashton-Miller JA. Racial differences in the structure and function of the stress urinary continence mechanism. Obstet Gynecol. 2000;95(5):713–7. PubMed PMID: 10775735. Pubmed Central PMCID: 1283097.

24. Ashton-Miller JA, DeLancey JO. Functional anatomy of the female pelvic floor. Ann N Y Acad Sci. 2007;1101:266–96. PubMed PMID: 17416924.

25. Caine M. Peripheral factors in urinary continence. J Urol (Paris). 1986;92(8):521–30.

26. Jackson SR, Brookes S, Abrams P. Measuring urethral blood flow using Doppler ultrasonography. BJU Int. 2000;86(7):910–7.

27. Siracusano S, Bertolotto M, d'Aloia G, Silvestre G, Stener S. Colour Doppler ultrasonography of female urethral vascularization in normal young volunteers: a preliminary report. BJU Int. 2001;88(4):378–81. PubMed PMID: 11564025.

28. Siracusano S, Bertolotto M, Cucchi A, Lampropoulou N, Tiberio A, Gasparini C, et al. Application of ultrasound contrast agents for the characterization of female urethral vascularization in healthy pre- and postmenopausal volunteers: preliminary report. Eur Urol. 2006;50(6):1316–22. PubMed PMID: 16831513.

29. Wieczorek AP, Wozniak MM, Stankiewicz A, Santoro GA, Bogusiewicz M, Rechberger T, et al. Quantitative assessment of urethral vascularity in nulliparous females using high-frequency endovaginal ultrasonography. World J Urol. 2011;29(5):625–32. PubMed PMID: 21796481.

30. Wieczorek AP, Wozniak MM, Stankiewicz A, Bogusiewicz M, Santoro GA, Rechberger T, Scholbach J. The assessment of normal female urethral vascularity with Color Doppler endovaginal ultrasonography: preliminary report. Pelviperineology. 2009;28:59–61.

31. Lone F. (2012) Vascularity of the Urethra in urinary continent women using colour Doppler high-frequency endovaginal ultrasonography (EVUS). 37th Annual Meeting of International Urogynaecological Association (IUGA), Brisbane, Australia, 4–8 September 2012.

32. Chaudhari VV, Patel MK, Douek M, Raman SS. MR imaging and US of female urethral and periurethral disease. Radiographics. 2010;30(7):1857–74. PubMed PMID: 21057124.

33. Albers P, Foster RS, Bihrle R, Adams MC, Keating MA. Ectopic ureters and ureteroceles in adults. Urology. 1995;45(5):870–4. PubMed PMID: 7747379.

34. Wang S, Lang JH, Zhou HM. Symptomatic urinary problems in female genital tract anomalies. Int Urogynecol J Pelvic Floor Dysfunct. 2009;20(4):401–6. PubMed PMID: 19093064.

35. Tunn R, Schaer G, Peschers U, Bader W, Gauruder A, Hanzal E, et al. Updated recommendations on ultrasonography in urogynecology. Int Urogynecol J Pelvic Floor Dysfunct. 2005;16(3):236–41. PubMed PMID: 15875241.

36. Yang JM, Huang WC, Yang SH. Transvaginal sonography in the diagnosis, management and follow-up of complex paraurethral abnormalities. Ultrasound Obstet Gynecol. 2005;25(3):302–6. PubMed PMID: 15693039.

37. Kawashima A, Sandler CM, Wasserman NF, LeRoy AJ, King Jr BF, Goldman SM. Imaging of urethral disease: a pictorial review. Radiographics. 2004;24 Suppl 1:S195–216. PubMed PMID: 15486241.

38. Huang WC, Yang SH, Yang SY, Yang E, Yang JM. Vaginal abscess mimicking a cystocele and causing voiding dysfunction after burch colposuspension. J Ultrasound Med. 2009;28(1):63–6. PubMed PMID: 19106358.

39. Rostaminia G, White DE, Quiroz LH, Shobeiri SA. Visualization of periurethral structures by 3D endovaginal ultrasonography in midsagittal plane is not associated with stress urinary incontinence status. Int Urogynecol J. 2013;24(7):1145–50. doi: 10.1007/s00192-012-1990-x. Epub 2012 Nov 24. PubMed PMID: 23179501.

40. Yang JM, Yang SH, Huang WC. Two- and three-dimensional sonographic findings in a case of distal urethral obstruction due to a paraurethral tumor. Ultrasound Obstet Gynecol. 2005;25(5):519–21. PubMed PMID: 15846764.

41. Schaer GN, Perucchini D, Munz E, Peschers U, Koechli OR, Delancey JO. Sonographic evaluation of the bladder neck in continent and stress-incontinent women. Obstet Gynecol. 1999;93(3):412–6. PubMed PMID: 10074990.

42. Dietz HP. Ultrasound imaging of the pelvic floor. Part I: two-dimensional aspects. Ultrasound Obstet Gynecol. 2004;23(1):80–92. PubMed PMID: 14971006.

43. Huang WC, Yang JM. Bladder neck funneling on ultrasound cystourethrography in primary stress urinary incontinence: a sign associated with urethral hypermobility and intrinsic sphincter deficiency. Urology. 2003;61(5):936–41. PubMed PMID: 12736011.

44. Tunn R, Goldammer K, Gauruder-Burmester A, Wildt B, Beyersdorff D. Pathogenesis of urethral funneling in women with stress urinary incontinence assessed by introital ultrasound. Ultrasound Obstet Gynecol. 2005;26(3):287–92. PubMed PMID: 16082725.

45. Dietz HP, Clarke B, Herbison P. Bladder neck mobility and urethral closure pressure as predictors of genuine stress incontinence. Int Urogynecol J Pelvic Floor Dysfunct. 2002;13(5):289–93. PubMed PMID: 12355287.

46. Petros PP, Von Konsky B. Anchoring the midurethra restores bladder-neck anatomy and continence. Lancet. 1999;354(9183):997–8. PubMed PMID: 10501364.

47. Hall RJ, Rogers RG, Saiz L, Qualls C. Translabial ultrasound assessment of the anal sphincter complex: normal measurements of the internal and external anal sphincters at the proximal, mid-, and distal levels. Int Urogynecol J Pelvic Floor Dysfunct. 2007;18(8):881–8. PubMed PMID: 17221149.

48. Khullar V, Salvatore S, Cardozo L, Bourne TH, Abbott D, Kelleher C. A novel technique for measuring bladder wall thickness in women using transvaginal ultrasound. Ultrasound Obstet Gynecol. 1994;4(3):220–3. PubMed PMID: 12797185.

49. Khullar V, Cardozo LD, Salvatore S, Hill S. Ultrasound: a noninvasive screening test for detrusor instability. Br J Obstet Gynaecol. 1996;103(9):904–8. PubMed PMID: 8813311.

50. Klauser A, Frauscher F, Strasser H, Helweg G, Kolle D, Strohmeyer D, et al. Age-related rhabdosphincter function in female urinary stress incontinence: assessment of intraurethral sonography. J Ultrasound Med. 2004;23(5):631–7. PubMed PMID: 15154529. quiz 8–9.

51. Perucchini D, DeLancey JO, Ashton-Miller JA, Galecki A, Schaer GN. Age effects on urethral striated muscle. II. Anatomic location of muscle loss. Am J Obstet Gynecol. 2002;186(3):356–60. PubMed PMID: 11904591.

52. Perucchini D, DeLancey JO, Ashton-Miller JA, Peschers U, Kataria T. Age effects on urethral striated muscle. I. Changes in number and diameter of striated muscle fibers in the ventral urethra. Am J Obstet Gynecol. 2002;186(3):351–5. PubMed PMID: 11904590.

53. Wieczorek AP, Woźniak MM, Stankiewicz A. Ultrasonography. In: Santoro GA, Wieczorek AP, Bartram CI, editors. Pelvic floor disorders: imaging and multidisciplinary approach to management. Dordrecht: Springer; 2010. p. 175–87.

54. Santoro GA, Wieczorek AP, Woźniak MM, Stankiewicz A. Endoluminal ultrasonography. In: Santoro GA, Wieczorek AP, Bartram CI, editors. Pelvic floor disorders: imaging and multidisciplinary approach to management. Dordrecht: Springer; 2010. p. 389–403.

55. Dietz HP, Wilson PD. Anatomical assessment of the bladder outlet and proximal urethra using ultrasound and videocystourethrography. Int Urogynecol J Pelvic Floor Dysfunct. 1998;9(6):365–9. PubMed PMID: 9891957.

56. Gordon D, Pearce M, Norton P, Stanton SL. Comparison of ultrasound and lateral chain urethrocystography in the determination of bladder neck descent. Am J Obstet Gynecol. 1989;160(1):182–5. PubMed PMID: 2643321.

57. Kociszewski J, Rautenberg O, Kolben S, Eberhard J, Hilgers R, Viereck V. Tape functionality: position, change in shape, and outcome after TVT procedure–mid-term results. Int Urogynecol J. 2010;21(7):795–800. PubMed PMID: 20204326. Pubmed Central PMCID: 2876268.

58. Kociszewski J, Rautenberg O, Perucchini D, Eberhard J, Geissbuhler V, Hilgers R, et al. Tape functionality: sonographic tape characteristics and outcome after TVT incontinence surgery. Neurourol Urodyn. 2008;27(6):485–90. PubMed PMID: 18288705.

59. Chantarasorn V, Shek KL, Dietz HP. Sonographic appearance of transobturator slings: implications for function and dysfunction. Int Urogynecol J. 2011;22(4):493–8. PubMed PMID: 20967418.

60. Santoro GA, Wieczorek AP, Dietz HP, Mellgren A, Sultan AH, Shobeiri SA, et al. State of the art: an integrated approach to pelvic floor ultrasonography. Ultrasound Obstet Gynecol. 2011;37(4):381–96. PubMed PMID: 20814874.

61. Prasad SR, Menias CO, Narra VR, Middleton WD, Mukundan G, Samadi N, et al. Cross-sectional imaging of the female urethra: technique and results. Radiographics. 2005;25(3):749–61. PubMed PMID: 15888623.

62. Defreitas GA, Wilson TS, Zimmern PE, Forte TB. Three-dimensional ultrasonography: an objective outcome tool to assess collagen distribution in women with stress urinary incontinence. Urology. 2003;62(2):232–6. PubMed PMID: 12893325.

63. Santoro GA, Shobeiri SA, Scholbach J, Chlebiej M, Wieczorek AP. Technical innovations in pelvic floor ultrasonography. In: Santoro GA, Wieczorek AP, Bartram CI, editors. Pelvic floor disorders: imaging and multidisciplinary approach to management. Dordrecht: Springer; 2010. p. 103–14.

64. Reddy AP, DeLancey JO, Zwica LM, Ashton-Miller JA. On-screen vector-based ultrasound assessment of vesical neck movement. Am J Obstet Gynecol. 2001;185(1):65–70. PubMed PMID: 11483906.

3D Endovaginal Imaging of the Anorectal Structures

6

Dena E. White and S. Abbas Shobeiri

Learning Objectives

1. Briefly review anatomic structures relevant to sonographic imaging of the anorectal structures
2. Discuss techniques of 2D transperineal and 2D/3D endovaginal imaging of the anorectal structures
3. Discuss clinical applications of 2D transperineal and 2D/3D endovaginal imaging of the anorectal structures

6.1 Introduction

Posterior compartment pathologies, including rectocele, enterocele, rectal intussusception, and pelvic floor dyssynergy, are common in the urogynecologic population and are related to bothersome symptoms, including discomfort from prolapse, obstructed defecation, incomplete bowel emptying, and the need to splint with bowel movements. At times difficult to diagnose on clinical examination, many of these disorders have historically been difficult to fully evaluate and treat optimally due to

technological limitations. Neither 3D endoanal ultrasonography (EAUS) nor MRI defecography can simultaneously evaluate both functional diseases and posterior compartment anatomy [1–3].

3D endovaginal ultrasonography has emerged as an imaging technique capable of visualizing important anorectal structures while allowing for functional evaluation of common disorders. By allowing visualization of structures within the axial, sagittal, and coronal planes of the rendered 3D volume rendered from 3D endovaginal imaging (3D EVUS), one can evaluate the internal and external anal sphincters (IAS and EAS), the rectovaginal septum (RVS), and the anorectal angle (ARA), as well as perform dynamic imaging by asking the patient to perform a Valsalva maneuver during the ultrasound examination [4]. Similarly, transperineal ultrasound (TPUS) has been shown to be useful in the anatomic and functional evaluation of posterior compartment prolapse [5, 6].

In this chapter, we will discuss the techniques and clinical applications of both 3D EVUS and TPUS as they relate to evaluation of the anorectal disorders.

6.2 Sonographic Anatomy

6.2.1 Transperineal Imaging

3D TPUS imaging using GE and Phillips abdominal probes (Fig. 6.1) has been extensively studied as an alternative to EAUS, largely as an

D.E. White, M.D. • S.A. Shobeiri, M.D. (✉)
Department of Obstetrics and Gynecology, Section of
Female Pelvic Medicine and Reconstructive Surgery,
University of Oklahoma Health Sciences Center,
WP 2410, 920 Stanton L. Young Blvd., Oklahoma
City, OK 73104, USA
e-mail: abbas-shobeiri@ouhsc.edu

S.A. Shobeiri (ed.), *Practical Pelvic Floor Ultrasonography: A Multicompartmental Approach
to 2D/3D/4D Ultrasonography of Pelvic Floor*, DOI 10.1007/978-1-4614-8426-4_6,
© Springer Science+Business Media New York 2014

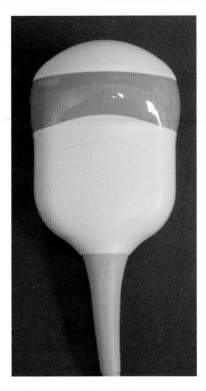

Fig. 6.1 GE RAB4-8-RS 4–8 MHz probe used for 3D transperineal imaging of the pelvic floor. © Shobeiri

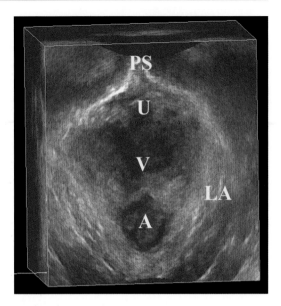

Fig. 6.2 Normal pelvic floor anatomy as seen on 3D transperineal imaging. *PS* pubic symphysis, *U* urethra, *V* vagina, *A* anus, *LA* levator ani. © Shobeiri

attempt to minimize patient discomfort and to allow for functional evaluation of anorectal structures. More about this is presented on the chapter on transperineal ultrasonography. Using TPUS technology, it is possible to evaluate the anatomy and biometry of the pelvic floor (Fig. 6.2) as well as the anal sphincter complex, including the evaluation of defects within the internal and/or external anal sphincter [7–9]. Additionally, it is capable of visualizing the perineal body and the levator plate in the midsagittal plane [7, 10]. It is capable of visualizing the superficial transverse perineal muscle or the anterior longitudinal length of the external anal sphincter.

6.2.2 Endovaginal Imaging

3D EVUS can provide a detailed anatomic depiction of normal posterior compartment structures, and the comparison of these structures to those seen on cadaveric specimens established the basis for the reliable use of this technology in the

evaluation of the critical anatomy in this compartment [11]. Additionally, the ARA, which is important in functional assessments, can be visualized and measured [5]. For the beginner sonographer, evaluation of the axial, sagittal, and coronal planes of the rendered 3D volume makes it possible to fully assess the structural and functional anatomy of the anorectum.

Axial Plane

The axial plane allows for visualization of the internal and external anal sphincters. The anal mucosa is visualized at the 6 o'clock position, with the internal anal sphincter creating a hypoechoic ring around the anus. The external anal sphincter can be seen as the more hyperechoic structure surrounding the internal anal sphincter (Fig. 6.3). In 360° imaging with a BK 2052 or 8838 probe, this plane also allows for the evaluation of the levator ani subdivisions, which is discussed in the levator ani imaging chapter. In posterior 3D imaging, important information about the levator plate anatomy can be obtained.

Sagittal Plane

The midsagittal plane gives a longitudinal view of the perineal body, external anal sphincter (main

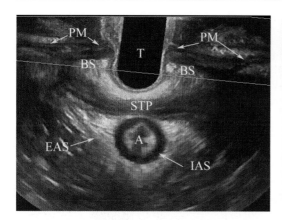

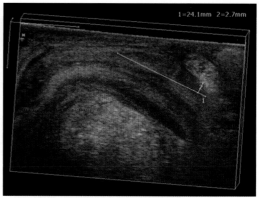

Fig. 6.3 Axial view of the anal sphincter complex as seen on 3D EVUS. *T* transducer, *STP* superficial transverse perinea, *A* anus, *EAS* external anal sphincter, *IAS* internal anal sphincter, *PM* perineal membrane, *BS* bulbospongiosus muscle. © Shobeiri

Fig. 6.5 3D EVUS image of the posterior compartment in the midsagittal plane in a patient with normal anatomy. The internal anal sphincter measurements (length and width) are shown. © Shobeiri

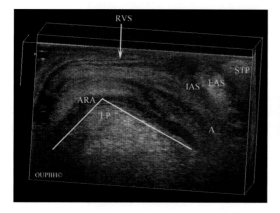

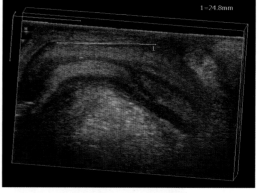

Fig. 6.6 3D EVUS image of the posterior compartment in the midsagittal plane in a patient with normal anatomy. The rectovaginal septum length is shown. © Shobeiri

Fig. 6.4 3D EVUS image of the posterior compartment in the midsagittal plane in a patient with normal anatomy. *A* anus, *RVS* rectovaginal septum, *LP* levator plate, *IAS* internal anal sphincter, *EAS* external anal sphincter, *STP* superficial transverse perinea, *ARA* anorectal angle. © Shobeiri

and subcutaneous sections), internal anal sphincter, and RVS (Figs. 6.4, 6.5, and 6.6). The levator plate can also be measured in this plane, allowing for dynamic imaging of this structure both at rest and with Valsalva or squeeze (Figs. 6.7, 6.8, and 6.9). The ARA can also be measured (Fig. 6.10), which may be important in the evaluation of pelvic floor dyssynergy [5, 12].

Coronal Plane

The coronal plane allows the visualization and measurement of both internal and external anal

sphincter thickness (Fig. 6.11a, b). This view also allows visualization of the intricate LAM anatomy which creates a collection funnel to allow for passage of bowel contents.

6.3 Techniques and Literature Review

6.3.1 Translabial Ultrasound

The posterior compartment imaging always starts with translabial 2D imaging of the posterior compartment. Translabial ultrasound examinations

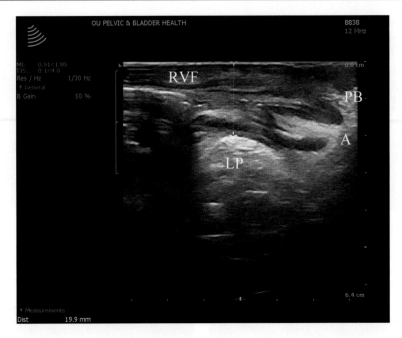

Fig. 6.7 Normal levator plate as visualized in the mid-sagittal plane in 3D EVUS imaging. In this image, the patient is at rest with the transducer in the vagina in a neutral position. *LP* levator plate, *PB* perineal body, *A* anus, *RVF* rectovaginal fascia. © Shobeiri

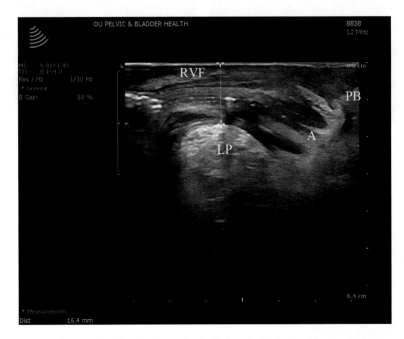

Fig. 6.8 Normal levator plate as visualized in the midsagittal plane in 3D EVUS imaging. Here, the patient has been asked to squeeze her pelvic floor. *LP* levator plate, *PB* perineal body, *A* anus, *RVF* rectovaginal fascia. © Shobeiri

should be performed with the patient in the dorsal lithotomy position, with hips flexed and abducted. A convex transducer is positioned on the perineum between the mons pubis and anal margin (Fig. 6.12). We use a BK 3D convex 8802 frequency 4.3–6 MHz probe with a focal range of

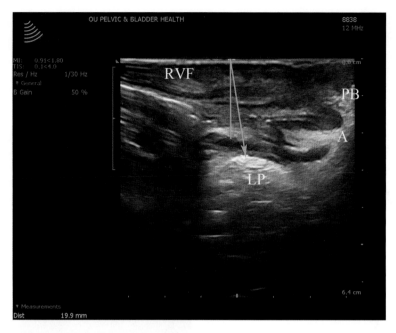

Fig. 6.9 Normal levator plate as visualized in the midsagittal plane in 3D EVUS imaging. During imaging, the patient is performing a Valsalva maneuver. *LP* levator plate, *PB* perineal body, *A* anus, *RVF* rectovaginal fascia. © Shobeiri

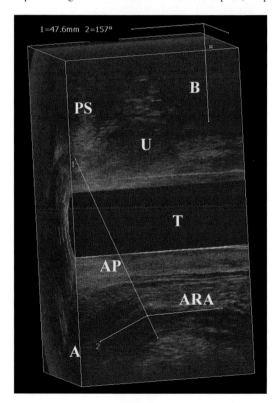

Fig. 6.10 3D EVUS image of the posterior compartment in the midsagittal plane in a patient with normal anatomy. The anorectal angle is measured as shown. *PS* pubic symphysis, *U* urethra, *T* transducer, *A* anus, *ARA* anorectal angle, *AP* anteroposterior line of minimal levator hiatus. © Shobeiri

6–114 mm (Fig. 6.13) as further described in the instrumentations and techniques chapter. However, it is possible to use any curved-array transducer with frequencies of 3.5–8 MHz [13, 14]. These probes are readily available in any urologist's or gynecologist's office and offer a good introduction to dynamic pelvic floor imaging. Depending on the setting of the machine, the image may be upside down on the machine, and most machines have the capability to display the image as if the patient is standing with the left sagittal plane in view (Fig. 6.13). The transducer is covered with ultrasound gel and covered with a glove, a plastic wrap, or a cover. The pubic symphysis will be on the bottom right of the screen and the levator plate should be visualized on the lower left. During the examination, dynamic imaging is obtained by asking the patient to perform a Valsalva maneuver. It is important, when performing TLUS or TPUS, to avoid excessive pressure on the perineum or inappropriate angle of the transducer (and thus the ultrasound beam) to the anal canal. For more information on transperineal imaging, please refer to the chapter dedicated to this topic.

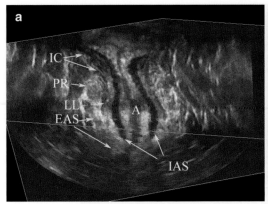

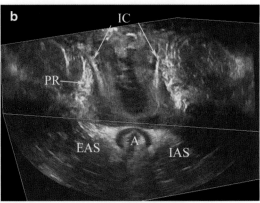

Fig. 6.11 (**a**) Midcoronal of view of the anal canal (**b**) demonstrating the role of the levator ani muscles in funneling of the anorectum. Iliococcygeus (IC) creates the collection area, pouborectalis (PR) the neck, longitudinal ligament (LL) the body, and the internal anal sphincter (IAS)/external anal sphincter (EAS) the outlet of the funnel. (2) a more anterior view of the funnel demonstrates overlapping relationship of PR to sheath like structure of IC. © Shobeiri

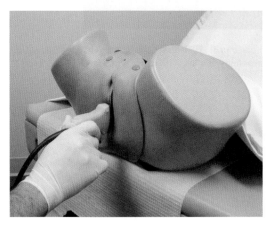

Fig. 6.12 Appropriate positioning of the BK 3D convex 8802 transducer in transperineal imaging. © Shobeiri

Clinical Applications

Rectocele. Although many clinicians use the term "rectocele" to refer to any prolapse of the posterior vaginal wall, regardless of underlying anatomic considerations, a true rectocele is defined as herniation of the anterior rectal wall into the vagina and is typically seen during defecation [14]. It is thought to result from a defect in the RVS, although this has not been consistently demonstrated in the literature [15]. Defecography is considered the gold standard imaging technique for evaluation of true rectocele [16], but TPUS has been demonstrated to be an acceptable alternative in the evaluation of true rectocele as well as enterocele and rectal intussusception [5, 6].

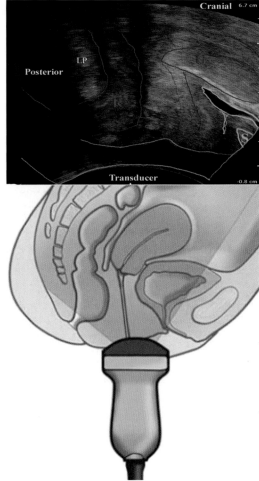

Fig. 6.13 BK 3D convex 8802 transducer. © Shobeiri

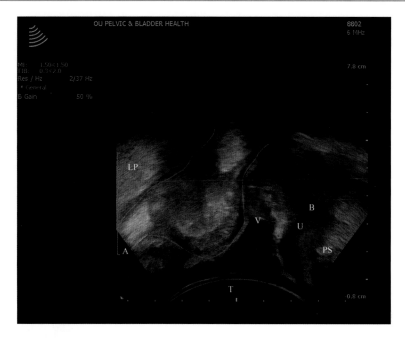

Fig. 6.14 3D TPUS image of a rectocele (outlined in *green*). On POP-Q examination, this rectocele was identified as a stage 2 rectocele. *LP* levator plate, *A* anus, *V* vagina, *B* bladder, *U* urethra, *PS* pubic symphysis. © Shobeiri

By obtaining transperineal images in the midsagittal plane and asking the patient to perform a Valsalva maneuver, one is capable of actively visualizing the downward displacement of the rectum. Its extent can be measured as the maximal depth of protrusion on Valsalva beyond the inferior symphyseal margin (Fig. 6.14). A descent of greater than 10 mm is considered diagnostic of rectocele on ultrasound imaging [5]. However, to date, no studies have demonstrated an association between extent of prolapse and clinical symptoms [17–19].

Enterocele. An enterocele is a hernia of the most inferior point of the abdominal cavity into the vagina or rectovaginal space (pouch of Douglas) and typically contains small bowel or sigmoid colon. It is often indistinguishable from rectocele on clinical examination [20]. However, it is important to distinguish between the two when planning surgical intervention. As with a true rectocele, defecography has classically been the imaging modality of choice. However, TPUS may be used as an alternative imaging technique [21].

On TPUS, it is possible to visualize the displacement of small bowel into the vagina with Valsalva (Fig. 6.15). Peristalsis is often seen in the enterocele, and hyperechoic stool which is typical of a rectocele or a sigmoidocele is not visualized. If there is stool present, we call the herniation a sigmoidocele. The differentiation between an enterocele and sigmoidocele is important as redundant sigmoid colon will continue to cause defecatory dysfunction even after repair of the prolapse. The role of levator ani muscles in pathogenesis of prolapse can be easily seen during functional 2D transperineal imaging. A patient with a stage 2 prolapse can easily reduce her prolapse by recruitment of her levator ani muscles (Fig. 6.16).

Rectal intussusception. Rectal intussusception refers to the condition where the rectal wall telescopes into the rectal lumen and can involve the rectal mucosa or full thickness of the rectal wall. Symptoms typically occur when the intussusception has extended into or beyond the anal canal and usually include obstructed defecation,

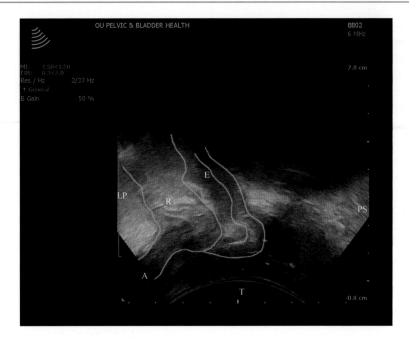

Fig. 6.15 3D TPUS image of a rectocele and enterocele (outlined in *green*). This image was captured while the patient was asked to perform a Valsalva maneuver. *LP* levator plate, *E* enterocele, *R* rectocele, *A* anus, *T* transducer, *PS* pubic symphysis. © Shobeiri

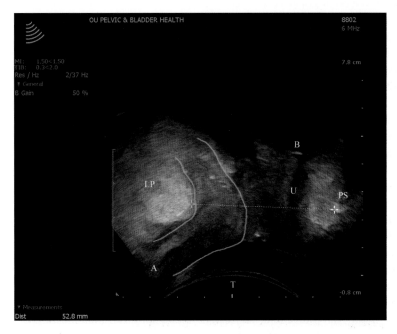

Fig. 6.16 3D TPUS image of the enterocele (outlined in *green*) of the patient in Fig. 6.15. This image was captured while the patient was asked to squeeze her pelvic floor muscles, resulting in reduction of the enterocele. *LP* levator plate, *A* anus, *T* transducer, *PS* pubic symphysis, *B* bladder, *U* urethra. © Shobeiri

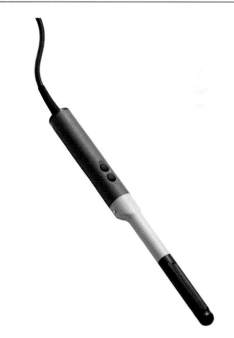

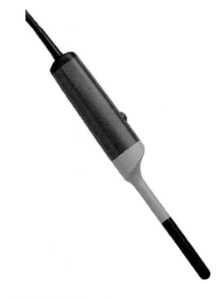

Fig. 6.18 BK 8838 transducer

Fig. 6.17 BK 8848 transducer

incomplete emptying, and need to splint to have a bowel movement. On dynamic TPUS, rectal intussusception is rarely visualized unless frank rectal prolapse has developed.

6.3.2   Endovaginal Ultrasound

3D EVUS imaging is performed with the patient in dorsal lithotomy position with the hips flexed and abducted. The patient is recommended to have a comfortable volume of urine in the bladder. No rectal or vaginal contrast is required. A BK Medical Ultra Focus or Flex Focus machine (Peabody, MA, USA) and an 8848 (Fig. 6.17) or 8838 12 mHz transducer (Fig. 6.18) are inserted in a neutral position to a length of 6 cm, taking care to avoid excessive pressure on surrounding structures and inadvertently distorting the anatomy. When obtaining 3D volumes, the hand should be rested to avoid shaking of the transducer. If using an 8848 transducer, the groove on the probe is faced posteriorly. If the 8838 is used, the probe is rotated to show the posterior view. Either probe is capable of dynamic imaging. Dynamic endovaginal technique may have

limited utility with POPQ stage above 2 since the probe will be pushed out with Valsalva. If 3D imaging is desired, the 8848 needs to be mounted on a mechanical mover as described in the chapter on instrumentations and techniques. With the 8848 probe, radial scans are taken every 0.25° for 179°, starting at the 3 o'clock position and ending at the 9 o'clock position, for a total of 720 scans from which a 3D volume is rendered. If the 8838 probe is used, you can obtain a 360° volume encompassing both the anterior and posterior compartments. The transducer can be adjusted to obtain 3D volumes to your specifications. Of course, for the best high-definition volume, you must choose the narrowest angle which is every 0.25° to obtain 720 scans in 45 s. Both transducers can obtain excellent data volumes. The 8838 probe has the inherent advantage of obtaining anterior, posterior, and levator ani evaluation all in one step. We believe evaluation of the levator ani muscles, the ARA, and the levator plate position is an important part of posterior compartment evaluation. Levator ani trauma can occur during vaginal delivery and must be evaluated in women who present postpartum with complaints of unresolving pelvic pain or pelvic floor disorders such as fecal incontinence and pelvic organ prolapse. An ARA, measured by 3D endovaginal

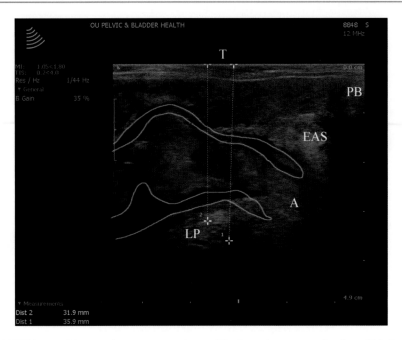

Fig. 6.19 3D EVUS image of the posterior compartment in the midsagittal plane in a patient with a rectocele (margins of rectum are in outlined in *green*). This image was captured while the patient was performing a Valsalva maneuver. *T* transducer, *PB* perineal body, *LP* levator plate, *IAS* internal anal sphincter, *EAS* external anal sphincter. © Shobeiri

ultrasound technique, greater than 170° has been positively associated with both fecal incontinence and obstructive defecatory symptoms. Similarly, a levator plate descent angle of greater than 9° has been associated with obstructive defecatory symptoms (unpublished data).

3D EVUS with the 2052 probe has been shown to reliably visualize and measure normal internal and external anal sphincters. This is the standard probe used in endoanal imaging of the anal sphincter complex. However, using this same probe endovaginally has been shown to be 100 % specific and predictive for imaging normal external anal sphincters and 83 % specific for imaging normal internal anal sphincters. However, it is not as accurate in detection of sphincter defects (unpublished data). For this reason, we recommend doing an initial sphincter evaluation with the less-invasive endovaginal route, but if there is any question of the presence of a defect, then further endoanal imaging is warranted.

Clinical Applications

Rectocele. Rectocele can be evaluated in the midsagittal plane by asking the patient to perform a Valsalva maneuver during endovaginal imaging (Figs. 6.19 and 6.20). This allows one to visualize the downward descent of the rectum with Valsalva and the ability to recruit the levator plate with levator contractions. Rectocele depth has been measured in relation to a line perpendicular to the expected contour of the anterior rectal wall, but a rectocele is not a 2D structure and this measurement does not have a clinical utility. A recognized limitation of EVUS in the evaluation of rectocele is the potential of the probe to reduce or prevent prolapse while in the vagina.

Enterocele. Like rectocele, enterocele is best evaluated by dynamic endovaginal ultrasonography in the midsagittal plane. It is visualized as loops of peristalsing small bowel herniating into the rectovaginal space (Fig. 6.21). An enterocele can be distinguished from sigmoidocele on endovaginal imaging by its content. Small loops of bowel are hypoechoic with fluid in them while the rectal and sigmoid contents are solid and hyperechoic.

Intussusception. Rectal intussusception has been traditionally overdiagnosed with radiologic

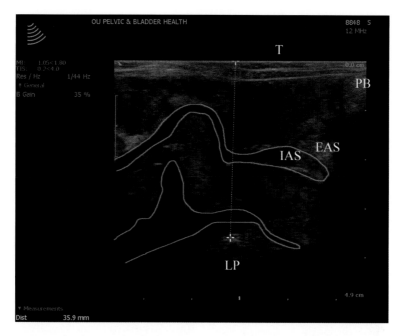

Fig. 6.20 3D EVUS image of the posterior compartment in the midsagittal plane in a patient with a rectocele (margins of rectum are in outlined in *green*). This image was captured while the patient was squeezing her pelvic floor, resulting in reduction of the rectocele. *T* transducer, *PB* perineal body, *LP* levator plate, *A* anus, *EAS* external anal sphincter. © Shobeiri

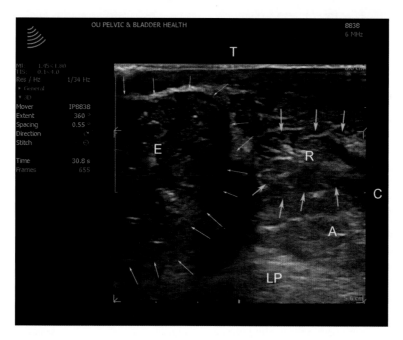

Fig. 6.21   3D EVUS image of an enterocele, seen as herniation of small bowel into the rectovaginal space. *E* enterocele, *A* anal canal, *LP* levator plate, *R* rectocele. © Shobeiri

examinations perhaps of high incidence of coexistence of rectoceles and defecatory dysfunction. Rectoceles may invaginate rectally and give the appearance of an intussusception. Therefore, in the presence of a rectocele, endovaginal imaging may make more sense as the probe reduces the

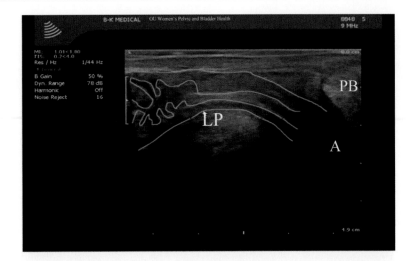

Fig. 6.22 3D EVUS image of intussusception (rectum is outlined in *green*) as seen in the midsagittal plane. *LP* levator plate. © Shobeiri

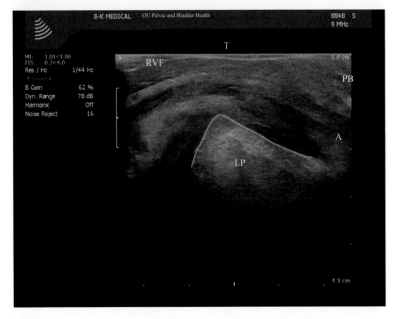

Fig. 6.23 3D EVUS image of a patient with pelvic floor dyssynergy. This image was taken in the midsagittal plane during a Valsalva maneuver. Despite this maneuver, she is unable to relax her pelvic floor muscles. *PS* pubic symphysis, *U* urethra, *T* transducer, *A* anus, *LP* levator plate, *LPDA* levator plate descent angle. © Shobeiri

rectocele and detects if a true intussusception exists. In dynamic 3D EVUS imaging, rectal intussusception is identified in the sagittal view as an invagination of the rectal wall into the lumen (Fig. 6.22).

Pelvic floor dyssynergy. Women with posterior compartment abnormalities often complain of

obstructed defecation, incomplete bowel emptying, dyspareunia, and dysfunctional voiding. The ARA is measured as the angle between the anal and rectal canal axis (Fig. 6.10). Evaluation of the ARA both at rest and with straining can suggest a failure of the normal relaxation of the levator ani muscles [14] (Fig. 6.23). During straining, the levator plate drops; the ARA may narrow while

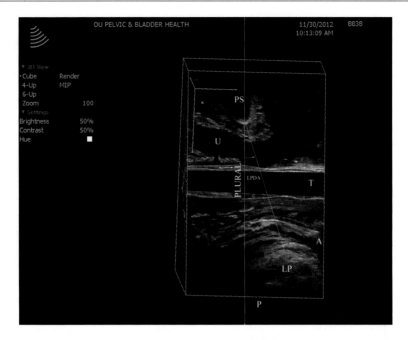

Fig. 6.24 3D EVUS image in the midsagittal plane in a patient with a levator ani defect. Note that the levator plate is distant to the pubic symphysis as a result of detachment of the levator ani from the pubic bone. *PS* pubic symphysis, *B* bladder, *U* urethra, *T* transducer, *LP* levator plate. © Shobeiri

the anteroposterior dimension of the levator hiatus shortens as the anorectum is elevated, often referred to as levator coactivation. While levator coactivation is commonly seen in young nulliparous patients with normal pelvic floor anatomy, persistent coactivation may be a sign of pelvic floor dyssynergy [22].

Other findings in the posterior pelvic floor compartment. In addition to the clinically visible posterior compartment disorders such as rectocele and dyssynergy, 3D EVUS is capable of characterizing abnormalities of the deeper structures in the pelvic floor that likely affect clinical presentation. In the midsagittal plane of 3D EVUS, the relationship of the levator plate to the pubic symphysis can be evaluated and may suggest levator ani deficiency. In a normal patient, the levator plate lies cephalad to the pubic symphysis and the PLURAL line (Fig. 6.24). In patients with defecatory dysfunction, the levator plate is caudad to the PLURAL line (Fig. 6.25). Such patients often require posterior anal pressure

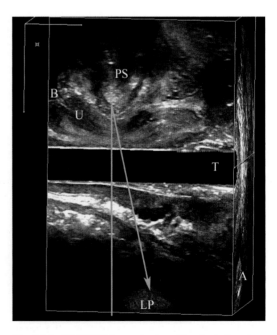

Fig. 6.25 3D EVUS image in the midsagittal plane in a patient with levator ani defect. Note the relationship of the levator plate to the pubic symphysis. *PS* pubic symphysis, *U* urethra, *T* transducer, *A* anus, *LP* levator plate, *LPDA* levator plate descent angle. © Shobeiri

applied with fingers to elevate the dysfunctional levator plate. Descent of the levator plate is a function of levator ani deficiency, levator ani separation from the pubic bone, or fascial weakness (Fig. 6.26). Patients with posterior compartment disorders, including levator ani defects, posterior compartment prolapse, and defecatory dysfunction, may also have abnormalities in measurements of the minimal levator hiatus and flattening of the levator plate (Fig. 6.27). The levator plate collapse is not as readily seen with TPUS (Fig. 6.28). Therefore, this is another area in which endovaginal imaging offers an advantage due to proximity of the probe to the area of interest. If a 360° transducer such as 8838 is used, measurements of the levator ani deficiency and the levator plate descent angle and the ARA can be obtained concurrently (Fig. 6.29). 360° imaging with this probe gives vivid images of the midsagittal view because the probe's crystals are lined up to obtain the images in sagittal plane.

Finally, as seen in other chapters, the synthetic mesh that has previously been placed in the posterior

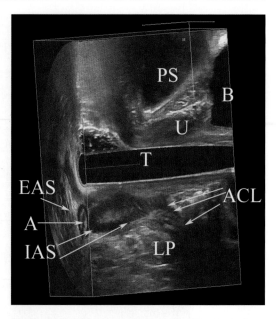

Fig. 6.26 3D EVUS image in the midsagittal plane, taken with the levator ani at rest. Note the flattened levator plate and rectum, as well as the distance of the levator plate from the probe. *T* transducer, *R* rectum, *A* anus, *LP* levator plate, *EAS* external anal sphincter. © Shobeiri

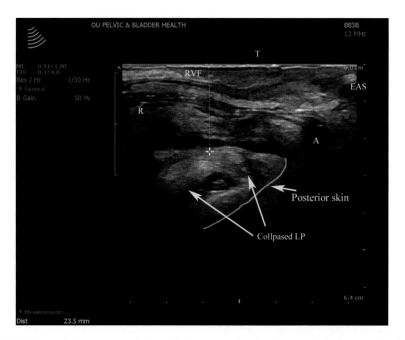

Fig. 6.27 3D EVUS image in the midsagittal plane of the same patient as in Fig. 6.26, but now attempting to recruit her muscles. Note the flattened levator plate and rectum, as well as the distance of the levator plate from the probe. *T* transducer, *R* rectum, *A* anus, *LP* levator plate, *EAS* external anal sphincter. © Shobeiri

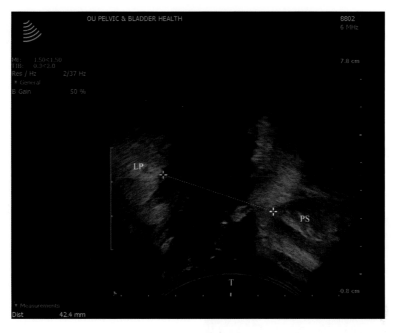

Fig. 6.28 3D TPUS image of the same patient as in Fig. 6.26, taken at rest. Note that the AP is distant to the MLH. *LP* levator plate, *PS* pubic symphysis, *T* transducer. © Shobeiri

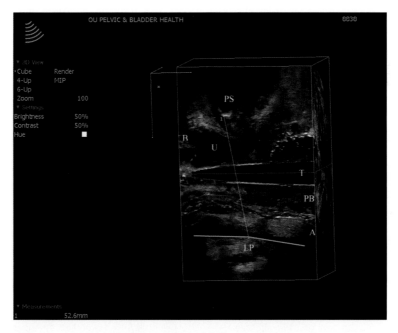

Fig. 6.29 3D TPUS image of the same patient as in Fig. 6.26, taken while squeezing her levator ani. Note that the AP is distant to the MLH. *LP* levator plate, *PS* pubic symphysis, *T* transducer. © Shobeiri

compartment can be easily visualized on 3D EVUS imaging. The use of rendering on the desktop software brings the mesh out of the black and white shadows such that the full extent of it can be seen (Fig. 6.30). Using 3D EVUS to characterize mesh can aid in preoperative planning if there is a need to perform a procedure for a mesh complication (Fig. 6.31). It can also aid in locating the slings intraoperatively, reducing operating times due to the ability to find the mesh more quickly and efficiently.

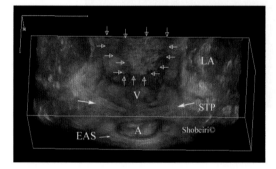

Fig. 6.30 3D EVUS image in the midsagittal plane of the same patient as in Fig. 6.26. Note the flattened anorectal angle. *PS* pubic symphysis, *T* transducer, *B* bladder, *U* urethra, *A* anus, *LP* levator plate, *PB* perineal body. © Shobeiri

6.4 Conclusions

Prior to advances in transperineal and endovaginal ultrasound imaging techniques, anatomic and functional evaluation of the anorectum was limited. Defecography, while known to be useful in the evaluation of posterior compartment disorders, can be time consuming, cause significant patient discomfort, expose the patient to irradiation, and require bowel preparation in advance of the study. TPUS and EVUS can be used as alternatives in the evaluation of these disorders. However, it should be recognized that there are certain limitations. Both TPUS and EVUS are operator dependent, with the technique used impacting the images available for evaluation. It also must be performed in the dorsal lithotomy position, which is a deviation from the normal, functional position of patients in relation to defecation. When evaluating prolapse, the presence of the transducer may distort the anatomy and limit the visualization of prolapse. However, taking a multimodal approach to imaging, by performing both TPUS and EVUS in addition to EAUS, increases the diag-

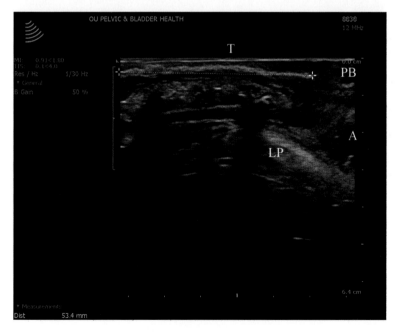

Fig. 6.31 3D EVUS image in the midsagittal plane of a patient with prior mesh placement for posterior compartment prolapse. *T* transducer, *A* anus, *LP* levator plate, *PB* perineal body. © Shobeiri

nostic ability of ultrasound imaging and has helped solidify its place in the initial assessment of women with posterior compartment disorders.

References

1. Dain L, Auslander R, Rosen T, Segev Y, Goldschmidt E, Abramov Y. Urodynamic findings in women with pelvic organ prolapse and obstructive voiding symptoms. Int J Gynaecol Obstet. 2010;111(2):119–21.
2. Olsen AL, Smith VJ, Bergstrom JO, Colling JC, Clark AL. Epidemiology of surgically managed pelvic organ prolapse and urinary incontinence. Obstet Gynecol. 1997;89(4):501–6.
3. Smith FJ, Holman CD, Moorin RE, Tsokos N. Lifetime risk of undergoing surgery for pelvic organ prolapse. Obstet Gynecol. 2010;116(5):1096–100.
4. Santoro GA, Wieczorek AP, Bartram C. Pelvic floor disorders: imaging and multidisciplinary approach to management. 1st ed. Milan: Springer; 2010. p. 729.
5. Dietz HP, Steensma AB. Posterior compartment prolapse on two-dimensional and three-dimensional pelvic floor ultrasound: the distinction between true rectocele, perineal hypermobility and enterocele. Ultrasound Obstet Gynecol. 2005;26(1):73–7.
6. Beer-Gabel M, Teshler M, Barzilai N, Lurie Y, Malnick S, Bass D, et al. Dynamic transperineal ultrasound in the diagnosis of pelvic floor disorders: pilot study. Dis Colon Rectum. 2002;45(2):239–45. discussion 45–8.
7. Weinstein MM, Pretorius DH, Jung SA, Nager CW, Mittal RK. Transperineal three-dimensional ultrasound imaging for detection of anatomic defects in the anal sphincter complex muscles. Clin Gastroenterol Hepatol. 2009;7(2):205–11.
8. Huang WC, Yang SH, Yang JM. Three-dimensional transperineal sonographic characteristics of the anal sphincter complex in nulliparous women. Ultrasound Obstet Gynecol. 2007;30(2):210–20.
9. Oom DM, West RL, Schouten WR, Steensma AB. Detection of anal sphincter defects in female patients with fecal incontinence: a comparison of 3-dimensional transperineal ultrasound and 2-dimensional endoanal ultrasound. Dis Colon Rectum. 2012;55(6):646–52.
10. Valsky DV, Messing B, Petkova R, Savchev S, Rosenak D, Hochner-Celnikier D, et al. Postpartum evaluation of the anal sphincter by transperineal three-dimensional ultrasound in primiparous women after vaginal delivery and following surgical repair of third-degree tears by the overlapping technique. Ultrasound Obstet Gynecol. 2007;29(2):195–204.
11. Shobeiri SA, White D, Quiroz LH, Nihira MA. Anterior and posterior compartment 3D endovaginal ultrasound anatomy based on direct histologic comparison. Int Urogynecol J. 2012;23(8):1047–53.
12. Steensma AB, Oom DM, Burger CW, Schouten WR. Assessment of posterior compartment prolapse: a comparison of evacuation proctography and 3D transperineal ultrasound. Colorectal Dis. 2010;12(6): 533–9.
13. Dietz HP. Ultrasound imaging of the pelvic floor. Part I: two-dimensional aspects. Ultrasound Obstet Gynecol. 2004;23(1):80–92.
14. Dietz HP, Beer-Gabel M. Ultrasound in the investigation of posterior compartment vaginal prolapse and obstructed defecation. Ultrasound Obstet Gynecol. 2012;40(1):14–27.
15. Dietz HP. Can the rectovaginal septum be visualized by transvaginal three-dimensional ultrasound? Ultrasound Obstet Gynecol. 2011;37(3):348–52.
16. Harvey CJ, Halligan S, Bartram CI, Hollings N, Sahdev A, Kingston K. Evacuation proctography: a prospective study of diagnostic and therapeutic effects. Radiology. 1999;211(1):223–7.
17. Halligan S, Bartram CI. Is barium trapping in rectoceles significant? Dis Colon Rectum. 1995;38(7):764–8.
18. Infantino A, Masin A, Melega E, Dodi G, Lise M. Does surgery resolve outlet obstruction from rectocele? Int J Colorectal Dis. 1995;10(2):97–100.
19. Kenton K, Shott S, Brubaker L. The anatomic and functional variability of rectoceles in women. Int Urogynecol J Pelvic Floor Dysfunct. 1999;10(2): 96–9.
20. Hock D, Lombard R, Jehaes C, Markiewicz S, Penders L, Fontaine F, et al. Colpocystodefecography. Dis Colon Rectum. 1993;36(11):1015–21.
21. Beer-Gabel M, Assoulin Y, Amitai M, Bardan E. A comparison of dynamic transperineal ultrasound (DTP-US) with dynamic evacuation proctography (DEP) in the diagnosis of cul de sac hernia (enterocele) in patients with evacuatory dysfunction. Int J Colorectal Dis. 2008;23(5):513–9.
22. Orno AK, Dietz HP. Levator co-activation is a significant confounder of pelvic organ descent on Valsalva maneuver. Ultrasound Obstet Gynecol. 2007;30(3): 346–50.

Endovaginal Imaging of Vaginal Implants

7

Aparna Hegde and G. Willy Davila

Learning Objectives

1. Understand the utility of multicompartment endovaginal 3D imaging in the visualization of retropubic and transobturator slings and the diagnosis and planning of future treatment in patients with failed slings
2. Understand the utility of multicompartment endovaginal 3D imaging in the visualization of mesh used in prolapse surgery
3. Understand the utility of multicompartment endovaginal 3D imaging in the visualization of biologic grafts
4. Understand the utility of multicompartment endovaginal 3D imaging in the visualization of bulking agents injected for the treatment of stress urinary incontinence and prognostication of outcomes following the procedure

A. Hegde, M.D., M.S. (✉)
Founder, Delhi Pelvic Health Institute, Former IUGA fellow, Cleveland Clinic, Florida, FL, USA
e-mail: aparnag.hegde@gmail.com

G.W. Davila, M.D., F.A.C.O.G.
Section of Urogynecology and Reconstructive Pelvic Surgery, Department of Gynecology, Cleveland Clinic Florida, Weston, FL 33331, USA

7.1 Introduction

Synthetic and biologic grafts are important tools in the armamentarium of the pelvic floor surgeon. The introduction of the tension-free vaginal tape (TVT) in 1996 [1], followed by the transobturator tape (TOT) in 2001 [2], has led to a remarkable increase in the use of synthetic material in the surgical treatment of stress urinary incontinence in the last decade. Similarly, the use of graft materials in the surgical management of pelvic organ prolapse (POP) has evolved from autologous muscle and fascia to the use of synthetic grafts of varying composition and pore size and xenografts from various animal sources with varying methods of preparation. None of the graft materials are without problems, and therefore, imaging of the synthetic materials following surgery is evolving into a valuable diagnostic tool in the treatment algorithm for the patient.

MRI and X-ray imaging have been found to be inferior in their ability to visualize graft materials when compared with ultrasound [3–5]. A study, which compared the efficacy of introital sonography and magnetic resonance imaging in the visualization of the TVT tape, found that the depiction of the tape by MRI was limited overall and particularly poor in visualizing the tape in a sub- or paraurethral location [3]. Synthetic grafts cannot be imaged by X-rays. Even in a research setting, X-ray imaging of synthetic grafts is tedious and requires marking of the tape intraoperatively,

S.A. Shobeiri (ed.), *Practical Pelvic Floor Ultrasonography: A Multicompartmental Approach to 2D/3D/4D Ultrasonography of Pelvic Floor*, DOI 10.1007/978-1-4614-8426-4_7,
© Springer Science+Business Media New York 2014

either with metal clips (titanium clips) or an X-ray-proof string [4]. In contrast, most of the modern synthetic implant materials are highly echogenic and easily visualized on ultrasound [6]. Also, in the last decade, various urethral bulking agents have been used in treating female stress urinary incontinence. However, success rates are highly variable [7]. Bulking agents such as Macroplastique (MPQ; Uroplasty, Minnetonka, MN) can be clearly visualized on ultrasound, and therefore, ultrasound imaging may be helpful in improving treatment outcomes [8].

Three-dimensional (3D) ultrasound improves on two-dimensional ultrasound by allowing visualization of the grafts and the bulking materials in planes that cannot be assessed by conventional imaging techniques [9]. Real-time manipulation of the high-resolution 3D data volume obtained in sagittal, coronal, and axial planes enables the examiner to document the implant along its entire intrapelvic course. With experience, the data volume can be manipulated using a combination of oblique and straight planes and rendered volumes to follow the intrapelvic course of grafts even when it is very tortuous. Two-dimensional dynamic examination in the midsagittal or axial view during Valsalva, squeeze, and cough maneuvers allows real-time assessment of the in vivo functional behavior of the graft during periods of stress.

Multicompartment 3D imaging combines detailed anatomical examination with a combination of probes (transperineal scan with the 8802 probe, endovaginal 180° scan with the 8848 probe, and 360° endovaginal scan with the 2052 or 8838 probe) with dynamic functional assessment to obtain a complete anatomic and functional understanding of all the pelvic floor compartments. Multicompartment imaging provides the "full picture" which is critical in the management of pelvic floor dysfunction as it is often complex and involves more than one anatomical component and more than one pelvic floor function. Multicompartment imaging summates the benefits and compensates for the drawback of each probe to provide us a comprehensive high-resolution functional and anatomic assessment

of the graft and surrounding tissue from various angles. Examination with one probe confirms the diagnosis obtained through the other while helping to differentiate between artifacts and true pathology.

In the last decade, research on the use of 3D ultrasound for the visualization of vaginal implants has focused mainly on the transperineal route. However, 3D endovaginal ultrasound imaging (3D EVUS), especially multicompartment imaging, is proving to be a useful tool at our center to evaluate outcomes of surgery with implants, delineate the reason for complications or failure, and plan treatment, especially in patients with a complicated treatment history. This chapter is an attempt to share our experience and discuss future directions of research in endovaginal imaging as it pertains to synthetic tapes and grafts and bulking agents. For the purposes of this chapter, a BK Pro Focus UltraView machine, with a variety of transperineal (8802) and endovaginal (8848 and 2052 probes), was used as discussed in the chapter on instrumentation and techniques. Though the primary focus of the chapter is endovaginal imaging, we shall touch upon transperineal imaging where necessary to provide a comprehensive review about our current understanding of imaging for synthetic implants.

7.2 Multicompartment Endovaginal Imaging in the Visualization of Slings

Multicompartment imaging following sling surgery is indicated for various reasons. Imaging may be useful to determine the type of sling surgery performed in patients who do not remember or do not know the exact nature of the surgery. It may be useful to determine the location, function, and in vivo biomechanical characteristics of the sling during the follow-up visit [6]. Clinically, complications such as recurrence of stress incontinence, voiding dysfunction, erosion, and postoperative irritative bladder symptoms may benefit from imaging assessment [6].

7.2.1   3D Imaging of Retropubic (Pubovaginal and Midurethral) and Transobturator Slings

We perform multicompartment 3D EVUS for the imaging of retropubic and transobturator slings with the 8848 and the 2052 probes. The technique of 180° scan of the anterior compartment using the 8848 probe and 360° scan with the 2052 probe and the pelvic floor structures seen are explained elsewhere in this book. However, we will mention a few important details regarding the technique as it pertains to imaging of implants.

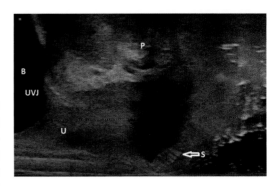

Fig. 7.1 180° scan of anterior compartment: midurethral retropubic sling seen as a hyperechogenic structure beneath midurethra. *B* bladder, *U* urethra, *P* pubic symphysis, *UVJ* urethrovesical junction, *S* midurethral retropubic sling

7.2.2   Technical Details of Performing 3D EVUS to Visualize Slings

7.2.2.1 180° Scan of the Anterior Compartment

Before performing the 180° 3D scan with the 8848 probe, it is important to peruse the 2D image in the midsagittal plane to ensure that the probe has been inserted correctly to obtain a satisfactory 3D data volume. Firstly, it is important to ensure that the probe has been inserted in the vagina in the neutral position in order to prevent compression of the anterior compartment structures. Secondly, it is also important to ensure that the midsagittal 2D image includes a portion of the bladder at its cephalad perimeter so as to ensure that the urethrovesical junction is included in the 3D scan. At the same time, it is important to ensure that the external urethral meatus is in view at the caudad end of the image so that the urethra is imaged in its entirety. If too much of the bladder is included in the image, the external urethral meatus may extend beyond the caudad boundary of the scan. The sling, whether retropubic or transobturator, is seen as a hyperechogenic horizontal structure beneath the urethra in the midsagittal 2D image (Fig. 7.1). The location will vary depending on the type of sling surgery,

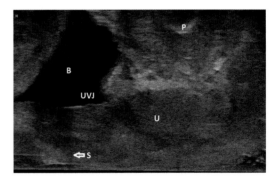

Fig. 7.2 180° scan of anterior compartment: retropubic sling seen proximal to the urethrovesical junction. *B* bladder, *U* urethra, *P* pubic symphysis, *UVJ* urethrovesical junction, *S* retropubic sling

bladder neck or midurethral. However, in a patient with poor outcome following sling surgery, the sling may not have fixated suburethrally and hence may be located proximally beneath the bladder. Hence if the sling is not seen as described above, beneath the urethra, it is important to extend the probe towards the vaginal apex so that the region between the vaginal wall and bladder can be imaged to locate the sling (Fig. 7.2). In such a situation, it may be useful to image the bladder and the urethra in two separate 3D data volumes so that all important details are captured for offline analysis and are available as a permanent record for the future.

7.2.2.2 360° Scan

Similarly, while scanning with the 2052 probe, it is important to ensure that the probe is inserted in the vagina in the neutral position and has been inserted cephalad enough to capture all important details. Though normally the cephalad extent of the 3D scan should begin just proximal to the urethrovesical junction so that in the sagittal cut of the data volume, a small portion of the bladder is seen narrowing into the urethrovesical junction, it must be kept in mind that in the case of slings that have not fixated suburethrally and hence are located proximally beneath the bladder, the 3D scan may need to begin even more cephalad. At the same time, it is necessary to ensure that the caudad extent of the 3D data volume is beyond the external urethral meatus so that the urethra is imaged along its entire length. Hence often it may be necessary to capture two 3D data volumes along the length of the urethra to ensure that all important structures are included. Increasing the depth may help to include the entire extent needed in a single data volume, but it must be remembered that increasing the depth reduces the resolution and decreases the image size.

7.2.3 Manipulation of the 3D Data Volume to Trace the Intrapelvic Course of Slings, Retropubic, and Transobturator

The 180° 3D data volume of the anterior pelvic compartment (probe 8848) can be manipulated in the sagittal, axial, or coronal planes. However to track the intrapelvic course of a sling, it is preferable to begin with manipulation in the sagittal plane. It is important to first orient to the egocentric coordinates, i.e., the relative directions of the data volume, or more simply put, it is important to first understand which sagittal surface of the data volume denotes the left of the patient and which surface, the right. Depending on how the 3D external mover moves the probe, the 3D scan may begin on the left or right of the patient. If the 3D external mover is programmed to begin the

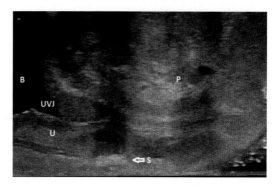

Fig. 7.3 180° scan of anterior compartment: transobturator sling seen as a hyperechogenic structure beneath midurethra. *B* bladder, *U* urethra, *P* pubic symphysis, *UVJ* urethrovesical junction, *S* transobturator sling

scan on the left of the patient, then the data volume is constructed progressively in real time during scanning from the left to the right.

As one begins manipulating the 3D data volume in the sagittal plane, the arm of the sling on that side progressively comes into vision. The arm of the sling, in case of retropubic slings, can be seen, exhibiting a mesh-like weave, extending until the pubic symphysis. In the case of transobturator sling, the arm can be seen extending at a more obtuse angle beyond the pubic symphysis. The sling can be tracked behind the urethra in the midsagittal plane and then can be seen extending on the other side to the pubic symphysis in case of retropubic slings or beyond the pubic symphysis at a more obtuse angle in case of transobturator slings.

The location of the sling behind the urethra in the midsagittal plane will vary depending on the type of sling. In case of TVT slings (Fig. 7.1) and transobturator slings (Fig. 7.3), the sling will be seen as a hyperechogenic horizontal structure beneath the midurethra, and in the case of a bladder neck sling, it can be seen beneath the proximal urethra with its proximal end at the urethrovesical junction (Fig. 7.4).

The intrapelvic course of the slings can be tracked more easily when the rendered volume of the data volume is manipulated (Fig. 7.5). Often one may need to manipulate the data volume in oblique parasagittal planes to be able to track the sling course better.

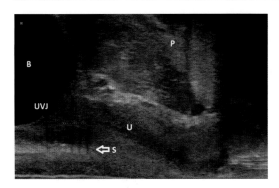

Fig. 7.4 180° scan of anterior compartment: pubovaginal sling seen at bladder neck. *B* bladder, *U* urethra, *P* pubic symphysis, *UVJ* urethrovesical junction, *S* pubovaginal sling

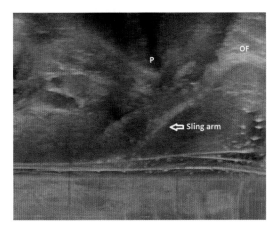

Fig. 7.5 180° scan of anterior compartment: rendered volume, single incision sling arm seen on the right of the patient extending beyond the pubic symphysis until the obturator foramen. *P* pubic symphysis, *OF* obturator foramen

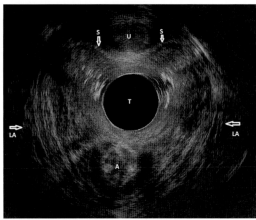

Fig. 7.6 360° scan: retropubic sling seen hugging the urethra in a u-shape. *U* urethra, *A* anal canal, *LA* levator ani muscles, *T* probe, *S* midurethral retropubic sling

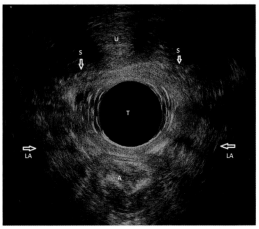

Fig. 7.7 360° scan: transobturator sling seen extending hammock-like to the obturator foramina bilaterally. *U* urethra, *A* anal canal, *LA* levator ani muscles, *T* probe, *S* transobturator sling

Manipulation of the 3D data volume obtained with the 2052 probe can also be done in the axial, sagittal, and coronal planes. However, transobturator and retropubic slings can be more easily differentiated in the axial plane. Manipulation in the axial plane adds to the information obtained from sagittal manipulation of the data volume obtained via the 8848 probe as we are able to look at the sling from a different angle. The retropubic sling can be seen in the axial plane in a u-shaped curve hugging the urethra (Fig. 7.6), while the transobturator sling can be seen extending hammock-like to the obturator foramina bilaterally (Fig. 7.7). The slings can be seen better when the rendered

volume of the data volume is manipulated. We may also need to manipulate the data volume in oblique planes to follow the course of the sling until its insertion points bilaterally.

7.2.4 2D Dynamic Functional Assessment of the Slings and Its Correlation with Outcome

The in vivo behavior of the sling during periods of stress, namely, cough, Valsalva, and squeeze maneuvers, can be assessed by recording 20 s 2D cineloops in the midsagittal plane or the axial plane using the 8848 probe (endovaginal ultrasound of the anterior compartment) or the 8802 probe (transperineal ultrasound). These cineloops can also be stored for offline analysis and are available as a permanent record of in vivo sling behavior.

Dynamic assessment of the sling in the midsagittal plane helps to understand whether the urethra moves in a concordant manner with the sling during cough and Valsalva maneuvers. We are currently conducting a study in which we are comparing results of dynamic assessment of the sling performed with the transperineal 8802 probe and endovaginal 8848 probe with continence outcomes in the case of Monarc (American Medical Systems, Minnetonka, MN), TVT (Ethicon, Bridgewater, New Jersey), and I-STOP pubovaginal sling (CL Medical, Lyon, France) 1 year after surgery. Our experience has helped us understand that when the urethra and the sling don't move in a concordant fashion, i.e., the urethra moves independent of the sling, the outcome is poor. It may be that the sling has not fixated itself well to the suburethral connective tissue or that the sling has been inserted too loosely and therefore, even though the sling has scarred in following surgery, the urethra and surrounding tissue move independent of it. Therefore even if the midurethral or bladder neck sling is confirmed on static 2D and 3D ultrasound to be placed in the correct location, dynamic assessment may show that the urethra moves independent of it on dynamic assessment. In some patients with failed slings, the urethrovesical junction is sometimes even seen to move distal to the sling on dynamic assessment. Therefore the sling does not have the desired functional effect and may fail.

Kociszewski et al. correlated the dynamic changes in TVT sling shape seen on transperineal ultrasound with outcomes following TVT sling surgery in 72 women [10]. They found that 98 % of patients, in whom the tape was flat at rest along its width in the midsagittal plane and curved into a c-shape during straining, were continent after surgery. There was improvement in one case (2 %) and none of these patients was classified as failure. However, in 39 % of the patients, no change was visible in the sling shape along its width on straining in the midsagittal plane. In the 11 % of patients in whom the tape position was flat along its width at rest and during straining (i.e., too far away from the urethra), the failure rate was highest at 25 %. In the 28 % of patients in whom the sling was c-shaped along its width at rest and on straining, the failure rate was 10 %.

In our experience, the deformability of the sling on Valsalva (flat at rest along its width and deformed to a c-shape on Valsalva), the concordance of urethral movement with the sling and the location of the sling are all correlated with outcomes following sling surgery. Our data (unpublished) suggests that the best outcomes following transobturator sling surgery are found to be associated with concordance of urethral movement with the sling, followed by midurethral location of the sling and deformability of the sling on dynamic assessment in that order. A patient in whom the sling does not deform on Valsalva (i.e., does not curve into a c-shape from flat at rest along its width) may still have a successful outcome if the sling is located in the correct location (midurethral) at rest and the urethra moves in a concordant manner with the sling. Conversely, a patient, in whom the sling deforms on Valsalva, may still have a poor outcome if the urethra moves in a discordant manner with the sling and/or the sling is not located beneath midurethra.

7.2.5 Diagnosis and Planning of Future Treatment in the Case of Failed Sling Surgery

In patients who have poor outcomes following sling surgery, multicompartment 3D imaging can often be invaluable in delineating the cause for failure and also plan future treatment. There are various scenarios we encounter in such patients at our center which we shall discuss in this section.

7.2.5.1 Unknown Sling Type

Often the patient is unaware of the exact nature of the previous sling surgery. 2D imaging cannot delineate the type of sling on either transperineal ultrasound or endovaginal ultrasound. A midure-thral sling, whether retropubic or transobturator, will appear as a hyperechogenic horizontal structure behind the midurethra (Figs. 7.1 and 7.3). A bladder neck sling, which is located correctly at the urethrovesical junction, should ideally be easy to distinguish from a midurethral sling based on location. But in patients with poor outcome following surgery, a midurethral sling is often found to be located too proximally. Therefore a sling that is found to be located under proximal urethra may not necessarily be a bladder neck sling, but could be a midurethral sling.

Multicompartment 3D imaging including dynamic functional assessment is very useful in determining the type of sling that was inserted in such patients. As described above, the intra-pelvic course of the sling can be tracked by manipulating the 3D data volume. The sling can be examined in the three different data volumes obtained with transperineal ultrasound, 180° endovaginal scan with the 8848 and/or 360° scan, and hence the diagnosis obtained through one probe can be confirmed through the other. Rendered volumes can be used to track the sling better.

Dynamic functional assessment also helps to distinguish slings based on elasticity and deform-ability. At our center, we use an inelastic retropu-bic sling (I-STOP, CL Medical, Lyon, France) placed at the bladder neck in patients with intrin-sic sphincter deficiency. The I-STOP sling has lower elasticity and lower deformability as com-pared to other slings [11]. We find that an I-STOP sling lies flat at rest (Fig. 7.4) against the urethra and, on dynamic assessment, it moves with the urethra and constricts the bladder neck without deforming or bending into a c-shape along its width. This is concordant with its mechanism of action, which is by increasing resistance at the bladder neck during periods of stress as opposed to that of elastic midurethral slings, which act by causing dynamic compression. Thus it is easy to distinguish the I-STOP sling from other slings that have higher elasticity and greater deformabil-ity (TVT (Ethicon, Bridgewater NJ), Monarc (American Medical Systems, Minnetonka, MN), SPARC (American Medical Systems, Minnetonka, MN), etc.).

It is also possible to distinguish different types of materials, with the previous generation IVS being much less echogenic than the TVT [6]. Because the I-STOP sling is less deformable, it appears fatter and wider than TVT or Monarc slings. Also since the SPARC sling carries a central suture that prevents pretensioning [12], it generally seems flatter and wider than TVT sling [6].

7.2.5.2 Determining the Location of a Failed Sling

Confirming the location of the sling may be useful preoperatively if sling takedown surgery is planned. Determining the location of the failed sling may help to elucidate the reasons for failure of the surgery. There is controversy whether loca-tion of the sling is important to ensure conti-nence. Several authors contend that location of the midurethral sling does not have any impact on the outcome following surgery [4, 13, 14]. From a theoretical point of view, Dietz et al. contend that since midurethral slings work by "dynamic compression," i.e., kinking or compression of the urethra against the posteroinferior contour of the pubic symphysis whenever intraabdominal pressure is raised, it should not matter much for success as to whether the obstruction affects proximal or distal urethra [6].

However, urethral pressure profile measure-ments and lateral urethrocystography have con-firmed that the urethral zone between the point of maximal urethral closure pressure and the urethral knee is crucial for continence mechanism. This zone, termed as the high-pressure zone of the ure-thra, has been calculated to lie between 53 and 72 % of the functional urethral length, where pubourethral ligaments attach [1]. We conducted an unmatched case-control study of 100 patients who underwent transobturator sling surgery (Monarc, American Medical Systems, Minnetonka, MN) at our center to determine the association of static and dynamic location of tran-sobturator slings with outcomes 1–2 years follow-ing surgery [15]. These 100 patients constituted two groups: group A ($n=50$) who had successful outcomes and group B ($n=50$) who had poor out-comes 1–2 years following surgery. Treatment outcome was determined based on a composite measure of "failure": presence of urine leakage on a standardized cough stress test (CST) at 250 mL and a "yes" answer to question 3 of the UDI-6 validated questionnaire. All the enrolled patients underwent 3D EVUS of the anterior pelvic compartment by a fellow who was blinded to the treatment outcomes. The sling location was significantly more proximal in group B as compared to group A ($p < 0.001$). In group A, while only 50 % of the slings were located beneath the "high-pressure zone," 20 % were located at the junction of proximal and midurethra. On dynamic assessment during cough and Valsalva, the urethra moved concordant with the sling in 44 (88 %) patients in group A and only in 21 (42 %) of patients in group B ($p < 0.001$). The urethrovesical junction moved distal to the sling on dynamic assessment in nine (18 %) patients in group B and none of the patients in group A ($p < 0.001$). Thus in our study, transobturator slings were found to be located more proximally on 3D EVUS in patients with sling surgery when compared with patients with successful outcomes. Also dynamic functional assessment of the sling helped understand in vivo sling behavior in patients with poor outcome following surgery.

Kociszewski et al. [10] found using transperineal ultrasound in 72 women, that a TVT tape located between 50 and 80 % of the urethral length was associated with a success rate of 91 %, whereas the other tape positions failed in 36 % of the patients ($p = 0.0085$). In another study of 61 patients who had poor outcome following sling surgery (49 patients had undergone transobturator sling surgery and the remaining, a retropubic procedure), 3D EVUS was performed with the 8848 probe [16]. Only 21.3 % of the patients had the tape positioned between 50 and 75 % of the urethral length. The tape was found below 50 % of the functional urethral length in 73.8 % of the patients examined and above 75 % of functional urethral length in 4.9 % of the patients [16].

Is this change in position observed a natural progression or iatrogenic? The position of TVT sling has not been observed to change much over time [17, 18]. A gradual caudal displacement of the TVT has been described, but it is concordant with the distal movement of the surrounding tissues, particularly in women who have undergone concomitant anterior repair. It therefore may reflect recurrence or progression of prolapse rather than natural tape movement [6]. One possible explanation is that the sling was inserted proximally rather than in the midurethral location at the time of surgery. In a study of 102 women who underwent TVT sling surgery, urethral length was measured by preoperative introital ultrasonography, and suburethral incision was initiated at one-third of the sonographically measured urethral length [19]. Six months following surgery, the TVT sling was found in the target range of 50–70 % of the urethral length in 88.2 % of patients. 91.1 % of the patients were cured and 6.9 % of the patients showed improved continence symptoms.

If location of the sling is important, does stitching the sling in place after insertion help? Rechberger et. al. randomly allocated 463 patients with SUI to treatment with a standard transobturator sling procedure (232 patients) or to a transobturator sling procedure with additional 2-point tape fixation with absorbable sutures (231 patients). Both the subjective cure rate (85.15 % vs. 75.77 %) and the objective cure rate (85.37 % vs. 75.59 %) were significantly more in the tape-fixation group [20]. Among patients with intrinsic sphincter deficiency, the outcomes were significantly better in the tape-fixation group when compared with the control group (95.1 % vs. 73.8 % cured or improved; $p = 0.0011$).

However, does suture-fixating the sling at the time of implantation ensure that the sling will remain in the desired location a year after surgery? We conducted an unmatched case-control study of 80 patients returning to our center for the 1-year follow-up visit following sling surgery for SUI [21]. The study group A consisted of 40 patients who had undergone transobturator sling surgery (Monarc, American Medical Systems, Minnetonka MN) in which the sling was not suture-secured to the midurethra. Forty patients had undergone a suburethral pubovaginal sling procedure during which the tape was suture-fixated to the proximal urethra (I-STOP, CL Medical, Lyon, France) and constituted the control group B. All the enrolled patients underwent

3-dimensional endovaginal ultrasound of the anterior pelvic compartment at the 1-year follow-up visit by a fellow who was blinded to the type of sling surgery performed. Only 14 (35 %) patients had the sling in the desired location in group A as compared to 31 (77.5 %) patients in group B ($p<0.001$). The odds of the sling being located at the desired position was significantly more in group B when compared with group A (OR, 2.21; 95 % CI, 1.027–4.77, $p=0.04$). Thus, we found that suture-fixating the sling tape in place during implantation may ensure that the sling is in the desired location 1 year following sling surgery. In order to understand whether the transobturator route of the surgery was a potential confounder to the study results, we expanded the study to include 40 patients who had undergone TVT (Ethicon, Bridgewater, NJ) sling surgery in a third group (unpublished data). In the TVT group also, only 14 (35 %) patients had the sling in the desired midurethral location when compared to 31 (77.5 %) in the I-STOP group. Based on tape percentile (the distance of the midpoint of the sling from the urethrovesical junction divided by the urethral length), the tape location in the patients who had undergone transobturator sling surgery was more proximal than that in patients who had undergone TVT sling surgery; however, it was not statistically significant ($p=0.254$). There may be other confounders that we have not accounted for, including the difference in elasticity and flexibility of the slings; however, the study results do suggest that suture-fixating the tape in place during implantation may help to ensure desired sling location a year following surgery. We are now conducting a pilot study where we are stitching Monarc slings in place after insertion, and we will compare location of the slings in these patients with those in whom the sling has not been stitched in place.

7.2.5.3 Planning of Treatment in Patients with Complicated Treatment History

Many patients who are referred to a center with incontinence have a complicated treatment history. Many have history of multiple sling surgeries

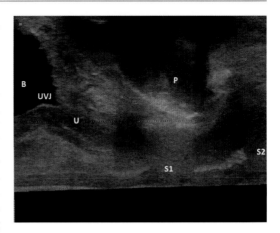

Fig. 7.8 180° scan of anterior compartment: multiple previous sling surgeries. *B* bladder, *U* urethra, *P* pubic symphysis, *UVJ* urethrovesical junction, *S1* midurethral retropubic sling, *S2* transobturator sling displaced distally

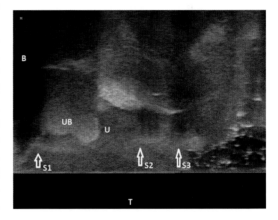

Fig. 7.9 180° scan of anterior compartment: previous three sling surgeries and MPQ injection. *B* bladder, *U* urethra, *UB* urethral bulking agent, *T* probe, *S1* prolene patch sling, *S2* midurethral retropubic sling, *S3* transobturator sling

(Fig. 7.8) or multiple previous sling surgeries followed by multiple bulking agent injections (Fig. 7.9).

Multicompartment 3D imaging is useful in understanding the location of the slings and bulking agent injections and plan future treatment. For example, in a patient with a previous sling and bulking agent injection in whom symptoms have improved but not completely cured, multicompartment imaging may show that the sling is in the right location; however, the bulking agent is not distributed circumferentially around the urethra.

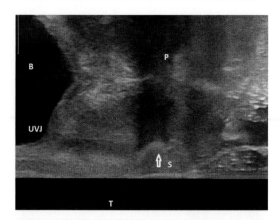

Fig. 7.10 180° scan of the anterior compartment: transobturator sling too close to the urethral lumen. *B* bladder, *U* urethra, *P* pubic symphysis, *UVJ* urethrovesical junction, *S* transobturator sling, *T* probe

In such a patient, one may decide to inject the bulking agent in the bare area around the urethra where the bulking agent is not present. Conversely, one may see multiple slings; however none of them may be located in the appropriate location. Dynamic functional assessment also aids in planning future treatment by helping understand the in vivo behavior of the slings inserted previously.

7.2.5.4 Planning of Treatment in Patients with Voiding Dysfunction Following Sling Surgery

Voiding dysfunction following sling surgery can often pose a diagnostic and treatment conundrum. While it is often severe enough for the future treatment plan to be clear, the symptoms and signs are frequently indeterminate. Urodynamic parameters may also be borderline. In such a scenario, ultrasound examination including dynamic assessment may provide useful information to help make the correct diagnosis and plan future treatment. 3D EVUS with the 8848 probe may show the sling to be too close to the urethral lumen thus causing obstruction (Fig. 7.10). Multicompartment imaging, particularly with transperineal ultrasound, helps to confirm the diagnosis and also clarify that the reduced distance between the sling and the urethral lumen is not due to compression of the

anterior compartment structures caused by the insertion of the probe in the vagina. Dynamic functional assessment may allow a real-time assessment of the obstruction of the urethra during Valsalva. Often patients with voiding dysfunction have Valsalva voiding thereby compounding the obstruction.

There is no consensus in literature on the sonographic diagnosis of urethral obstruction caused by the sling, but there are many studies that confirm using transperineal ultrasound that a reduced sling–symphysis pubis distance and a reduced sling–urethral lumen distance are associated with voiding dysfunction. Chantarasorn et al. measured the tape gap, i.e., the distance between the sling and symphysis pubis at maximal Valsalva in 92 patients who had undergone Monarc sling (American Medical Systems, Minnetonka, MN) surgery and found that patients who had voiding dysfunction had significantly reduced tape gap (9.91 mm as compared to 11.31 mm in patients without voiding dysfunction, $p=0.014$) [22]. Yang et al., in a study of 56 women who had undergone Monarc (American Medical Systems, Minnetonka, MN) transobturator sling surgery, found that compared to the patients who did not, the women who reported de novo or worsening voiding dysfunction postoperatively had larger resting sTA (symphysis pubis-tape angle, i.e., the angle between a line from the center of the tape to the inferior border of the symphysis pubis and the midline of the symphysis pubis in the sagittal plane) and higher incidence of urethral encroachment at rest [23]. Urethral encroachment was defined as the presence, in the sagittal plane, of an indentation in the urethral outer wall beside the tape, with a plateau-like elevation of the inner wall and narrowing of the echolucent urethral core, which encompassed the lumen and surrounding tissues [23]. Kociszewski et al., in their study on the dynamic changes in TVT shape at rest and during straining mentioned earlier in the chapter, also studied whether the sling–urethral lumen distance was correlated with symptomatology following surgery. They found that the best outcome following surgery was obtained in the patients in whom the tape was at least 3 mm from the urethral lumen. Complications such as voiding dysfunction and frequency/urgency with or without incontinence were only seen in patients with a distance between the tape and urethral lumen of less than 3 mm [10]. They contend that the c-shape along its width that the tape assumes on Valsalva indicates that tension is being exerted. They therefore extrapolated that a TVT tape that is already c-shaped along its width at rest is an indication of too much tension exerted on the urethra and therefore may be associated with voiding dysfunction. This is supported by Dietz et al. who also stated that most suburethral tapes can assume a tight c-shape, in particular on Valsalva [6]. The more pronounced this effect is at rest, the tighter one may assume the tape to be [6]. However, the c-shape seen at rest may be a reflection of tape bending or twisting following insertion and not necessarily a tight sling placement. A loosely placed tape can also assume a c-shape along its width, and therefore, it is the distance of the tape from the urethral lumen at rest that would seem more predictive of voiding dysfunction than the presence of a c-shaped tape at rest.

7.2.6 Comparison of Transperineal and Endovaginal Ultrasound in the Imaging of Slings

We conducted a prospective cohort study of 100 patients who underwent transobturator sling surgery (Monarc, American Medical Systems, Minnetonka MN) in whom both transperineal ultrasound and 3D EVUS of the anterior pelvic compartment were performed at the 1-year follow-up visit [24]. A composite outcome measure was used to determine treatment failure: positive urine leakage on a standardized CST (250 mL) and a positive answer to question 3 of UDI-6 validated questionnaire. The 3D volumes obtained were analyzed to determine sling location in the midsagittal view. Seventy of the patients included in the study had successful outcome at the 1-year follow-up visit (group A), and 30 patients had failed sling surgery (group B). Based on concordance of sling location using the

two approaches, the location was called concordant proximal, concordant midurethral, or concordant distal if the location of the sling using the two approaches were both proximal, midurethral, or distal, respectively. The location was called discordant type 1 if the sling was found to be more proximal using 3D EVUS as compared to transperineal ultrasound and discordant type 2 if the sling was found to be more distal using 3D EVUS as compared to transperineal ultrasound. The number of patients with concordant midurethral location of the sling on both transperineal and endovaginal ultrasound was significantly more in group A as compared to group B ($p < 0.001$). The relative risk of failing sling surgery in patients with discordant type 1 profile of sling location was 4.01 (95 % CI 2.47 – 6.52; $p < 0.001$) that in patients who did not have discordant type 1 profile.

On dynamic assessment of the sling with transperineal ultrasound, in all the 14 patients with discordant type 1 profile at rest, the urethra was seen to move distally dissonant to the movement of the sling. In six patients, the urethrovesical junction moved distal to the sling. However, in all patients with concordant midurethral sling location at rest as seen using the two probes, the sling and urethra moved in a concordant manner ($p < 0.001$). Thus, patients in whom sling seems to be located more proximally on endovaginal ultrasound as compared to transperineal ultrasound are more likely to have poor outcome following sling surgery. In the patients who have a good outcome following surgery, the sling is seen at the same location with both probes. There are two possible explanations for the above finding: It may be that the sling has not fixated in place properly or that the sling has been inserted loosely at the time of surgery and therefore the bladder, urethra, and their surrounding tissues can move independent of the sling. In other words, the bladder and urethra move when the 8848 probe is inserted into the vagina. However, the sling does not move with them as there is no tissue bridge connecting the sling with the urethra.

Endovaginal ultrasound can also diagnose tape bunching or twisting (Fig. 7.11a, b) and asymmetry. There is some literature on the utility

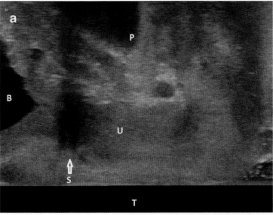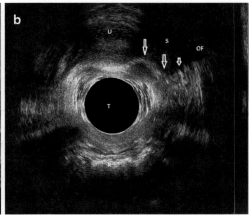

Fig. 7.11 (**a**) 180° scan of the anterior compartment: transobturator sling bunched and shifted proximally. *B* bladder, *U* urethra, *P* pubic symphysis, *T* probe, *S* transobturator sling. (**b**) 360° scan: 3D data volume manipu- lated in an oblique plane to demonstrate single incision sling twisted near its insertion. *U* urethra, *R* rectum, *T* probe, *OF* obturator foramen, *S* single incision sling

of 3D ultrasound in understanding the reasons for postoperative de novo urgency; however it is not conclusive. De novo urge symptoms have been found to increase significantly when the TVT tape was positioned less than 3 mm from the urethral lumen [10]. Conversely another study found significantly higher rates of urgency incontinence if the tape gap (distance of the tape from symphysis pubis) was higher. Tape location has not been found to be associated with postoperative de novo urgency incontinence [22].

7.3 Multicompartment Endovaginal Imaging in the Visualization of Meshes Used in Pelvic Organ Prolapse Surgery

Before the recent FDA notification [25], there was a worldwide trend towards mesh implantation, especially for recurrent prolapse [6]. Synthetic mesh use in POP surgery is often associated with complications such as mesh erosion [26], contraction, and pain [27]. Multicompartment imaging is useful in determining the location and function of synthetic implants (Fig. 7.12a, b). Ultrasound can be used to image both older materials such as Marlex and Mersilene as well as the currently used prolene and combination meshes such as Vypro [6]. The advantage of 3D ultrasound,

as stated before, is the fact that the 3D data volume can be manipulated using a combination of straight and oblique planes to determine the intrapelvic course of mesh implants.

Multicompartment imaging has several uses when synthetic mesh implants are considered. It can help clarify the symptoms of pain and erosion associated with mesh implants. It is also useful in patients with a history of mesh surgery in whom the exact nature of the surgery or the site of mesh placement is unknown. Imaging can be performed preoperatively to understand the intrapelvic course of the mesh implant in order to plan mesh revision surgery better. It can also be performed following mesh removal surgery to determine if there is any mesh left behind. Dynamic functional assessment of the pelvis can also help to understand function and location of the mesh. In one patient who underwent mesh revision surgery following Avaulta anterior repair due to mesh erosion into the urethra, 3D EVUS of the anterior pelvic compartment following surgery revealed that though the mesh eroding into the urethra had been removed, there was still a piece of mesh in the urethral wall that could erode out into the urethral lumen in the future. Lastly, anterior mesh kits like Perigee are not attached to the apex, and the resultant "gap" in support leads to failure of the repair which can be diagnosed on transperineal ultrasound (Fig. 7.12c).

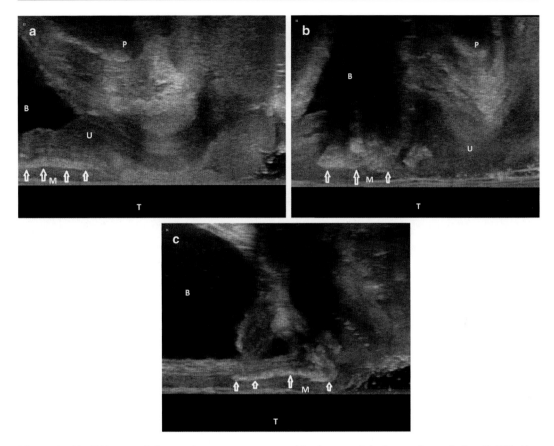

Fig. 7.12 (**a**) 180° scan of the anterior compartment: mesh in the anterior vaginal wall. *B* bladder, *P* pubic symphysis, *U* urethra, *M* mesh. (**b**) 180° scan of the anterior compartment: mesh in the anterior vaginal wall associated with edema mesh in the anterior vaginal wall. *B* bladder, *P* pubic symphysis, *U* urethra, *M* mesh. (**c**) Transperineal ultrasound: mesh in the anterior vaginal wall detached from the apex. *B* bladder, *M* mesh, *T* probe

Shek et al. used 3D transperineal ultrasound to audit transobturator mesh repair for large and/or recurrent cystocele [28]. The implant was visible in all 48 women at an average follow-up of 11 months [6]. In five women, the mesh axis changed markedly on Valsalva with more than 90° of rotation of the cranial margin in a ventro-caudal direction, implying dislodging of the superior anchoring arms [6].

7.4   Multicompartment Endovaginal Imaging in the Visualization of Biologic Grafts

In the last few years, our group has started assessing the use of biologic grafts for POP surgery, especially the use of composite synthetic tape-biologic graft (non-cross-linked porcine dermis graft) kits for combined apical and anterior/posterior repair. The composite kit enables us to provide sturdy support to the apex with the synthetic tape (mimicking level I ligamentous support) and biological graft augmentation to the anterior/posterior wall, while avoiding the complications associated with vaginally implanted synthetic mesh materials. Given the recent FDA notification [25], biologic xenografts may have a significant role to play in selected patients with POP. Unpublished data from our center on the use of the InteXen LP graft in the Apogee and Elevate synthetic tape-biological graft combined kit has shown encouraging 1-year outcomes following combined apical/anterior and apical/posterior repairs.

The behavior of biologic grafts after implantation is not clearly understood. Non-cross-linked

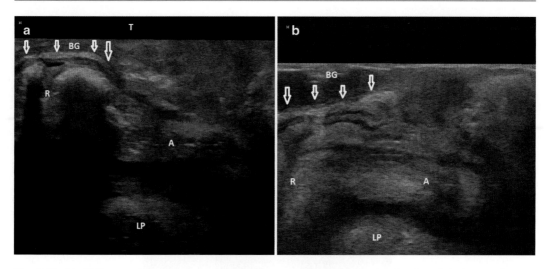

Fig. 7.13 (**a**) 180° scan of the posterior compartment: non-cross-linked porcine dermis graft in the posterior vaginal wall. *R* rectum, *A* anal canal, *BG* biologic graft, *LP* levator plate. (**b**) 180° scan of the posterior compartment: non-cross-linked porcine dermis graft in the posterior vaginal wall. *R* rectum, *A* anal canal, *BG* biologic graft, *LP* levator plate

biologic grafts are designed to provide a scaffold of acellular material to facilitate the infiltration and subsequent replacement of graft tissue with regenerated functional host tissue. The time frame in which this replacement of graft tissue occurs is crucial. Early resorption could lead to weaker repair and delayed resorption could be associated with the increased complications that the biologic grafts are meant to avoid, namely, erosion, dyspareunia, and contraction. Histopathological examination of implanted graft material at different time periods following surgery would be ideal to understand graft behavior in vaginal tissue. However, given the ethical issues underlying such a study, examination of the implanted tissue using ultrasound is a prudent alternative.

We conducted a prospective cohort study in 48 patients who had undergone multicompartment POP correction with a composite synthetic tape-biologic graft kit, to document whether non-cross-linked porcine dermis graft could be visualized on ultrasound and to determine the time frame of integration of the graft with host tissue. Postoperatively, patients visiting the clinic for their 3–4- or 6–7- or 10–12-month follow-up were examined with 3D EVUS of the anterior or posterior pelvic compartments with the BK 8848 probe [29]. The non-cross-linked porcine dermis graft was identified as a hyperechogenic layer between the vaginal wall and bladder/urethral wall or between the vaginal wall and anorectal muscularis (Fig. 7.13a, b) in patients who had undergone combined apical–anterior wall repair and apical–posterior wall repair, respectively. The median thickness of the graft was found to be 1.1 (range: 0.9–2) mm. Median length of the graft in patients who had undergone anterior repair was 20.35 (range: 16.37–23.12) mm, and those who had undergone posterior repair was 40.61 (34.12–48.25) mm. The graft was visualized in all patients at the 3–4-month period and 6–7-month period and in only 4.17 % patients at the 10–12-month period following surgery. Thus non-cross-linked porcine dermis grafts become completely incorporated into host tissue in most patients by the end of the first year after surgery. This study was encumbered by the fact that different groups of women were examined at the different follow-up milestones following surgery. We are therefore currently following up this study with a prospective study in which we are following the same group of women with 3D EVUS at 3-, 6-, and 9-month intervals.

7.5 Multicompartment Endovaginal Imaging in the Visualization of Bulking Agents

Transurethral injection of bulking agents is a viable alternative to surgery for patients with persistent or recurrent stress urinary incontinence due to intrinsic sphincter deficiency [8]. However, success rates following the procedure are highly variable [7]. The optimal site for injection and the amount to be injected are still unclear. The decision to perform repeat injections is largely empirical and is generally based on patient reporting on the post-procedure impact on continence [30]. Thus, identifying the optimal site of injection and other intraoperative clinical parameters that can reliably predict outcomes following the injection is highly desirable and may improve the cost-effectiveness of the procedure [8]. Bulking agents like MPQ (Uroplasty, Minnetonka, MN) [8] and collagen [30, 31] can be easily visualized with the help of ultrasound. 3D ultrasound allows for more accurate and precise volume estimation than the conventional B-mode imaging, particularly for structures that are irregularly shaped [32].

We performed 360° 3D EVUS in 100 treatment naïve patients following MPQ injection (Uroplasty, Minnetonka, MN) to identify sonographic parameters that are associated with successful outcomes [8]. The location, volumes, periurethral distribution, and the distance of the hyperechoic densities from the urethrovesical junction were assessed. The distance of the injected MPQ from the urethrovesical junction was determined by calculating the mean of the distance of the proximal limit of the left and right injected volumes from the urethrovesical junction (Fig. 7.14). For assessment of the periurethral distribution, the 3D data volume was manipulated to determine the axial plane in which the instillation of MPQ was maximal. The area of each quadrant filled with MPQ was determined in the selected axial plane [8]. Each quadrant was considered to be adequately filled if more than 50 % of the area of the quadrant in the

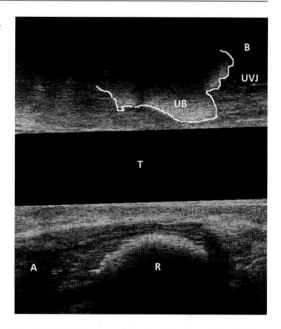

Fig. 7.14 360° scan: midurethral location of the bulking agent marked out. *T* probe, *R* rectum, *A* anal canal, *UVJ* urethrovesical junction, *UB* urethral bulking agent, *B* bladder

selected axial plane was filled with MPQ. The 3D data volume for each patient was then assessed to determine the number of quadrants adequately filled with MPQ: If more than 50 % of the area of 3 consecutive quadrants or all 4 quadrants were filled with MPQ, the patient was considered to have "circumferential" distribution. If less than 50 % of the area of three consecutive quadrants or only 2 or 1 quadrant were filled with MPQ, the patient was considered to have "partial" distribution (Fig. 7.15a–c). For assessment of location of the injected MPQ, the urethra was divided along its length into three equal sections in the sagittal plane: proximal, middle, and distal [8]. The site of injection was considered to be proximal urethra, midurethra, or both if more than 50 % of the area of either or both was filled with MPQ instillation (Fig. 7.14).

The patients were divided into two groups: A ($n=72$), patients who had good clinical outcomes, and B ($n=28$), patients who were not improved or worsened. The two groups were compared with respect to the measured ultrasound parameters. Group A had a greater proportion of

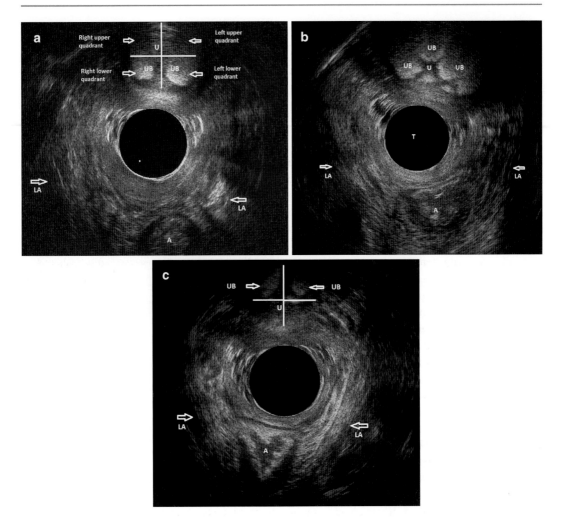

Fig. 7.15 (**a**) 360° scan: measuring the periurethral distribution of Macroplastique instillation. *A* anal canal, *LA* levator ani muscles, *U* urethra. (**b**) 360° scan: circumferentially distributed Macroplastique. *T* probe, *UB* urethral bulking agent, *LA* levator ani muscles, *U* urethra, *A* anal canal. (**c**) 360° scan: partially distributed Macroplastique. *LA*: levator ani muscles, *A* anal canal, *U* urethra, *UB* urethral bulking agent

women with MPQ located in proximal urethra, while midurethral location was found to be significantly more in group B ($p = 0.036$). The odds of a circumferential periurethral distribution in group A were 13.62 times the odds in group B (95 % CI: 5.12–56.95). When the location of the injection and the type of periurethral distribution were considered together, it was found that when the site of injection was proximal, the odds for circumferential distribution in group A were significantly greater than that in group B (odds ratio (95 % CI): 22 (3.05–203.49), $p < 0.001$). Thus proximally located MPQ and circumferential

periurethral distribution of MPQ are individually associated with successful outcomes following the injection. The combination of circumferentially distributed and proximally located MPQ is associated with best short-term clinical outcomes [8].

Previously, in a study of 23 women with transperineal ultrasound carried out before and after periurethral collagen injections, it was reported that short-term continence status was related to the height of the "collagen bumps" on either side of the bladder neck. Continence was not achieved in the study if the "bumps" were located less than

10 mm from the bladder neck [33]. In another study of 31 women, in whom transperineal ultrasound was performed 3 months after the first periurethral collagen implant, a distance of collagen from the bladder neck of less than 7 mm was found to be associated with positive outcomes. The threshold of 7 mm was found to have a sensitivity of 83.3 %, specificity of 85.7 %, positive predictive value of 93.7 %, and negative predictive value of 66.6 % [34]. Although these studies support instillation of the material in the proximal urethra, description of the implants in terms of the distance from the urethrovesical junction may not be adequate as it does not take into account the extent to which the proximal urethra is filled with the implant. For example, the implant may be only 3 mm in distance from the urethrovesical junction; however, it may only fill 10 % of the proximal urethra and the rest of the implant may be placed mostly in the midurethra. In our study, we did not find any statistically significant difference in the distance of the MPQ implants from the urethrovesical junction between groups [8].

Other studies have also commented on periurethral distribution of bulking agents and its correlation with clinical success [8]. In a retrospective study of 46 women in whom 3D transperineal ultrasound was performed 4–12 weeks following the periurethral collagen injection, DeFreitas et al. [30] found that a significantly greater proportion of women with a good clinical outcome had circumferentially distributed collagen on ultrasound (62 %) compared with the women who did not benefit from the treatment (20 %, p00.006) [8]. Conversely, a significantly greater proportion of women who did not benefit from the treatment had a partial distribution (68 %) compared with the women with a good clinical outcome (29 %, p=0.0169). Radley et al. performed transurethral 3D ultrasound in nine patients after MPQ injection. They reported that in the 6 women with good outcome, echogenic MPQ foci were seen to almost completely encircle the urethra, whereas in the 3 women with persistent stress incontinence, urethral encirclement was incomplete, and large gaps were observed between echogenic areas [35]. However, in these two studies, the criteria used to define distributions were not based on actual area measurements that are replicable [8]. In the paper by DeFreitas et al., the term "asymmetric" was used to describe an ultrasound finding in which collagen was located in one area around the urethra predominantly, either right, left, anterior, or posterior. Equal distribution of the collagen between the left and right sides of the urethra was termed "symmetric," and "circumferential" was used when the collagen was distributed in a circular or horseshoe configuration [8, 30]. Our study provides standard criteria based on area cutoffs to define circumferential and partial distribution that can be reliably reproduced and used in both further studies and in practice. Poon et al. [32] reported that the volume of the injected material on ultrasound at which continence improvement was achieved following collagen injection spanned a fairly broad range, from 1 cm^3 to more than 5 cm^3. Thus, they argued that more than measuring the volume of the implant, 3D ultrasound assessment is necessary to determine how well the periurethral submucosal space is circumferentially "filled" in a given patient. This study corroborates this fact: It was the distribution of injected material in the various quadrants considered together that was found to correlate with clinical outcomes. Volume measurements are not helpful as the same volume of injected material can often occupy two quadrants in one patient and three in another [8].

Determination of periurethral distribution on 3-dimensional endovaginal ultrasound following MPQ injection has several potential benefits. This study suggests that circumferential periurethral distribution on ultrasound can be used as an intra-procedure parameter to predict short-term clinical outcomes. In a patient with partial distribution seen on ultrasound performed immediately after the injection, MPQ may be injected in an unfilled quadrant submucosally in the same visit so that circumferential distribution is obtained. Hence repeat injections can be avoided or the number of repeat injections needed may be reduced, thus reducing patient bother and also the cumulative costs of the procedure. An ultrasound examination can also be performed during the follow-up visit in a patient with unsatisfactory

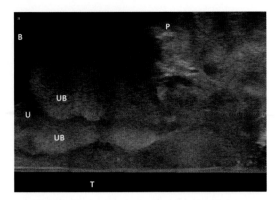

Fig. 7.16 180° scan of the anterior compartment: Macroplastique circumferentially distributed around proximal urethra. *B* bladder, *U* urethra, *UB* urethral bulking agent, *T* probe, *P* pubic symphysis

improvement. The need for a repeat injection can be determined, and the quadrants where the material needs to be injected could be mapped out. An ultrasound can be performed immediately after the repeat procedure to confirm the improved periurethral distribution of the MPQ [8]. We did not follow up our patients in group B with repeat injections to convert the partial distribution into circumferential distribution. DeFreitas et al. had performed repeat collagen injections in seven of their 27 patients who failed to improve after their first collagen treatment and converted them from an asymmetric to a circumferential distribution. Of these seven women, six had a good clinical response [30].

In centers with access to 3-dimensional endovaginal ultrasound examination, circumferential distribution of the injection can be ensured in addition to confirming that the MPQ has been injected in a proximal location. Also multicompartmental scanning can be done; namely, 180° anterior pelvic compartment scanning can be performed with 8848 probe [8] to confirm the findings of the 360° scan (Fig. 7.16).

7.6 Conclusions and Future Research

As is evident in this chapter, multicompartment imaging can be very useful in the diagnosis and treatment of patients with complications related to synthetic materials, both synthetic slings used

for incontinence surgery and synthetic mesh used for prolapse surgery. 3D EVUS can be used to image biologic grafts and also to document the timeline of integration of biologic grafts into host tissue. The 3D EVUS may have prognostic value following bulking agent injection for incontinence. Assessment of the 3D data volumes obtained using the different probes and 2D dynamic assessment films adds entirely new spectra to understanding functional anatomy in the patient. The convenience with which pre- and posttreatment imaging data can be obtained and archived can help us maintain a visual record of the patients' pelvic floor treatment history. Thus multicompartment 3D imaging adds multiple dimensions to the diagnosis and treatment of the urogynecology patient, especially in patients in whom synthetic implants have been used. Perhaps, this is the most important contribution of this technology: allowing the surgeon to better understand the goals of reconstructive surgery and avoid many common pitfalls.

But this is just the beginning. The potential uses can possibly make 3D multicompartmental imaging the diagnostic standard for management of problems related to synthetic implants. However, there is very limited evidence currently supporting the routine use of endovaginal ultrasound imaging in such patients. It is necessary to conduct research where the efficacy of endovaginal ultrasound in imaging and diagnosing problems is established and compared to that of transperineal ultrasound. There needs to be a consensus on the terminology and various measurements that can be made so that diagnosis using 3D EVUS can be standardized and diagnostic criteria established. Prospective studies are needed to validate the results of various retrospective studies in literature, especially prospective randomized studies where treatment with/without 3D EVUS is compared to understand effectiveness of the use of 3D EVUS in routine practice. Given the improved understanding of functional anatomy obtained with the 2D dynamic assessment films, ultrasound imaging may be able to significantly enhance our understanding of the mechanism of action of various slings used and therefore potentially help develop better treatments.

Eventually, whether this technology becomes a part of routine practice will depend on cost-effectiveness, availability of teaching resources, and improved understanding of its clinical value.

References

1. Ulmsten U, Hendriksson L, Johnson P, Varhos G. An ambulatory surgical procedure under local anaesthesia for treatment of female urinary incontinence. Int Urogynecol J Pelvic Floor Dysfunct. 1996;7:81–6.
2. Delorme E. Transobturator urethral suspension: mini-invasive procedure in the treatment of stress urinary incontinence in women. Prog Urol. 2001;11:1306–13.
3. Schuettoff S, Beyersdorff D, Gauruder-Burmester A, Tunn R. Visibility of the polypropylene tape after tension-free vaginal tape (TVT) procedure in women with stress urinary incontinence: comparison of introital ultrasound and magnetic resonance imaging in vitro and in patients. Ultrasound Obstet Gynecol. 2006;27(6):687–92.
4. Kaum HJ, Wolff F. TVT: on midurethral tape positioning and its influence on continence. Int Urogynecol J. 2002;13(2):110–5.
5. Halaska M, Otcenasek M, Martan A, Masata J, Voight R, Seifert M. Pelvic anatomy changes after TVT procedure assessed by MRI. Int Urogynecol J. 1999;10(S1):S87–8.
6. Dietz HP. Imaging of implant materials. In: Dietz HP, Hoyte LPJ, Steensma AB, editors. Atlas of pelvic floor ultrasound. London: Springer; 2008.
7. Davila W. Nonsurgical outpatient therapies for the management of female stress urinary incontinence: long-term effectiveness and durability. Adv Urol. 2011;2011:1–14.
8. Hegde A, Smith AL, Aguilar VC, Davila GW. Three-dimensional endovaginal ultrasound examination following injection of Macroplastique for stress urinary incontinence: outcomes based on location and periurethral distribution of the bulking agent. Int Urogynecol J. 2013;24(7):1151–59.
9. Santoro GA, Wieczorek AP, Stankiewicz A, Wozniak MM, Bogusiewicz M, Rechberger T. High resolution 3D endovaginal ultrasonography in the assessment of pelvic floor anatomy: a preliminary study. Int Urogynecol J. 2009;20:1213–22.
10. Kociszewski J, Rautenberg O, Perucchini D, Eberhard J, Geissbuhler V, Hilgers R, Viereck V. Tape functionality: sonographic tape characteristics and outcome after TVT incontinence surgery. Neurourol Urodyn. 2008;27:485–90.
11. Jijon A, Hegde A, Arias B, Aguilar V, Davila GW. An inelastic retropubic suburethral sling in women with intrinsic sphincter deficiency. Int Urogynecol J.; 2012 Dec 11 (Epub ahead of print).
12. Dietz HP, Foote AJ, Mak HL, Wilson PD. TVT and Sparc suburethral slings: a case-control series. Int Urogynecol J. 2004;15(2):129–31.
13. Ng CC, Lee LC, Han WH. Use of 3D ultrasound scan to assess the clinical importance of midurethral placement of the tension-free vaginal tape (TVT) for treatment of incontinence. Int Urogynecol J. 2005;16(3):220–5.
14. Dietz HP, Mouritsen L, Ellis G, Wilson PD. How important is TVT location? Acta Obstet Gynecol Scand. 2004;83(10):904–8.
15. Hegde A, Nogueiras M, Aguilar V, Davila GW. Correlation of static and dynamic location of the transobturator sling with outcomes as described by 3 dimensional endovaginal ultrasound. Abstract. 38th Annual meeting of the International Urogynecological Association, Dublin, Ireland; 2013, in press.
16. Bogusiewicz M, Stankiewicz A, Monist M, Wozniak M, Wiezoreck A, Rechberger T. Most of the patients with suburethral sling failure have tapes located outside the high-pressure zone of the urethra. Int Urogynecol J. 2012;23 Suppl 2:S68–9.
17. Lo TS, Horng SG, Liang CC, Lee SJ, Soong YK. Ultrasound assessment of mid-urethra tape at three-year follow-up after tension-free-vaginal tape procedure. Urology. 2004;63(4):671–5.
18. Dietz HP, Mouritsen L, Ellis G, Wilson PD. Does the tension-free vaginal tape stay where you put it? Am J Obstet Gynecol. 2003;188(4):950–3.
19. Kociszewski J, Rautenberg O, Kuszka A, Eberhard J, Hilger R, Viereck V. Can we place tension-free vaginal tape where it should be? The one-third rule. Ultrasound Obstet Gynecol. 2012;39:210–4.
20. Rechberger T, Futyma K, Jankiewicz K, Adamiak A, Bogusiewicz M, Bartuzi A, Miotla P, Skorupski P, Tomaszewski J. Tape fixation: an important surgical step to improve success rate of anti-incontinence surgery. J Urol. 2011;186(1):180–4.
21. Hegde A, Nogueiras M, Aguilar V, Davila GW. Should a suburethral sling be suture-fixated in place at the time of implantation? Abstract. 38th annual meeting of the International Urogynecological Association, Dublin, Ireland; 2013, in press.
22. Chantarasorn V, Shek KL, Dietz HP. Sonographic appearance of transobturator slings: implications for function and dysfunction. Int Urogynecol J. 2011;22:493–8.
23. Yang JM, Yang SH, Huang WC, Tzeng CR. Correlation of tape location and tension with surgical outcome after transobturator suburethral tape procedures. Ultrasound Obstet Gynecol. 2012;39:458–65.
24. Hegde A, Nogueiras M, Aguilar V, Davila GW. Is there concordance in the location of the transobturator sling as determined by transperineal and endovaginal 3 dimensional ultrasound?: correlation with outcomes. Abstract. 38th annual meeting of the International Urogynecological Association, Dublin, Ireland; 2013, in press.
25. FDA Safety Communication. UPDATE on serious complications associated with transvaginal placement of surgical mesh for pelvic organ prolapse. Silver Spring, MD: Food and Drug Administration (US), Center for Devices and Radiological Health. Available at http://www.fda.gov/MedicalDevices/

Safety/AlertsandNotices/ucm262435.htm. Accessed 13 July 2011.

26. Gauruder-Burmester A, Koutouzidou P, Rohne J, Gronewold M, Tunn R. Follow-up after polypropylene mesh repair of anterior and posterior compartments in patients with recurrent prolapse. Int Urogynecol J Pelvic Floor Dysfunct. 2007;18(9):1059–64.

27. Iglesia CB, Sokol AI, Sokol ER, Kudish BI, Gutman RE, Peterson JL, Shott S. Vaginal mesh for prolapse. Obstet Gynecol. 2010;116:293–303.

28. Shek K, Dietz HP, Rane A. Transobturator mesh anchoring for the repair of large or recurrent cysto-cele. In: ICS annual scientific meeting, Christchurch, New Zealand. Abstract; 2006.

29. Hegde A, Aguilar VC, Davila GW. Non-cross-linked porcine dermis graft becomes completely integrated with host tissue over a period of 12 months. In: IUGA annual scientific meeting, Brisbane, Australia. Abstract; 2012.

30. DeFreitas G, Wilson T, Zimmern P, Forte T. 3D ultra-sonography: an objective outcome tool to assess col-lagen distribution in women with stress urinary incontinence. Urology. 2003;62:232–6.

31. Poon CI, Zimmern PE, Wilson TS, Defreitas GA, Foreman MR. Three-dimensional ultrasonography to assess long-term durability of periurethral colla-gen in women with stress urinary incontinence due to intrinsic sphincter deficiency. Urology. 2005;65: 60–4.

32. Athansiou S, Khullar V, Boos K, Salvatore S, Cardozo L. Imaging of the urethral sphincter with three-dimensional ultrasound. Obstet Gynecol. 1999;94: 295–301.

33. Benshushan A, Brzezinski A, Shoshani O, Rojansky N. Periurethral injection for the treatment of urinary incontinence. Obstet Gynecol Surv. 1998;53: 383–8.

34. Khullar V, Cardozo LD, Abbott D, Hillard T, Norman S, Bourne T. The mechanism of continence achieved with GAX collagen as determined by ultrasound (abstract). Neurourol Urodyn. 1993;78:439–40.

35. Radley S, Chapple C, Mitsogiannis I, Glass K. Transurethral implantation of Macroplastique for the treatment of female stress urinary incontinence sec-ondary to urethral sphincter deficiency. Eur Urol. 2001;39:383–9.

Endovaginal Imaging of Pelvic Floor Cysts and Masses

8

Ghazaleh Rostaminia and S. Abbas Shobeiri

Learning Objectives

Become familiar with the utility of 3D endovaginal ultrasonography for the assessment of pelvic floor cysts and masses such as Bartholin Gland cyst/abscess, skene Gland cyst/abscess, urethral diverticulum, gartner duct cyst, leiomyoma, malignant vaginal masses, rectovaginal septum endometrioma, vaginal hematomas and endometriomas.

8.1 Introduction

The utility of sonography in the evaluation of anatomy of the female internal organs is well established, but little has been reported on the characterization of vulvovaginal masses. Vaginal Gartner duct cysts [1], solid masses [2, 3], urethral diverticulum [4–7], and Bartholin glands [8, 9] have been reported by varied 2-dimensional

G. Rostaminia, M.D., • S.A. Shobeiri, M.D., (✉)
Section of Female Pelvic Medicine and Reconstructive Surgery, University of Oklahoma Health Sciences Center, WP 2410, 920 Stanton L. Young Blvd., Oklahoma City, OK 73104, USA
e-mail: abbas-shobeiri@ouhsc.edu

ultrasonography techniques. There are case reports of varied masses evaluated by magnetic resonance imaging (MRI) or computed tomography (CT) scanning [10–12].

3D endovaginal ultrasound technique has been described previously for identification of levator ani muscles and authenticated its interobserver and interdisciplinary reproducibility [13, 14]. The aim of this chapter is to demonstrate the utility of 3D endovaginal ultrasonography (3D EVUS) for visualization of variety of vaginal masses seen by this technique.

8.2 Text

8.2.1 3D Endovaginal Ultrasound Technique

Unlike the other transducers that utilize end-fire probes for visualization of female reproductive organs, the probes used in this article are side-fire to visualize vaginal walls and the structures lateral to it. BK Medical Ultraview ultrasound machine (Peabody, MA) with an 8848 or a 2052 automatic transducer with 3D imaging technology can be used for acquisition of images as outlined in chapter on instrumentation and techniques. The transducers are the size of an average index finger (2 cm in diameter) which is important since many patients with vaginal pathology may present with pain or pressure.

S.A. Shobeiri (ed.), *Practical Pelvic Floor Ultrasonography: A Multicompartmental Approach to 2D/3D/4D Ultrasonography of Pelvic Floor*, DOI 10.1007/978-1-4614-8426-4_8,
© Springer Science+Business Media New York 2014

Ample ultrasound gel should be used to avoid air artifact. The scanning with a 2052 probe is performed in a standardized fashion from 6 cm cephalad the hymen to 3 cm caudad to the hymenal ring depending on the location of the mass [13]. With each scan, a length of 6 cm is scanned in 60 s with axial images obtained every 0.2 mm with cumulative 300 scans from which a 3D-rendered volume is calculated. The 8838 transducer scans a 360° angle for a length of 6 cm. The 3D volume is obtained rotational computer-controlled acquisition of 1,400 radial 2D images every 0.25° to encompass the bladder and urethra and the anorectum. These probes can also be utilized in 2D or 3D in color Doppler modes for evaluation of vascular structures in selected cases. Echogenic structures or hypoechoic structures suspicious for being vaginal masses can be easily evaluated. Each 3D volume can be digitally catalogued for future analysis on a desktop computer.

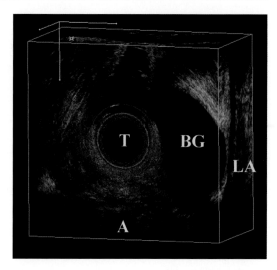

Fig. 8.1 Left Bartholin gland cyst. Axial view with 360° endovaginal ultrasound probe. *A* anus, *BG* Bartholin gland, *LA* levator ani muscle, *T* transducer. © Shobeiri

8.2.2 Bartholin Gland Cyst/Abscess

Bartholin glands are paired vulvovaginal, tubular alveolar glands lined by mucous-secreting epithelium, drained by ducts approximately 2.5 cm in length which exit at the junction of the hymenal ring and labia minora on the posterolateral aspect of the vagina. The ducts, lined by transitional epithelium, are prone to obstruction at their vestibular orifice, resulting in accumulation of secretion and subsequent cystic dilatation. Although such obstructions can result from gonococcal infection, other infections and trauma more commonly explain the occlusion. Bartholin gland cysts account for 2 % of all gynecologic visits per year. Most Bartholin duct cysts are asymptomatic. When symptoms do occur, most patients complain of discomfort during coitus or pain while sitting or walking. The treatment of Bartholin gland cysts has evolved from a complicated, bloody procedure requiring general anesthesia to, most recently, a simple puncture of the cyst and placement of a drain performed in the office. Although treatments for Bartholin gland cysts seem simple on the surface, recurrent cysts as well as differentiating simple cysts from abscesses

or malignancy can complicate treatment for this common problem [15].

3D Endovaginal Ultrasound Appearance of Bartholin Gland Cyst

Sonographic findings of these lesions vary and may include anechoic, hypoechoic, or echogenic texture with variable combinations of this pattern. Usually the anechoic center is surrounded by irregular echogenic layers thought to represent an inflammatory reaction in the adjacent tissue. Occasionally debris and septations may be noted within the anechoic center structure [8]. Internal growth and septations are worrisome for malignancy (Figs. 8.1 and 8.2).

8.2.3 Skene Gland Cyst/Abscess

Paraurethral Skene glands are considered the homologue of the prostate in females [16, 17]. Controversy exists on the function of Skene's glands, their role in sexual function, female orgasm and ejaculation, and even their anatomy. Infection in these glands was described with gonorrheal infection in 1672 by Regnier de Graaf (1641–1693), which was long before Skene described them in 1880. Asymptomatic cysts of the duct or gland are uncommon and when infection occurs can cause pain, dysuria, vaginal

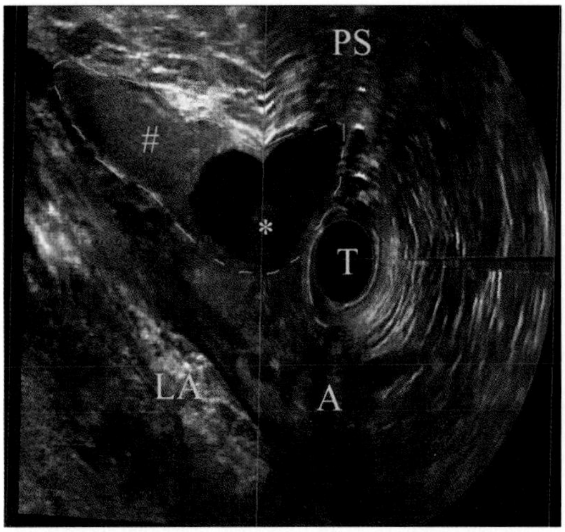

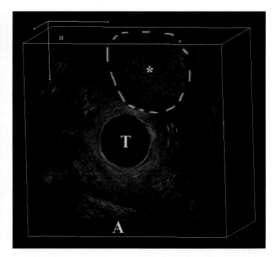

Fig. 8.2 Right Bartholin gland cyst. Axial and sagittal view with 360° endovaginal probe. Internal echo can be seen in cyst. In sagittal view cephalad extension of cyst can be evaluated. *A* anus, *LA* levator ani muscle, *PS* pubic symphysis, *T* transducer, # internal echo of cyst, * Bartholin gland cyst. © Shobeiri

Fig. 8.3 Skene gland mass. Axial view with 360° endovaginal probe. *A* anus, *T* transducer, * Skene gland mass. © Shobeiri

discharge, and dyspareunia. On examination a palpable painful mass is present next to the distal urethra and purulent material can be expressed from the ductal orifice. Skene's abscesses can be distinguished from urethral diverticulum, which is usually more proximal and communicates with the urethra through a diverticular orifice. When doubt exists, imaging with positive pressure urography using a Trattner's catheter, ultrasound, or MRI can be helpful [18].

3D Endovaginal Ultrasound Appearance of Skene Gland Cyst

Skene glands are group of tubular glands that lie on the vaginal surface of the urethra. These paraurethral glands empty into the lumen at several points on the dorsal surface of the urethra; the majority of them are located in the middle to distal urethra, near the 3 o'clock and 9 o'clock positions [19]. Two prominent openings on the inner aspects of the external urethral orifice can be seen when the orifice is open. Obstruction of their terminal duct can result in cyst formation.

They represent smooth margins on ultrasound images. Depending on its contents, the cyst may show no internal echoes or echoes may diffusely line the interior of the cysts (Figs. 8.3 and 8.4).

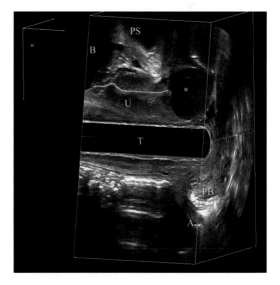

Fig. 8.4 Skene gland cyst. Midsagittal view with 360° endovaginal probe. *A* anus, *B* bladder, *PB* perineal body, *PS* pubic symphysis, *T* transducer, *U* urethra, * Skene gland cyst. © Shobeiri

8.2.4 Urethral Diverticulum

Urethral diverticulum in women may be more common than has been suspected and should be excluded in patients with chronic irritative voiding symptoms, post void dribbling, or dyspareunia. The pathogenesis of this condition is poorly understood, and these lesions represent a spec-

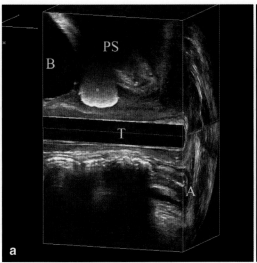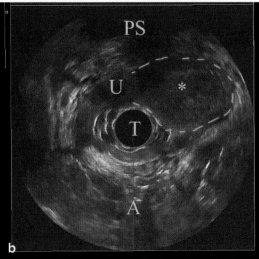

Fig. 8.5 (**a**) Left midsagittal view with 360° endovaginal probe of periurethral bulking agent at vesicourethral junction. *A* anus, *B* bladder, *PS* pubic symphysis, *T* transducer, * periurethral bulking material. © Shobeiri. (**b**) Axial view of a periurethral mass masquerading as a diverticulum. *A* anus, *PS* pubic symphysis, *T* transducer, * left periurethral mass with indistinct borders is outlined. © Shobeiri

trum of disorders ranging from isolated sub urethral cysts to herniation of the urethral lining into the vaginal mucosa. Urethral diverticula usually are small, varying from 3 mm to 3 cm in diameter. Although most diverticula lie posterior to the urethra, they also can be located laterally or anteriorly or even partially or completely surround the urethra (saddle diverticulum). Accurate diagnosis is based on history and clinical evaluation. Perineal ultrasound and MRI have been used for diagnosis. A diverticulum may fill during the voiding phase of urography or cystourethrography, presenting as a well-contained fluid collection adjacent to the urethra. Assessing urethral diverticula by sonography was first introduced by Lee and Keller [20]. Ultrasonography can be used to help differentiate solid from cystic sub urethral masses, to identify stones within diverticula, and to visualize intraluminal masses (e.g., carcinoma, nephrogenic adenoma, mesonephric adenocarcinoma) [21].

3D Endovaginal Ultrasound Appearance of Urethral Diverticulum

The majorities of urethral diverticula are located in the middle third of the urethra and involve the posterolateral wall [22]. Ultrasound shows a relatively echo-free cavity adjacent to the urethra with an orifice that communicates with the urethral lumen; it also may demonstrate inflammatory debris and/or surrounding inflammatory edema. Given that urethral diverticulum is very common, clinical acuity is needed to differentiate it from the other conditions (Figs. 8.5a, b and 8.6).

8.2.5 Gartner Duct Cyst

The distal mesonephric ducts in the female are resorbed but may persist as vestigial remnants in the anterolateral vaginal wall down to the hymen (Gartner's duct cysts) and between the layers of the broad ligament (paraovarian cysts). These cysts are usually small and asymptomatic and have been reported to occur in as many as 1 % of all women [23, 24]. Because the ureteral bud also develops from the Wolffian duct, it is not surprising that Gartner duct cysts have been associated with ureteral and renal abnormalities in addition to associated anomalies of the female genital tract [25–28]. Ultrasonography of the upper and lower urinary tract is a noninvasive useful initial

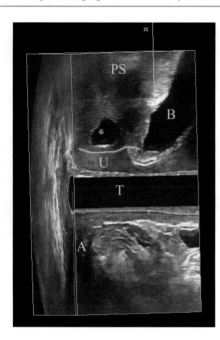

Fig. 8.6 Urethral diverticulum anterior to the urethra seen at midsagittal view with 360° endovaginal probe. This patient's complaint was pain and a palpable mass was not evident by physical examination. *A* anus, *B* bladder, *PS* pubic symphysis, *T* transducer, *U* urethral, * anterior urethral diverticulum. © Shobeiri

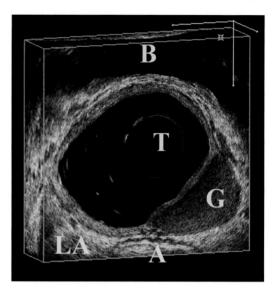

Fig. 8.7 Gartner duct cyst. Axial view with 360° endovaginal probe. *A* anus, *B* bladder, *G* Gartner duct cyst, *LA* levator ani muscle, *T* transducer. © Shobeiri

investigation. The Gartner duct cysts can be elusive and result in varied fistulas, including urethrovaginal fistulas [29].

Gartner duct cysts can have varied clinical presentations and 3D EVUS characteristics.

3D Endovaginal Ultrasound Appearance of Gartner Duct Cyst

Gartner's duct cysts will usually be incidental findings during pelvic ultrasonography. Of developmental origin, they may present anywhere along the lateral aspect of the female genital tract. When the cysts are of paraovarian origin, they will mimic other fluid-filled adnexal masses, and no specific diagnosis can be made. When alongside the vagina or cervix, however, their ultrasonographic appearance is probably characteristic (Figs. 8.7 and 8.8).

8.2.6 Leiomyoma of Vagina

Although uterine fibroids are common uterine benign neoplasms worldwide, and many treatment options exist for them, vaginal fibroid reports

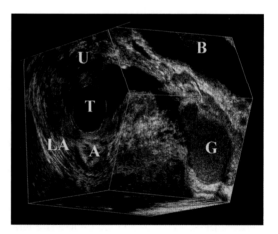

Fig. 8.8 Gartner duct cyst. Axial and sagittal view with 360° endovaginal probe. *A* anus, *B* bladder, *G* Gartner duct cyst, *LA* levator ani muscle, *T* transducer, *U* urethra. © Shobeiri

are scarce in the literature [30]. The boundaries of such mesodermal tumors are difficult to delineate, but most of the tumors are benign. Even recurrence does not signify malignant alteration. Vaginal leiomyoma presenting as a mass is most often diagnosed clinically and removed during surgery. An uncommon presentation may necessitate imaging studies. The lesion described can have MRI and ultrasound features similar to its uterine counterpart.

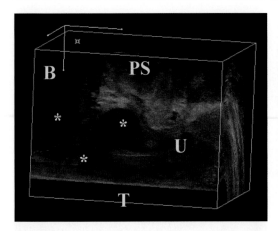

Fig. 8.9 Periurethral and endovesical leiomyoma. Midsagittal view with 180° endovaginal probe. Anterior compartment is visualized in this ultrasound image. *B* bladder, *PS* pubic symphysis, *T* transducer, *U* urethra, * leiomyoma. © Shobeiri

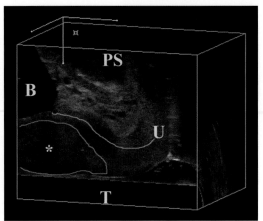

Fig. 8.10 Vaginal cancer. Midsagittal view with 180° endovaginal probe. *B* bladder, *PS* pubic symphysis, *T* transducer, *U* urethra, * vaginal mass. © Shobeiri

3D Endovaginal Ultrasound Appearance of Leiomyoma

Vaginal leiomyoma has variable consistency and can be cystic, semi-cystic, or solid. The ultrasound reveals the heterogeneous echo texture consistent with myomata (Fig. 8.9). The leiomyoma can occur anywhere along the vaginal tract; however the condition is very uncommon.

8.2.7 Malignant Vaginal Masses

Carcinoma of the vagina is uncommon, occurring in less than 2 % of patients with gynecologic malignancies. The most common histologic type of primary vaginal tumor is squamous carcinoma. As with cervical intraepithelial neoplasia and carcinoma, the human papilloma virus is probably responsible for the majority of vaginal carcinomas. Plentl and Friedman [31] found that 51 % of vaginal carcinoma lesions occur in the upper third part of the vagina, 30 % in the lower third, and 19 % in the middle third. In the lower third, lesions most often occur in the anterior wall, whereas in the upper third, lesions most often appear in the posterior vaginal wall. In general, invasive carcinoma of the vagina appears as either as a raised exophytic lesion or an ulcerative, depressed lesion in the vaginal wall. In either case the definitive diagnosis is made by biopsy of the lesion.

3D Endovaginal Ultrasound Appearance of Malignant Vaginal Masses

The early diagnosis of vaginal cancer is made in the course of the routine gynecologic examination. If the tumor has spread to surrounding structures, the predominantly hypoechoic tumor masses may appear as solid, irregularly exophytic nodules. Ultrasound cannot reliably distinguish between inflammatory and carcinomatous infiltration. CT scans are used to assess metastasis to inguinal lymph nodes. Ultrasound may be useful for assessing growth of the tumor into the bladder or the rectum and assessing its vascularity (Fig. 8.10).

8.2.8 Rectovaginal Septum Endometrioma

Rectovaginal endometriosis involves the connective tissue between the anterior rectal wall and the vagina and it often infiltrates both. When endometriosis infiltrates the rectum, it may cause not only pain but also gastrointestinal symptoms including dyschezia, hematochezia, diarrhea, and constipation. Rectovaginal endometriosis is difficult to assess by clinical examination and infiltration of the rectal wall can only be suspected in 40–68 % of the cases. Therefore, imaging techniques are mandatory during the preoperative workup. A rectovaginal septum endometrioma can present as a flat cystic lesion. Their location and size can be varied. Transrectal ultrasonography has a sensitivity and specificity of 97 % and 96 %, respectively, in the diagnosis of the presence of rectovaginal endometriosis. The sonographers can identify infiltration of the rectal and vaginal walls. The sensitivity and specificity in the diagnosis of uterosacral ligament infiltration are 80 % and 97 %, respectively [32].

Ultrasonography is a reliable and simple method for the assessment of rectovaginal endometriosis and provides information on location, extension, and infiltration of the lesions, which are important factors in selecting the appropriate surgical route [33].

Transvaginal ultrasonography combined with water contrast in the rectum is significantly more accurate than transvaginal ultrasound alone in determining the presence of endometriotic infiltration reaching at least the muscular layer of the rectal wall. The sensitivity of water-contrast transvaginal ultrasound in identifying rectal lesions is 97 %, the specificity 100 %, the positive predictive value 100 %, and the negative predictive value 91.3 %. Water-contrast transvaginal ultrasound is associated with a higher intensity of pain than transvaginal ultrasound alone [34].

3D Endovaginal Ultrasound Appearance of Rectovaginal Septum Endometrioma

Endometriotic lesions are detected as irregular hypoechoic structures at the level of the vaginal wall, often infiltrating the surrounding structures. When they infiltrate the rectal wall, fixing the rectal tract during Valsalva maneuver or pressure with the probe, they are interpreted as rectal endometriosis [35] (Fig. 8.11).

8.2.9 Vaginal Seroma and Hematoma

Vaginal hematomas may present as an emergency due to vaginal trauma. Vaginal hematomas and seromas are also a consequence of recently

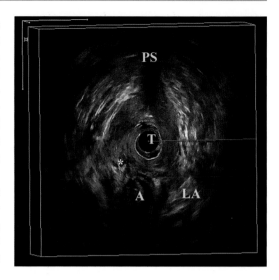

Fig. 8.11 Vaginal endometrioma. Axial view with 360° endovaginal probe. Rectovaginal septum endometrioma can be seen on *right side*. *A* anus, *LA* levator ani muscle, *PS* pubic symphysis, *T* transducer, * endometrioma. © Shobeiri

developed urogynecologic techniques. Seromas are seen in sling procedures [36] and insertion of vaginal grafts [37] and meshes [38]. They can develop in patients after posterior reconstruction with biologic grafts. Although one may criticize that hematomas are not true vaginal masses or cysts, they deserve mention here due to their interesting ultrasonic characteristics.

3D Endovaginal Ultrasound Appearance of Vaginal Seroma and Hematoma

Fluid collection can be seen as hypoechoic area in the area of interest. They can cause vaginal or rectal pressure. Sometimes patients present feeling as if they have recurrent vaginal prolapse. An ultrasound will reassure them that this is not the case. Postpartum hematoma in deep layers of levator ani muscle can be mistaken for levator ani avulsion. Serial ultrasounds can be helpful in evaluating hematomas and seromas. If they are associated with signs of infection or extremely bothersome symptoms, they will require drainage (Figs. 8.12 and 8.13).

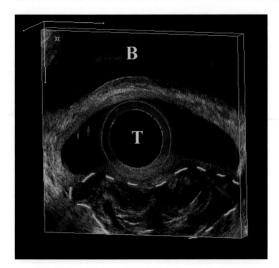

Fig. 8.12 Seroma in posterior vaginal wall around SIS causing rectal pressure and discomfort. Axial view with 360° endovaginal probe. *B* bladder, *T* transducer, *Dotted area* seroma around SIS. © Shobeiri

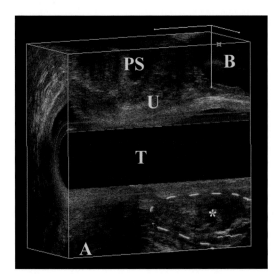

Fig. 8.13 Seroma in posterior vaginal wall around SIS causing rectal pressure and discomfort. Midsagittal view with 360° endovaginal probe. *A* anus, *B* bladder, *PS* pubic symphysis, *T* transducer, *U* urethra, * seroma around SIS. © Shobeiri

8.3 Conclusions and Key Points

3D EVUS may be utilized for the evaluation of vaginal cysts and masses. Although this seems to be a common sense approach to imaging, we have not found reports of this modality in the literature.

If the specialized ultrasound machine and expertise is available, the ease by which 3D EVUS can be performed in a clinical setting provides an opportunity to screen for vaginal masses in patients more quickly than is feasible with a CT scan or an MRI. Since the majority of these masses are in the vaginal side wall, a traditional 2D end-fire transvaginal probe may be less useful unless placed at the vaginal introitus. 3D EVUS can change the diagnosis in patients. This information can change the physicians proposed surgery and the patients' postoperative course expectations.

The reproducibility of 3D EVUS technique has already been published [14]. For those of us engaged in 3D imaging, we know the minor nuances of transducer application, but most of the work is done with the post-processing software that can manipulate the acquired data volume. The operator can quickly judge if the mass is cystic or solid, located next to the labia, urethra, or the rectum. The procedure takes less than 1 min to perform and can be taught proficiently.

The ability to visualize internal characteristics of vaginal cysts and masses is important because it can help us with management decisions. The use of 3D EVUS for visualization of pelvic floor structures has gained popularity [13, 39, 40]. The physicians and the sonographers can use this additional modality for diagnosis of more difficult problems.

References

1. Sherer DM, Abulafia O. Transvaginal ultrasonographic depiction of a Gartner duct cyst. J Ultrasound Med. 2001;20(11):1253–5. Epub 2002/01/05.eng.
2. McCarthy S, Taylor KJ. Sonography of vaginal masses. AJR Am J Roentgenol. 1983;140:1005–8. PubMed PMID: 6601411. English.
3. Kaur A, Makhija PS, Vallikad E, Padmashree V, Indira HS. Multifocal aggressive angiomyxoma: a case report. J Clin Pathol. 2000;53(10):798–9. PubMed PMID: 11064679. Pubmed Central PMCID: Source: NLM. PMC1731092. English.
4. Gerrard ER Jr, Lloyd LK, Kubricht WS, Kolettis PN. Transvaginal ultrasound for the diagnosis of urethral diverticulum. J Urol. 2003;169:1395–7. PubMed PMID: 12629370. English.
5. Romanzi LJ, Groutz A, Blaivas JG. Urethral diverticulum in women: diverse presentations resulting in

diagnostic delay and mismanagement. J Urol. 2000;164:428–33. PubMed PMID: 10893602. English.

6. Shobeiri SA, Rostaminia G, White D, Quiroz LH, Nihira MA. Visualization of vaginal pathologies by 3-Dimensional Endovaginal and Endoanal Ultrasonography: A Pictorial Essay. J Ultrasound Med. 2013;32(8):1499–507. doi: 10.7863/ultra.32.8.1499.

7. Rufford J, Cardozo L. Urethral diverticula: a diagnostic dilemma. BJU Int. 2004;94(7):1044–7. PubMed PMID: 15541125.

8. Abulafia O, Sherer DM. Bartholin gland abscess: sonographic findings. J Clin Ultrasound. 1997;25(1):47–9. PubMed PMID: 9010809. English.

9. Patil S, Sultan AH, Thakar R. Bartholin's cysts and abscesses. J Obstet Gynaecol. 2007;27:241–5. PubMed PMID: 17464802. English.

10. Wang S, Lang JH, Zhou HM. Venous malformations of the female lower genital tract. Eur J Obstet Gynecol Reprod Biol. 2009;145:205–8. PubMed PMID: 19520486. English.

11. Grenader T, Isacson R, Reinus C, Rosengarten O, Barenholz O, Hyman J, et al. Primary amelanotic melanoma of the vagina. Onkologie. 2008;31:474–6. PubMed PMID: 18787356. English.

12. Bujor A, Chen B. Metastatic mantle cell lymphoma presenting as a vaginal mass. A case report. Gynecol Obstet Invest. 2006;62:217–9. PubMed PMID: 16785735. English.

13. Shobeiri SA, Leclaire E, Nihira MA, Quiroz LH, O'Donoghue D. Appearance of the levator ani muscle subdivisions in endovaginal three-dimensional ultrasonography. Obstet Gynecol. 2009;114:66–72. PubMed PMID: 19546760.

14. Santoro GA, Wieczorek AP, Shobeiri SA, Mueller ER, Pilat J, Stankiewicz A, Battistella G. Interobserver and interdisciplinary reproducibility of 3D endovaginal ultrasound assessment of pelvic floor anatomy. Int Urogynecol J Pelvic Floor Dysfunct. 2011; 22:53–9.

15. Marzano DA, Haefner HK. The Bartholin gland cyst: past, present, and future. J Low Genit Tract Dis. 2004;8(3):195–204.

16. Zaviacic M. The adult human female prostata homologue and the male prostate gland: a comparative enzyme-histochemical study. Acta Histochem. 1985;77(1):19–31. Epub 1985/01/01.eng.

17. Zaviacic M, Jakubovska V, Belosovic M, Breza J. Ultrastructure of the normal adult human female prostate gland (Skene's gland). Anat Embryol. 2000; 201(1):51–61. Epub 1999/12/22.eng.

18. Dwyer PL. Skene's gland revisited: function, dysfunction and the G spot. Int Urogynecol J. 2012; 23(2):135–7. Epub 2011/09/09.eng.

19. Aspera AM, Rackley RR, Vasavada SP. Contemporary evaluation and management of the female urethral diverticulum. Urol Clin North Am. 2002;29(3):617–24. Epub 2002/12/13.eng.

20. Lee TG, Keller FS. Urethral diverticulum: diagnosis by ultrasound. AJR Am J Roentgenol. 1977;128(4): 690–1. Epub 1977/04/01.eng.

21. Lee JW, Fynes MM. Female urethral diverticula. Best Pract Res Clin Obstet Gynaecol. 2005;19(6):875–93. Epub 2005/09/27.eng.

22. Hahn WY, Israel GM, Lee VS. MRI of female urethral and periurethral disorders. AJR Am J Roentgenol. 2004;182(3):677–82. Epub 2004/02/21.eng.

23. Lee MJ, Yoder IC, Papanicolaou N, Tung GA. Large Gartner duct cyst associated with a solitary crossed ectopic kidney: imaging features. J Comput Assist Tomogr. 1991;15(1):149–51. Epub 1991/01/01.eng.

24. Scheible FW. Ultrasonic features of Gartner's duct cyst. J Clin Ultrasound. 1978;6(6):438–9. Epub 1978/12/01.eng.

25. Li YW, Sheih CP, Chen WJ. MR imaging and sonography of Gartner's duct cyst and single ectopic ureter with ipsilateral renal dysplasia. Pediatr Radiol. 1992;22(6):472–3. Epub 1992/01/01.eng.

26. Li YW, Sheih CP, Chen WJ. Unilateral occlusion of duplicated uterus with ipsilateral renal anomaly in young girls: a study with MRI. Pediatr Radiol. 1995;25 Suppl 1:S54–9. Epub 1995/11/01.eng.

27. Sheih CP, Li YW, Liao YJ, Chiang CD. Small ureterocele-like Gartner's duct cyst associated with ipsilateral renal dysgenesis: report of two cases. J Clin Ultrasound. 1996;24(9):533–5. Epub 1996/11/01.eng.

28. Rosenfeld DL, Lis E. Gartner's duct cyst with a single vaginal ectopic ureter and associated renal dysplasia or agenesis. J Ultrasound Med. 1993;12(12):775–8. Epub 1993/12/01.eng.

29. Dwyer PL, Rosamilia A. Congenital urogenital anomalies that are associated with the persistence of Gartner's duct: a review. Am J Obstet Gynecol. 2006;195(2):354–9. PubMed PMID: 16890546. Epub 2006/08/08.eng.

30. Ren X-L, Zhou X-D, Zhang J, He G-B, Han Z-H, Zheng M-J, et al. Extracorporeal ablation of uterine fibroids with high-intensity focused ultrasound. J Ultrasound Med. 2007;26:201–12.

31. Plentl AA, Friedman EA. Lymphatic system of the female genitalia. The morphologic basis of oncologic diagnosis and therapy. Major Probl Obstet Gynecol. 1971;2:1–223. Epub 1971/01/01.eng.

32. Fedele L, Bianchi S, Portuese A, Borruto F, Dorta M. Transrectal ultrasonography in the assessment of rectovaginal endometriosis. Obstet Gynecol. 1998; 91(3):444–8.

33. Dessole S, Farina M, Rubattu G, Cosmi E, Ambrosini G, Nardelli NB. Sonovaginography is a new technique for assessing rectovaginal endometriosis. Fertil Steril. 2003;79(4):1023–7.

34. Valenzano Menada M, Remorgida V, Abbamonte LH, Nicoletti A, Ragni N, Ferrero S. Does transvaginal ultrasonography combined with water-contrast in the rectum aid in the diagnosis of rectovaginal endometriosis infiltrating the bowel? Hum Reprod. 2008;23(5):1069–75. PubMed PMID: 18310049. Epub 2008/03/04.eng.

35. Saccardi C, Cosmi E, Borghero A, Tregnaghi A, Dessole S, Litta P. Comparison between transvaginal sonography, saline contrast sonovaginography and magnetic resonance imaging in the diagnosis of posterior

deep infiltrating endometriosis. Ultrasound Obstet Gynecol. 2012;40(4):464–9. Epub 2012/01/19.eng.

36. Kuuva N, Nilsson CG. A nationwide analysis of complications associated with the tension-free vaginal tape (TVT) procedure. Acta Obstet Gynecol Scand. 2002;81:72–7.

37. Konstantinovic ML, Ozog Y, Spelzini F, Pottier C, De Ridder D, Deprest J. Biomechanical findings in rats undergoing fascial reconstruction with graft materials suggested as an alternative to polypropylene. Neurourol Urodyn. 2010;29(3):488–93. PubMed PMID: 19618448. Epub 2009/07/21.eng.

38. Zimmerman CW, Theobald P, Braun NM. Exposure and erosion of vaginal meshes: etiology and treatment. London: Springer; 2011. p. 217–30.

39. Santoro G, Wieczorek A, Shobeiri S, Mueller E, Pilat J, Stankiewicz A, et al. Interobserver and interdisciplinary reproducibility of 3D endovaginal ultrasound assessment of pelvic floor anatomy. Int Urogynecol J. 2010;22:53–9.

40. Quiroz LH, Shobeiri SA, Nihira MA. Three-dimensional ultrasound imaging for diagnosis of urethrovaginal fistula. Int Urogynecol J. 2010;21:1031–3. PubMed PMID: 20069418.

Three-Dimensional Endoanal Ultrasonography of the Anorectal Region

9

Giulio A. Santoro and Sthela Murad-Regadas

Learning Objectvies
1. To understand the 3D-ultrasonography technique
2. To understand the normal 3D-endosonographic anatomy of the anorectal region
3. To understand the application of 3D-ultrasonography in the assessment of posterior compartment disorders

9.1   Introduction

Anorectal diseases require imaging for proper case management. At present, endoanal ultrasonography (EAUS) and endorectal ultrasonography (ERUS) have become important parts of diagnostic workup of patients with posterior compartment disorders (fecal incontinence, obstructed defecation, posterior vaginal wall prolapse, perianal fistulas, pelvic floor dyssynergy, and perianal pain)

and provide sufficient information for clinical decision-making in many cases [1–3]. However, with the currently available ultrasonographic equipment and techniques, a good deal of relevant information may remain hidden. The advent of high-resolution three-dimensional (3D) endoluminal ultrasound, constructed from a synthesis of standard two-dimensional cross-sectional images, promises to revolutionize diagnosis of anorectal disorders [4]. The anatomic structures in the pelvis, the axial and longitudinal extension of anal sphincter defects, the anatomy of the fistulous tract in complex perianal sepsis, and the presence of anterior rectal wall prolapse may be imaged in greater detail. This additional information will bring an improvement for both planning and conduct of surgical procedures [5].

This chapter is devoted to discussing the methods for generating and using the 3D-EAUS and 3D-ERUS particularly with regard to the advantages of these techniques in the diagnostic imaging of posterior compartment disorders.

G.A. Santoro, M.D., Ph.D. (✉)
Head Pelvic Floor Unit, 3rd Division of Surgery,
Regional Hospital, Piazzale Ospedale 1, 31100
Treviso, Italy
e-mail: giulioasantoro@yahoo.com

S. Murad-Regadas
Department of Surgery, School of Medicine of the
Federal University of Ceará, Fortaleza, Ceará, Brazil

Head Pelvic Floor Unit, Clinical Hospital, Federal
University of Ceará, Fortaleza, Ceará, Brazil

9.2   Ultrasonographic Techniques

Endoanal US may be performed with a high-multifrequency (9–16 MHz), 360° rotational mechanical probe (type 2050, B-K Medical, Herlev, Denmark) (Fig. 9.1) or a radial electronic probe (type AR 54 AW, frequency: 5–10 MHz, Hitachi Medical Systems, Japan) [1]. The difference

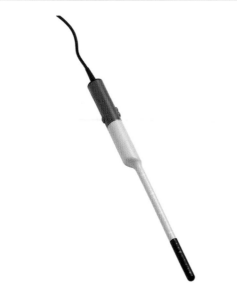

Fig. 9.1 High-multifrequency (9-16MHz), 360° rotational mechanical probe (type 2050, BK Medical, Herlev, Denmark

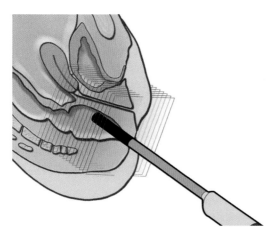

Fig. 9.2 Schematic illustration of the technique of three-dimensional endoanal ultrasonography performed by 2050 transducer (B-K Medical)

between these two transducers is that the 3D acquisition is freehand with the electronic transducer, whereas the mechanical transducer has an internal automated motorized system that allows an acquisition of 300 aligned transaxial 2D images over a distance of 60 mm in 60 s, without any movement of the probe within the tissue. The set of 2D images is instantaneously reconstructed into a high-resolution 3D image for real-time manipulation and volume rendering (Fig. 9.2). The 3D volume can also be archived for offline

analysis on the ultrasonographic system or on PC with the help of dedicated software [5].

Before the probe is inserted into the anus, a digital rectal examination should be performed. If there is an anal stenosis, the finger can check to determine whether it will allow easy passage of the probe. A gel containing condom is placed over the probe, and a thin layer of water-soluble lubricant is placed on the exterior of the condom. Any air interface will cause a major interference pattern. The patient should be instructed before the examination that no pain should be experienced. Under no circumstances should force be used to advance the probe. During examination, the patient may be placed in the dorsal lithotomy, in the left lateral or in the prone position. However, irrespective of the position, the transducer should be rotated so that the anterior aspect of the anal canal is superior (12 o'clock) on the screen, right lateral is left (9 o'clock), left lateral is right (3 o'clock), and posterior is inferior (6 o'clock). The length of recorded data should extend from the upper aspect of the "U"-shaped sling of the puborectalis (PR) to the anal verge.

9.3 Endosonographic Anatomy of the Normal Anal Canal

On ultrasound five hypoechoic and hyperechoic layers can be seen in the normal anal canal [6]. The ultrasonographer must have a clear understanding of what each of these five lines represent anatomically (Fig. 9.3):

1. The first hyperechoic layer, from inner to outer, corresponds to the interface of the transducer with the anal mucosal surface.
2. The second layer represents the subepithelial tissues and appears moderately reflective. The mucosa as well the level of dentate line is not visualized. The muscularis submucosae ani can be sonographically identified in the upper part of the anal canal as a low reflective band.
3. The third hypoechoic layer corresponds to the internal anal sphincter (IAS). The sphincter is not completely symmetric, either in thickness or termination. It can be traced superiorly into the circular muscle of the rectum, extending

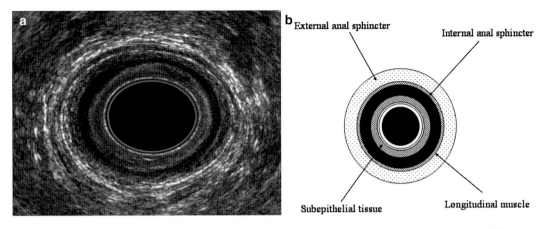

Fig. 9.3 (**a**) Normal ultrasonographic five-layer structure of the mid-anal canal. Axial image obtained by 2050 transducer (B-K Medical); (**b**) schematic representation

from the anorectal junction to approximately 1 cm below the dentate line. In older age groups, the IAS loses its uniform low echogenicity, which is characteristic of smooth muscle throughout the gut, to become more echogenic and inhomogeneous in texture.

4. The fourth hyperechoic layer represents the longitudinal muscle (LM). It presents a wide variability in thickness and not always is distinctly visible along the entire anal canal. The LM appears moderately echogenic, which is surprising as it is mainly smooth muscle; however, an increased fibrous stroma may account for this. In the intersphincteric space, the LM conjoins with striated muscular fibers from the levator ani, particularly the puboanalis, and a large fibroelastic element derived from the endopelvic fascia to form the "conjoined longitudinal layer" (CLL) (Fig. 9.4). Its fibroelastic component, permeating through the subcutaneous part of the external anal sphincter (EAS), terminates in the perianal skin.

5. The fifth mixed echogenic layer corresponds to the EAS. The EAS is made up of voluntary muscle that encompasses the anal canal. It is described as having three parts: (1) the deep part is integral with the PR. Posteriorly there is some ligamentous attachment. Anteriorly some fibers are circular and some decussate into the deep transverse perinei; (2) the superficial part has a very broad attachment to the underside of the coccyx via the anococcygeal

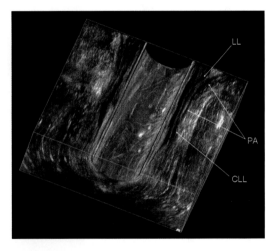

Fig. 9.4 Coronal image of the anal canal from three-dimensional reconstruction obtained by 2050 transducer (B-K Medical). The puboanalis (PA) joins the longitudinal muscle layer (LL) of the rectum to form the conjoined longitudinal layer (CLL)

ligament. Anteriorly there is a division into circular fibers and a decussation to the superficial transverse perinei; (3) the subcutaneous part lies below the IAS.

Ultrasound imaging of the anal canal can be divided into three levels of assessment in the axial plane (upper, middle, and lower levels) referring to the following anatomical structures (Fig. 9.5) [6]:

1. Upper level: the sling of the puborectalis (PR), the deep part of the EAS, and the complete ring of IAS

Fig. 9.5 (a) Three levels of assessment of the anal canal in the axial plane. Scan obtained by 2050 transducer (B-K Medical). *EAS* external anal sphincter, *IAS* internal anal sphincter, *PR* puborectalis; (**b**) three-dimensional reconstruction on the coronal plane

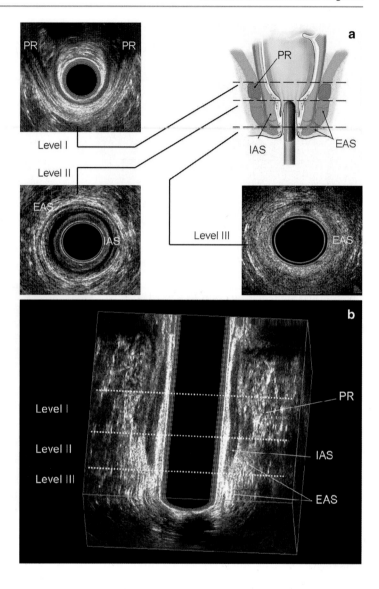

2. Middle level: the superficial part of the EAS (complete ring), the CLL, the IAS (complete ring), and the transverse perinei muscles
3. Lower level: the subcutaneous part of the EAS

The anal canal length is the distance measured between the proximal canal, where the PR is identified, and the lower border of the subcutaneous EAS. It is significantly longer in male than in female, as a result of a longer EAS, whereas there is no difference in PR length. The anterior part of the EAS differs between genders and anatomic studies showed that this difference is already present in fetal age. In males, the EAS is symmetrical at all levels; in females, it is shorter ante-

riorly, and there is no evidence of anterior ring high in the canal. In examining a female subject, the ultrasonographic differences between the natural gaps (hypoechoic areas with smooth, regular edges) and sphincter ruptures (mixed echogenicity, due to scarring, with irregular edges) occurring at the upper anterior part of the anal canal must be kept in mind. Three-dimensional longitudinal images are particularly useful to assess these anatomic characteristics of the EAS (Fig. 9.6) [7–10]. Williams et al. [7] reported that the anterior EAS occupied 58 % of the male anal canal compared with 38 % of the female canal ($P<0.01$). In female the PR occupied a significantly

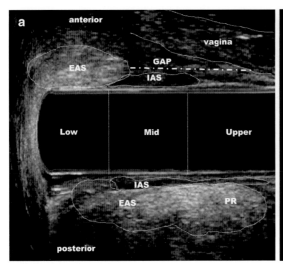
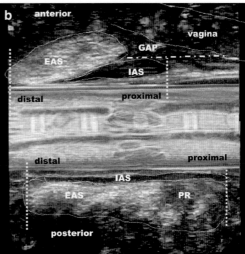

Fig. 9.6 (**a**) Female anal canal anatomic configuration. Three-dimensional reconstruction on the sagittal plane shows the asymmetrical shape of the anal canal and the positions of anal sphincters. The anterior anal canal (EAS and IAS) starts and ends more distally and the posterior anal canal (PR-EAS and IAS starts) starts and ends more proximally. *EAS* external anal sphincter, *IAS* internal anal sphincter, *PR* puborectalis muscle, *GAP* the area in the anterior quadrant without striated muscle, measured from the proximal edge of the posterior PR to the proximal edge of the anterior EAS; (**b**) render mode

larger proportion of the canal than in male (61 % vs. 45 %; $P=0.02$). There was no difference in the length of the IAS between male and female (34.4 vs. 33.2 mm) or the proportion of the anal canal that it occupied (67 % vs. 73 %; $P=0.12$).

Normal values for sphincter dimensions differ between techniques [6]. The importance to define the true values of sphincter muscle thickness is not very relevant, because the purpose of measuring anal sphincters is to distinguish a normal vs. abnormal measurement, regardless of the absolute values. Measurement should be taken at the 3, 6, 9, and 12 o'clock positions in the midlevel of the anal canal. The thickness of IAS varies from 1.8 ± 0.5 mm and increases with age owing the presence of more fibrous tissue as the absolute amount of muscle decreases, measuring 2.4–2.7 mm <55 years and 2.8–3.5 mm >55 years. Any IAS >4 mm thick should be considered abnormal whatever the patient's age; conversely a sphincter of 2 mm is normal in a young patient, but abnormal in an elderly one. The LM is 2.5 ± 0.6 mm in males and 2.9 ± 0.6 mm in females. The average thickness of the EAS is 8.6 ± 1.1 mm in males and 7.7 ± 1.1 mm in females. However, endosonography largely overestimates the size of the EAS due to its failure to recognize and separate

the LM. Frudinger et al. [11] reported a significant negative correlation of the EAS thickness with the patient's age at all anal canal levels. In particular, the anterior EAS part was found significantly thinner in older subjects.

Multiplanar EAUS has enabled detailed longitudinal measurement of the components of the anal canal (Figs. 9.6 and 9.7). Williams et al. [7] reported that the anterior EAS was significantly longer in men than women (30.1 vs. 16.9 mm; $P<0.001$). There was no difference in the length of the PR between men and women, indicating that the gender difference in anal canal length is solely due to the longer male EAS. The IAS did not differ in length between males and females. Regadas et al. [8] demonstrated the asymmetrical shape of the anal canal and also confirmed that the anterior EAS was significantly shorter in female. West et al. [12] reported similar results, with IAS and EAS volumes found larger in males than in females.

Regardless of the absolute values of the anal sphincter, the most relevant utility of EAUS applies in the detection of localized sphincter defects, where its benefit has been proved [13, 14]. It has been suggested that measuring sphincter thickness is important when EAUS cannot

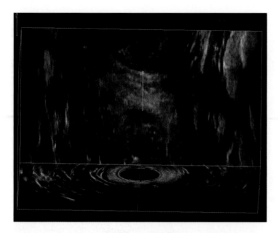

Fig. 9.7 Three-dimensional endoanal ultrasonography performed by 2050 transducer (B-K Medical). Measurement of the anterior length of the external sphincter in the coronal plane

depict any sphincter damage to exclude diffuse structural sphincter changes associated with idiopathic fecal incontinence, passive fecal incontinence, or obstructive defecation disorders. A postulated association between manometric function of the sphincters and their sonographic appearance, however, remained controversial in the literature. Some authors have found no correlation between muscle thickness and muscle performance, neither resting nor squeeze pressure. Scanning anal sphincter muscle may allow for determination of their integrity, but not for their morphometric properties.

9.4 Endosonographic Anatomy of the Rectum

The normal rectum is 11–15 cm long and has a maximum diameter of 4 cm. It is continuous with the sigmoid colon superiorly at the level of the third sacral segment and courses inferiorly along the curve of the sacrum to pass through the pelvic diaphragm and become the anal canal. It is surrounded by fibrofatty tissue that contains blood vessels, nerves, lymphatics, and small lymph nodes. The superior one-third is covered anteriorly and laterally by the pelvic peritoneum. The mid-dle one-third is only covered with peritoneum anteriorly, where it curves anteriorly onto the bladder in the male and onto the uterus in the female. The lower one-third of the rectum is below the peritoneal reflection and is related anteriorly to the bladder base, ureters, seminal vesicles, and prostate in the male and to the lower uterus, cervix, and vagina in the female.

The rectal wall consists of five layers surrounded by perirectal fat or serosa [15]. On ultrasound the normal rectal wall is 2–3 mm thick and is composed of a five-layer structure. Good visualization depends on maintaining the probe in the center lumen of the rectum and having adequate distension of a water-filled latex balloon covering the transducer to achieve good acoustic contact with the rectal wall. It is important to eliminate all bubbles within the balloon to avoid artifacts that limit the overall utility of the study. The rectum can be of varying diameters and therefore the volume of water in the balloon may have to be adjusted intermittently. The five layers represent (Fig. 9.8):

1. The first hyperechoic layer: the interface of the balloon with the rectal mucosal surface
2. The second hypoechoic layer: the mucosa and muscularis mucosae
3. The third hyperechoic layer: the submucosa
4. The fourth hypoechoic layer: the muscularis propria (in rare cases seen as two layers: inner circular and outer longitudinal layer)
5. The fifth hyperechoic layer: the serosa or the interface with the fibrofatty tissue surrounding the rectum (mesorectum). The mesorectum contains blood vessels, nerves, and lymphatics and has an inhomogeneous echo pattern. Very small, round to oval, hypoechoic lymph nodes should be distinguished from blood vessels which also appear as circular hypoechoic structures.

Endorectal US allows an accurate visualization of all pelvic organs adjacent to the rectum: the bladder, seminal vesicles, and prostate in male and the uterus, cervix, vagina, and urethra in female. Intestinal loops can also easily identified as elongate structures.

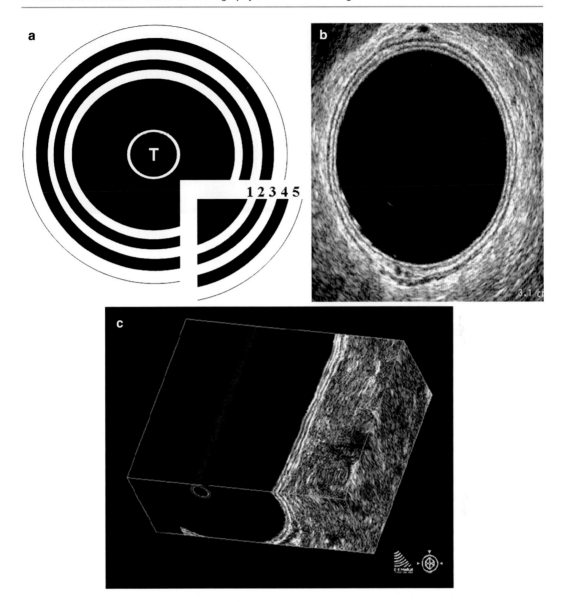

Fig. 9.8 (**a**) Schematic ultrasound representation of the rectal wall (*T* transducer); (**b**) the five layers in the axial plane correspond to (1) acoustic interface with mucosal surfaces, (2) mucosa, (3) submucosa, (4) muscularis pro- pria, and (5) serosa/perirectal fat interface; (**c**) three-dimensional reconstruction of the rectal wall in the coronal plane. Scans obtained by 2050 transducer (B-K Medical)

9.5 Clinical Application of 3D Endoanal/Endorectal Ultrasound

Clinical applications of pelvic floor ultrasonography [1] for both anatomical assessment and evaluation of function of posterior compartment disorders are reported in detail below.

9.5.1 Fecal Incontinence

Fecal incontinence (FI) is defined as the involuntary loss of feces (liquid or solid stool) and anal incontinence is defined as the complaint of involuntary loss of flatus or feces [13]. A meta-analysis revealed a rate of 11–15 % in the general population, although it may perhaps be underestimated [16].

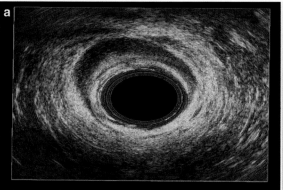 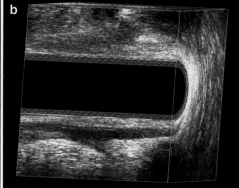

Fig. 9.9 (**a**) Internal anal sphincter lesion between 3 o'clock and 9 o'clock position following a left lateral internal sphincterotomy for fissure. (**b**) Anterior internal anal sphincter damage demonstrated with three-dimensional reconstruction in the sagittal plane. Scans obtained by 2050 transducer (B-K Medical)

Intact musculature including the PR, IAS, and EAS are prerequisites for fecal control, as is a functioning nerve supply to these muscles. Other factors contributing to FI include stool consistency, rectal sensitivity and capacity, and the anorectal angle (ARA). Any impairment to one or more of these factors may result in FI. Anal sphincter defects and pudendal nerve injury can occur during vaginal delivery and are by far the most common causes of FI, consequently making this problem more prevalent in women [16].

In patients with FI, therefore, it is fundamental to establish the underlying pathophysiology in order to choose the appropriate therapy (dietary or medications, biofeedback, sphincter repair, artificial bowel sphincter, graciloplasty, sacral nerve stimulation, injection of bulking agents). EAUS has become the gold standard for the morphological assessment of the anal canal [13, 14]. It can differentiate between incontinent patients with intact anal sphincters and those with sphincter lesions (defects, scarring, thinning, thickening, and atrophy). Tears are defined by an interruption of the circumferential fibrillar echo texture. Scarring is characterized by loss of normal architecture, with an area of amorphous texture that usually has low reflectivity. The operator should identify if there is a combined lesion of the IAS and EAS or if the lesion involves just one muscle. The number, circumferential (radial angle in degrees or in hours of the clock site), and

longitudinal (proximal, distal, or full length) extension of the defect should be also reported. In addition, 3D EAUS allows to measure length, thickness, area of sphincter defect in the sagittal and coronal planes, and volume of sphincter damage (Figs. 9.9, 9.10, 9.11, and 9.12) [5].

Using multiplanar EAUS, two scoring systems have been proposed to define the severity of the sphincter damage. Starck et al. [17] introduced a specific score, with 0 indicating no defect and 16 corresponding to a defect >180° involving the whole length and depth of the sphincters. Recently, Norderval et al. [18] reported a simplified system for analyzing defects, including fewer categories than the Starck score and not recording partial defects of the IAS. A maximal score of 7 denotes defects in both the EAS and the IAS exceeding 90° in the axial plane and involving more than half of the sphincter length. Both systems showed good intraobserver and interobserver agreement in classifying anal sphincter defects.

The presence of a sphincter defect, however, does not necessarily mean that it is the cause of FI, as many people have sphincter lesions without having symptoms of incontinence [19]. On the other hand, patients with FI and an apparent intact sphincter can have muscle degeneration, atrophy, or pudendal neuropathy. EAUS has an important role in detecting clinically occult anal sphincter injuries after a vaginal delivery [20].

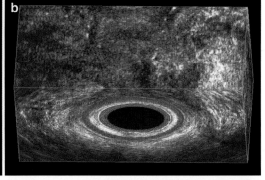

Fig. 9.10 (**a**) External sphincter lesion between 9 o'clock and 1 o'clock position due to obstetric trauma. (**b**) Anterior external anal sphincter damage demonstrated with three-dimensional reconstruction in the coronal plane. Scans obtained by 2050 transducer (B-K Medical)

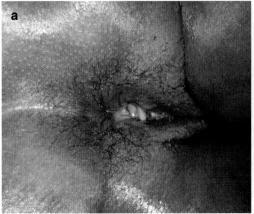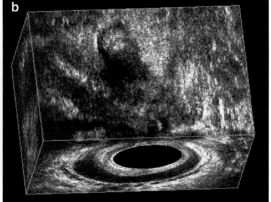

Fig. 9.11 (**a**) Fourth-degree anal sphincter lesion due to obstetric trauma. (**b**) Three-dimensional reconstruction demonstrates the combined anterior damage of the inter- nal and external anal sphincters in the coronal and axial planes. Scans obtained by 2050 transducer (B-K Medical)

In a meta-analysis of 717 vaginal deliveries, Oberwalder et al. [21] found an incidence of occult sphincter damage of 26.9 % among a sample of 462 primiparous women and a rate of 8.5 % new defects in the group of 255 multiparas. In one-third of these (29.7 %), postpartum sphincter damage was symptomatic. As shown in this meta-analysis, the probability that postpartum FI will be associated with anal sphincter defect is 77–83 %. This analysis included five studies where EAUS was the only imaging technique used. In another study, Oberwalder et al. [22] reported that FI related to sphincter lesions is likely to occur even in an elderly population of women who experienced vaginal deliveries earlier in life. They found that 71 % of women with late-onset FI (median age 61.5 years) had occult sphincter defects on EAUS.

Ultrasonographic imaging is useful to evaluate the result of treatments. Starck et al. [23] reported that the extent of endosonographic EAS defects after primary repair of obstetric sphincter tears increased over time and was related to FI. Scheer et al. [24] have demonstrated the value of EAUS and manometry in counselling women who previously sustained obstetric tears. Based on specific selection criteria, the majority of women delivered vaginally without deterioration in anal sphincter morphology and function or quality of life. Savoye-Collet et al. [25] noted improvement in FI in 86 % of patients in whom EAUS documented closure of the EAS defect

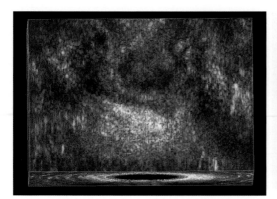

Fig. 9.12 External anal sphincter atrophy. Three-dimensional reconstruction in the coronal plane demonstrates a short anterior length (6.6 mm) of the external sphincter. Scans obtained by 2050 transducer (B-K Medical)

after anterior sphincter repair. In contrast, patients who had a persistent defect in the EAS still had significant FI. Dobben et al. [26] also found that patients with a persistent ultrasonographic EAS defect had a worse clinical outcome than those without an EAS defect.

Using 3D-EAUS, de la Portilla et al. [27] demonstrated that all the implants of silicone to treat FI were properly located in the intersphincteric space 3 months after injection. At 24 months, 75 % of implants were still properly located. They found that the continence deterioration suffered by most patients after the first year from the injection was not related to the localization and number of implants the patient had (Fig. 9.13).

9.5.2 Obstructed Defecation and Posterior Vaginal Wall Prolapse

Anorectal outlet obstruction, also known as obstruction defecation syndrome (ODS), is a pathological condition due to a variety of causes and is characterized by an impaired expulsion of the bolus after calling to defecate [13]. Patients complain of different symptoms, including incomplete evacuation with or without painful effort, unsuccessful attempts with long periods spent in bathroom, return visit to the toilette, use of perineal support, manual assistance (insertion of finger into the vagina or anal canal), straining,

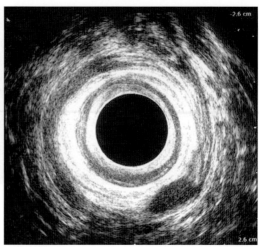

Fig. 9.13 Failure after bulking agent injection. Postoperative assessment with endoanal ultrasound demonstrated that the agent was positioned outside the external sphincter and not in the intersphincteric space. Scans obtained by 2050 transducer (B-K Medical)

and dependence on enema and/or laxatives. Other symptoms are pain at defecation; extreme straining to defecate; extended time at the toilet; perineal pain/discomfort when standing; feeling of incomplete evacuation; fragmented defecation; vaginal, perineal, or rectal digitation; use of laxatives or enemas; and fecal incontinence [13]. These symptoms often lead to a poor quality of life. Prevalence of the entire spectrum of constipation, of which ODS is part, accounts for 14.7 % in the US adult population while the true prevalence of ODS among the population is not known even if the feeling is that it is underestimated.

After ruling out pelvic and rectal tumor, the main distinction in the pathogenesis of ODS is between functional and mechanical causes. Failure to release the anal sphincters or paradoxical contraction of the PR muscle are considered the main and most frequent functional causes of ODS. In these patients, biofeedback can achieve reactivation of the inhibitory capacity of all pelvic floor muscles involved in defecation, with an improvement in symptoms of 50 %. The most relevant mechanical causes of ODS are rectocele, rectal intussusception, enterocele, genital prolapse, and descending perineum. It is fundamental to distinguish between rectal causes (rectocele and intussusception) and extrarectal causes (enterocele, genital prolapse, and descending perineum).

In recent years, alternatives to defecography, such as dynamic MRI and dynamic ultrasonography, have been developed for the evaluation of pelvic floor dysfunctions, with good correlation and the advantage of showing the entire pelvis [28–38]. Studies using dynamic ultrasound with different types of transducers (convex, endfire, biplanar probes) and different techniques (translabial, transperineal, introital ultrasound) have produced findings consistent with defecography to assess patients with ODS [31–38]. Murad-Regadas et al. [35–38] developed echodefecography, a 3D dynamic anorectal ultrasonography technique using a 360° transducer, automatic scanning, and high frequencies for high-resolution images to evaluate evacuation disorders affecting the posterior compartment (rectocele, intussusception, anismus) and the middle compartment (grade II or III sigmoidocele/enterocele). The standardization of the technique, parameters, and values of echodefecography makes the method reproducible [36–38]. Echodefecography was shown to correlate well with conventional defecography and was validated in a prospective multicenter study [36–38].

Echodefecography is performed with a 3D ultrasound device (Pro-Focus, endoprobe model 2052, B-K Medical®, Herlev, Denmark) with proximal-to-distal 6.0 cm automatic scans. By moving two crystals on the extremity of the transducer, axial and longitudinal images were merged into a single cube image, recorded and analyzed in multiple planes.

Following rectal enema, patients are examined in the left lateral position. Images are acquired by four automatic scans and analyzed in the axial, sagittal, and, if necessary, in the oblique plane. The result of the exam depends on the degree of cooperation obtained from the patient: scans 1, 2, and 4 use a slice width of 0.25 mm and last 50 s each; scan 3 lasts 30 s with a slice width of 0.35 mm:

Scan 1 (at rest position without gel): the transducer is positioned at 5.0–6.0 cm from the anal margin. It is performed to visualize the anatomic integrity of the anal sphincter musculature and to evaluate the position of the PR muscles and the EAS at rest. The angle

formed between a line traced along the internal border of the EAS/PR muscles (1.5 cm) and a line traced perpendicular to the axis of the anal canal is measured.

Scan 2 (at rest-straining-at rest without gel): the transducer is positioned at 6.0 cm from the anal verge. The patient is requested to rest during the first 15 s, strain maximally for 20 s, and then relax again, with the transducer following the movement. The purpose of the scan is to evaluate the movement of the PR and the EAS during straining, identifying normal relaxation, non-relaxation, or paradoxical contraction (anismus). The resulting EAS/PR muscle positions (represented by the angle size) are compared between scans 1 and 2. Normal relaxation is recorded if the angle increased by a minimum of 1°, whereas paradoxical contraction (anismus) is recorded if the angle decreased by a minimum of 1°. Non-relaxation is recorded if the angle changed less than 1° (Figs. 9.14 and 9.15).

Scan 3: the transducer is positioned proximally to the PR (anorectal junction). The scan started with the patient at rest (3.0 s), followed by maximum straining with the transducer in fixed position (the transducer does not follow the descending muscles of the pelvic floor). When the PR became visible distally, the scan is stopped. Perineal descent is quantified by measuring the distance between the position of the proximal border of the PR at rest and the point to which it had been displaced by maximum straining (PR descent). Straining time is directly proportional to the distance of perineal descent (Fig. 9.16). Even with patients in the lateral position, the displacement of the PR is easily visualized and quantified. On echodefecography, normal perineal descent during straining was defined as a difference in PR position of ≤2.5 cm and perineal descent >2.5 cm. The normal range values were established by comparing echodefecography findings with defecography

Scan 4: following injection of 120–180 mL ultrasound gel into the rectal ampulla, the transducer is positioned at 7.0 cm from the anal verge. The scanning sequence is the same as in Scan 2 (at

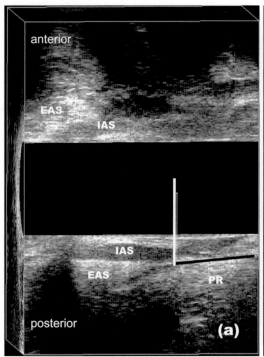

Fig. 9.14 (a) Angle measured at rest position in the sagittal plane (*lines*); (b) increased angle (normal relaxation) during straining (*lines*). *EAS* external anal sphincter, *IAS* internal anal sphincter, *PR* puborectalis. Scans obtained by 2050 transducer (B-K Medical)

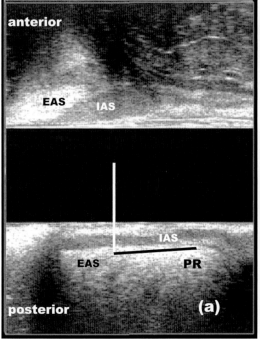

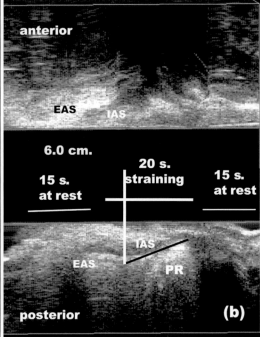

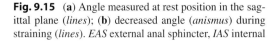

Fig. 9.15 (a) Angle measured at rest position in the sagittal plane (*lines*); (b) decreased angle (*anismus*) during straining (*lines*). *EAS* external anal sphincter, *IAS* internal anal sphincter, *PR* puborectalis. Scans obtained by 2050 transducer (B-K Medical)

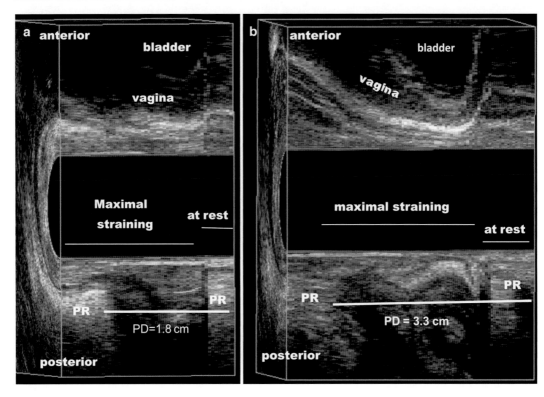

Fig. 9.16 Puborectal descent (PD) measured in the sagittal plane. (**a**) Normal perineal descent ≤2.5 cm; (**b**) pathologic perineal descent >2.5 cm. *PR* puborectalis. Scans obtained by 2050 transducer (B-K Medical)

rest, 15 s; strain maximally, 20 s; then relax again, with the transducer following the movement). The purpose of the scan is to visualize and quantify all anatomical structures and functional changes associated with voiding (rectocele, intussusception, grade II or III sigmoidocele/enterocele). In normal patients, the posterior vaginal wall displaces the lower rectum and upper anal canal inferiorly and posteriorly but maintains a straight horizontal position during defecatory effort. If rectocele is identified, it is classified as grade I (<6.0 mm), grade II (6.0–13.0 mm), or grade III (>13.0 mm) (Fig. 9.17). Measurements are calculated by first drawing two parallel horizontal lines along the posterior vaginal wall, with one line placed in the initial straining position and the other line drawn at the point of maximal straining. The distance between the two vaginal wall positions determined the size of the rectocele.

Intussusception is clearly identified by observing the rectal wall layers protruding through the rectal lumen. No classification is used to quantify intussusceptions (Fig. 9.18). Grade II or III sigmoidocele/enterocele is recognized when the bowel is positioned below the pubococcygeal line (on the projection of the lower rectum and upper anal canal).

Dynamic ultrasound scanning is a helpful tool in the evaluation of patients with obstructed defecation as it clearly shows the anatomical structures and mechanisms involved in defecation. It also demonstrates the anal canal anatomical integrity and is able to detect sphincter injury with high spatial resolution. In addition, the cube image acquired during the automatic scan is recorded in real time for subsequent analysis as may be necessary in many cases. It is quick, inexpensive, and well tolerated by patients without exposure to radiation.

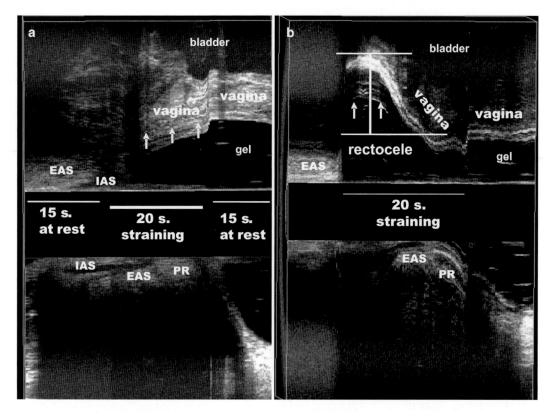

Fig. 9.17 (**a**) Patient without rectocele (*arrows*). Sagittal plane. Using gel in the rectum; (**b**) grade III rectocele (*arrows*). *EAS* external anal sphincter, *IAS* internal anal sphincter, *PR* puborectalis. Scans obtained by 2050 transducer (B-K Medical)

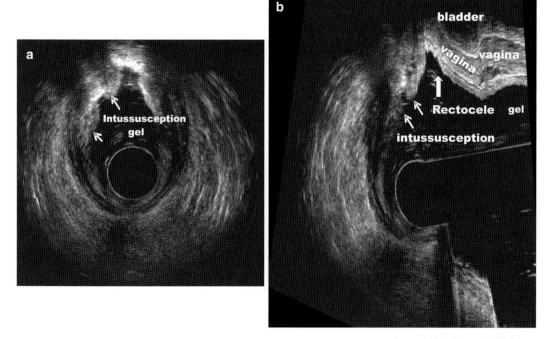

Fig. 9.18 (**a**) Anterior intussusception (*arrows*). Axial plane. Using gel into the rectum; (**b**) grade III rectocele and anterior intussusceptions (*arrows*). Sagittal with coronal plane. Scans obtained by 2050 transducer (B-K Medical)

9.5.3 Perianal Abscesses and Fistulas

The pathogenesis of anorectal abscesses and fistulae is generally attributed to an infection of the anal glands, usually located in the subepithelial position, the intersphincteric space, or the external sphincter, with ducts that enter at the base of the anal crypts of Morgagni at the dentate line level [39]. Infection of the glands can result in an abscess which can spread in a number of directions, usually along the path of least resistance, and can lead to the subsequent development of anal fistula.

Five presentations of anorectal abscess have been described [39]:

1. *Perianal abscess*, which is the most common type of anorectal abscess, occurring in 40–45 % of cases and is identified as a superficial, tender mass outside the anal verge. Physical examination reveals an area of erythema, induration, or fluctuance, and anoscopic examination can demonstrate pus exuding at the base of a crypt.
2. *Submucosal abscess*, which arises from an infected crypt in the anal canal and is located under the mucosa. Rectal examination may reveal a tender submucosal mass, which may not be readily apparent by anoscopy.
3. *Intersphincteric abscess*, which represents between 2 and 5 % of anorectal abscesses. In this condition, the infection dissects in the intersphincteric plane and can spread cephalad (high type) or caudal (low type).
4. *Ischioanal abscess*, which is seen in 20–25 % of patients and may present as a large, erythematous, indurated, tender mass of the buttock or may be virtually inapparent, the patient complaining only of severe pain or fever.
5. *Supralevator and pelvirectal abscesses*, which are relatively rare, comprising less than 2.5 % of anorectal abscesses. They may occur as a cephalad extension of an intersphincteric or transsphincteric abscess or may be associated with a pelvic inflammatory condition (Crohn's disease, diverticulitis, salpingitis) or pelvic surgery.

Anorectal fistula represents a communication between two epithelial surfaces: the perianal skin and the anal canal or rectal mucosa [39]. Any fistula is characterized by an internal opening, a primary tract, and an external or perineal opening. Occasionally the primary tract can present a secondary extension, or a fistula is without a perineal opening.

Parks et al. [39] classified the main tract of the fistula in relation to the sphincters into four types:

1. *Intersphincteric tract* (incidence between 55 and 70 %). An intersphincteric fistula passes through the internal sphincter and through the intersphincteric plane to the skin. Only the most superficial portions of the tract pass through the subcutaneous external sphincter. Secondary extension may be observed to proceed cephalad in the intersphincteric plane (high blind tract).
2. *Transsphincteric tract* (incidence between 55 and 70 %). A transsphincteric fistula passes through both the internal and external sphincters, into the ischioanal fossa, and to the skin. The level of the tract determines three types of transsphincteric fistula: high (traversing the upper two-thirds of the external sphincter), mid, or low. The height of the internal opening, however, does not always reflect the level at which a transsphincteric fistula crosses the EAS [40].
3. *Suprasphincteric tract* (incidence between 1 and 3 %). A suprasphincteric fistula courses above the puborectalis muscle and below the levator after initially passing cephalad as an intersphincteric fistula. It then transverses downward through the ischioanal fossa to the skin.
4. *Extrasphincteric tract* (incidence between 2 and 3 %). An extrasphincteric fistula is described by a direct communication between the perineum and rectum with no anal canal involvement.

Submucosal fistulae are those in which the tract is subsphincteric and does not involve or pass the sphincter complex. Anovaginal fistulae have an extension toward the vaginal introitus. Secondary tracks may develop in any part of the anal canal or may extend circumferentially in the intersphincteric, ischioanal, or supralevator spaces (horseshoe extensions). The term "complex" fistula is a modification of the Parks' classification, which describes fistulae whose treatment poses a higher risk for impairment of continence. According to the American Society of Colon and Rectal Surgeons (ASCRS) classification, an anal fistula may be termed "complex" when the tract crosses more than 30–50 % of the external sphincter (high transsphincteric, suprasphincteric, and extrasphincteric), is anterior in a female, has multiple tracts, and is recurrent, or the patient has preexisting incontinence, local irradiation, or Crohn's disease.

The configuration of perianal sepsis and the relationship of abscesses or fistulae with internal and external sphincters are the most important factors influencing the results of surgical management. Preoperative identification of all loculate purulent areas and definition of the anatomy of the primary fistulous tract, secondary extensions, and internal opening play an important role in adequately planning the operative approach in order to ensure complete drainage of abscesses, to prevent early recurrence after surgical treatment, and to minimize iatrogenic damage of sphincters and the risk of minor or major degrees of incontinence.

EAUS has been demonstrated to be a very helpful diagnostic tool in accurately assessing all fistula or abscess characteristics. It can be easily repeated while following patients with perianal sepsis to choose the optimal timing and modality of surgical treatment, to evaluate the integrity of or damage to sphincters after operation, and to identify recurrence of fistula. It also gives information about the state of the anal sphincters, which is valuable in performing successful fistula surgery. A fistula tract affecting minimal muscle can be safely excised, but where the bulk of external sphincter muscle is affected, it is best treated by seton drainage or mucosal advancement flap.

The ultrasound examination is generally started using 10–13 MHz, changing to 7 or 5 MHz to optimize visualization of the deeper structures external to the anal sphincters. The PR muscle, and EAS, CLL, and IAS should always be identified and used as reference structures for the spatial orientation of the fistula or abscess. An anal abscess appears as a hypoechoic dyshomoge-

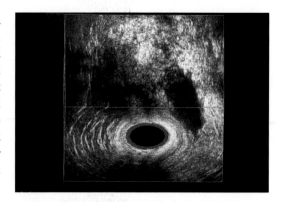

Fig. 9.19 Three-dimensional endoanal ultrasound with 2050 transducer (B-K Medical). Acute abscess in the left anterior perianal space presenting as an area of low reflectivity

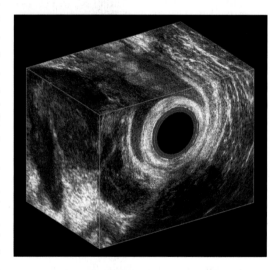

Fig. 9.20 Three-dimensional endoanal ultrasound with 2050 transducer (B-K Medical). Acute abscess in the right supralevator space

neous area, sometimes with hyperechoic spots within it, possibly in connection with a fistulous tract directed through the anal canal lumen. Abscesses are classified as superficial, intersphincteric, ischioanal, supralevator, pelvirectal, and horseshoe (Figs. 9.19 and 9.20).

An anal fistula appears as a hypoechoic tract, which is followed along its crossing of the subepithelium, internal or external sphincters, and through the perianal spaces. With regard to the anal sphincters, according to Parks' classification

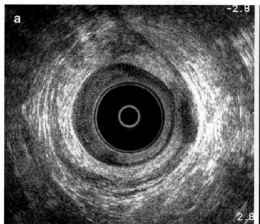 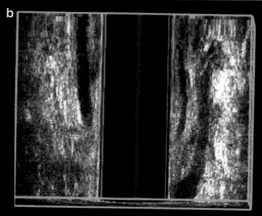

Fig. 9.21 Three-dimensional endoanal ultrasound with 2050 probe (B-K Medical). (**a**) A hypoechoic area is present in the left intersphincteric space (3 o'clock). (**b**) Reconstruction in the coronal plane confirms an inter-sphincteric tract, appearing as a band of poor reflectivity. The tract extends through the intersphincteric space without traversing the external anal sphincter

[39], the fistulous primary tract can be classified into four types:

(a) *Intersphincteric tract*, which is presented as a band of poor reflectivity within the longitudinal layer, causing widening and distortion of an otherwise narrow intersphincteric plane. The tract goes through the intersphincteric space without traversing the external sphincter fibers (Fig. 9.21).

(b) *Transsphincteric tract*, appearing as a poorly reflective tract running out through the external sphincter and disrupting its normal architecture. The point at which the main tract of the fistula traverses the sphincters defines the fistula level. The transsphincteric fistulae are divided into high, medium, or low, corresponding to the ultrasound level of the anal canal [40]. The low transsphincteric tract traverses only the distal external sphincter third at the lower portion of the medium anal canal. Medium transsphincteric tract traverses both sphincters, external and internal, in the middle part of the medium anal canal. High transsphincteric tract traverses both sphincters in the higher part of the medium anal canal, in the space below the puborectalis (Fig. 9.22).

(c) *Suprasphincteric tract*, which goes above or through the PR level. It can be very difficult to determine a suprasphincteric extension because EAUS is not able to visualize the precise position of the levator plate that lies in the same plane as the ultrasound beam.

(d) *Extrasphincteric tract*, which may be seen close to but more laterally placed around the external sphincter.

Differentiation between granulated tracts and scars is sometimes difficult. Straight tracts are easily identified, but smaller and oblique tracts are more difficult to image. Secondary tracts, when present, are related to the main one and are classified as intersphincteric, transsphincteric, suprasphincteric, or extrasphincteric. Similarly, horseshoe tracts, when identified, are categorized as intersphincteric, suprasphincteric, or extrasphincteric. The exact location (radial site and anal canal level) of the internal opening can be difficult to define, as the dentate line cannot be identified as a discrete anatomical entity on EAUS. It is assumed to lie at approximately mid-anal canal level, which is midway between the superior border of the PR muscle and the most caudal extent of the subcutaneous EAS. According to this, the site of the internal opening is categorized as being above, at, or below the dentate line or in the rectal ampulla. In addition, the site can also be characterized by the clock

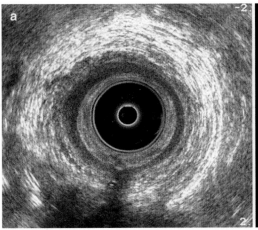

Fig. 9.22 Three-dimensional endoanal ultrasound with 2050 probe (B-K Medical). (**a**) A hypoechoic tract is traversing posteriorly the external anal sphincter. (**b**) Reconstruction in the sagittal plane confirms a posterior transsphincteric fistula

position, being classified from 1 o'clock to 12 o'clock. The internal opening can be identified as hypoechoic (when acute inflammation is present) or hyperechoic area (when chronically inflamed).

Initial experiences with EAUS reported a good accuracy for the selective identification of fistula (91.7 %) and abscess (75 %) configurations. However, a significant number of the internal openings (33.3 %) were not detected [41]. Worse results in the identification of the internal opening were reported by Poen et al. [42] (5.3 % accuracy) and Deen et al. [43] (11 % accuracy). The most probable reason for the poor results in the identification of internal openings by EAUS is the ultrasonographic criteria used. Seow-Choen et al. [44] described revised ultrasonographic criteria for identifying an internal opening, which included one or more of the following features: a hypoechoic breach of the subepithelial layer of the anorectum, a defect in the circular muscles of the IAS, and a hypoechoic lesion of the normally hyperechoic longitudinal muscle abutting on the normally hypoechoic circular smooth muscle. In spite of the improvement in accuracy (73 %) in identifying the internal openings, they found no significant difference between EAUS and digital examination. Cho [45] proposed the following endosonographic criteria to define the site of the internal opening:

Criteria 1. An appearance of a rootlike budding formed by the intersphincteric tract, which contacts the internal sphincter; Criteria 2. An appearance of a rootlike budding with an internal sphincter defect; and Criteria 3. A subepithelial breach connected to the intersphincteric tract through an internal sphincter defect. Using a combination of these three criteria, the author reported 94 % sensitivity, 87 % specificity, and 81 % and 96 % positive and negative predictive values, respectively.

The majority of problems while investigating primary tracts with EAUS occur because of the structural alterations of the anal canal and perianal muscles and tissues, which can overstage the fistula, or poor definition of the tract when filled with inflammatory tissue, which can downstage the fistula [46]. The disappointing results of EAUS in diagnosing the extrasphincteric fistulae could be due to the echogenicity of the fistulae, especially those with a narrow lumen, which is practically identical to the fat tissue in the ischioanal fossa, and to the short focal length of the transducer, which prevents imaging of fistula that are located at large distance from the anal canal. For this reason, performing ultrasonography after injecting 1.0–2.0 mL of 3 % hydrogen peroxide (HPUS) through the external opening of the fistula appears to be particularly useful [46].

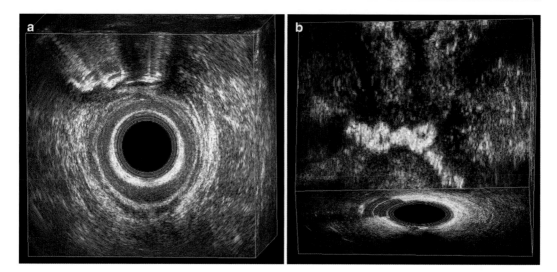

Fig. 9.23 Three-dimensional endoanal ultrasound with 2050 probe (B-K Medical). (**a**) After injection of hydrogen peroxide, the fistulous tract appears hyperechoic. (**b**) Reconstruction in the coronal plane

This technique allows identification of tracts whose presence has not been definitively established or distinction of an active fistulous tract from postsurgical or post-trauma scar tissue (Fig. 9.23). Gas is a strong ultrasound reflector, and after injection, fistula tracts become hyperechoic and the internal opening is identified as an echogenic breach at the submucosa. Because the injected hydrogen peroxide often results in bubbling into the anal canal, which then acts as a barrier to the ultrasound wave, injection should be performed in two phases: an initial injection of a small amount of hydrogen peroxide and a further injection at a greater pressure. A disadvantage inherent to hydrogen peroxide injection is the very strong reflection that occurs at a gas/tissue interface, which blanks out any detail deep to this interface. The bubbles produced by hydrogen peroxide induce acoustic shadowing deep to the tract, so all information deep to the inner surface of the tract is lost. The reported diagnostic accuracy of HPUS ranges from 71 to 95 % for primary tracts and from 63 to 96.1 % for secondary tracts, while that of standard EAUS ranges from 50 to 91.7 % for the primary tract and from 60 to 68 % for secondary tracts [47, 48]. The highest concordance is usually reported for primary transsphincteric fistulae, while the major diagnostic difficulty is still the adequate identification

of primary supra- and extrasphincteric fistulae. Injection can also contribute to a more accurate identification of the internal opening (HPUS accuracy ranging from 48 to 96.6 % vs. EAUS accuracy ranging from 5.3 to 93.5 %) [49].

The availability of 3D imaging has further improved the accuracy of EAUS [5]. With this technique, the operator can follow the pathway of the fistulous tract along all the desired planes (axial, coronal, sagittal, oblique). In addition, volume render mode can facilitate depiction of a tortuous fistula tract after hydrogen peroxide injection, due to the transparency and depth information [5]. Buchanan et al. [50] reported a good accuracy of 3D-EAUS in detecting primary tracts (81 %), secondary tracts (68 %), and internal openings (90 %) in 19 patients with recurrent or complex fistulae. The addition of hydrogen peroxide (3D-HPUS) did not improve these features (accuracies of 71 %, 63 %, and 86 %, respectively). Using 3D imaging, Ratto et al. [48] reported an accuracy of 98.5 % for primary tracts, 98.5 % for secondary tracts, and 96.4 % for internal openings, compared with 89.4 %, 83.3 %, and 87.9 %, respectively, when the 2D system was used. Our experience [49] on 57 patients with perianal fistulae confirmed that 3D reconstructions improved the accuracy of EAUS in the identification of internal opening compared to

2D-EAUS (89.5 % vs. 66.7 %; $P=0.0033$). Primary tracts, secondary tracts, and abscesses were similarly evaluated by both procedures.

Anal endosonography has some clear advantages related to the fact that it is relatively cheap and simple to perform, it is rapid and well tolerated by patients and, unlike MRI, can be performed easily in the outpatient clinic or even on the ward since the machines are easily portable. It is vastly superior to digital examination and is therefore well worth performing. The major advantage of MRI over EAUS is the facility with which it can image extensions that would otherwise be missed since they can travel several centimeters from the primary tract. It is especially important to search for supralevator extensions, since these are not only difficult to detect but pose specific difficulties with treatment. Complex extensions are especially common in patients with recurrent fistulae or those who have Crohn's disease. It should also be borne in mind that MRI and EAUS provide complementary and additive information, and there are no disadvantages to performing both procedures in the same patient where local circumstances, availability, and economics allow this.

References

1. Santoro GA, Wieczorek AP, Dietz HP, Mellgren A, Sultan AH, Shobeiri SA, Stankiewicz A, Bartram C. State of the art: an integrated approach to pelvic floor ultrasonography. Ultrasound Obstet Gynecol. 2011;37:381–96.
2. Groenendijk AG, Birnie E, Boeckxstaens GE, Roovens JP, Bonsel GJ. Anorectal function testing and anal endosonography in the diagnostic work-up of patients with primary pelvic organ prolapse. Gynecol Obstet Invest. 2009;67:187–94.
3. Groenendijk AG, Birnie E, de Blok S, Adriaanse AH, Ankum WM, Roovens JP, Bonsel GJ. Clinical-decision taking in primary pelvic organ prolapse; the effects of diagnostic tests on treatment selection in comparison with a consensus meeting. Int Urogynecol J. 2009;20:711–9.
4. Wieczorek AP, Stankiewicz A, Santoro GA, Wozniak MM, Bogusiewicz M, Rechberger T. Pelvic floor disorders: role of new ultrasonographic techniques. World J Urol. 2011;29:615–23.
5. Santoro GA, Fortling B. The advantages of volume rendering in three-dimensional endosonography of the anorectum. Dis Colon Rectum. 2007;50:359–68.
6. Santoro GA, Di Falco G. Endoanal and endorectal ultrasonography: methodology and normal pelvic floor anatomy. In: Santoro GA, Wieczorek AP, Bartram C, editors. Pelvic floor disorders imaging and a multidisciplinary approach to management. Milan: Springer; 2010. p. 91–102.
7. Williams AB, Cheetham MJ, Bartram CI, et al. Gender differences in the longitudinal pressure profile of the anal canal related to anatomical structure as demonstrated on three-dimensional anal endosonography. Br J Surg. 2000;87:1674–9.
8. Regadas FSP, Murad-Regadas SM, Lima DMR, et al. Anal canal anatomy showed by three-dimensional anorectal ultrasonography. Surg Endosc. 2007;21: 2207–11.
9. Bollard RC, Gardiner A, Lindow S, Phillips K, Duthie GS. Normal female anal sphincter: difficulties in interpretation explained. Dis Colon Rectum. 2002;45: 171–5.
10. Gold DM, Bartram CI, Halligan S, Humphries KN, Kamm MA, Kmiot WA. Three-dimensional endoanal sonography in assessing anal canal injury. Br J Surg. 1999;86:365–70.
11. Frudinger A, Halligan S, Bartram CI, Price AB, Kamm MA, Winter R. Female anal sphincter: age-related differences in asymptomatic volunteers with high-frequency endoanal US. Radiology. 2002; 224:417–23.
12. West RL, Felt-Bersma RJF, Hansen BE, Schouten WR, Kuipers EJ. Volume measurement of the anal sphincter complex in healthy controls and fecal-incontinent patients with a three-dimensional reconstruction of endoanal ultrasonography images. Dis Colon Rectum. 2005;48:540–8.
13. Haylen BT, de Ridder D, Freeman RM, Swift SE, Berghmans B, Lee J, Monga A, Petri E, Rizk DE, Sand PK, Schaer GN. An International Urogynecological Association (IUGA)/International Continence Society (ICS) joint report on the terminology for female pelvic floor dysfunction. Int Urogynecol J. 2010; 21:5–26.
14. Santoro GA. Which method is best for imaging of anal sphincter defects? Dis Colon Rectum. 2012; 55:646–52.
15. Santoro GA, Di Falco G. Endosonographic anatomy of the normal rectum. In: Santoro GA, Di Falco G, editors. Benign anorectal diseases. Diagnosis with endoanal and endorectal ultrasonography and new treatment options. Milan: Springer; 2006. p. 55–60.
16. Macmillan AK, Merrie AE, Marshall RJ, Parry BR. The prevalence of fecal incontinence in community-dwelling adults: a systematic review of the literature. Dis Colon Rectum. 2004;47:1341–9.
17. Starck M, Bohe M, Valentin L. Results of endosonographic imaging of the anal sphincter 2–7 days after

primary repair of third or fourth-degree obstetric sphincter tears. Ultrasound Obstet Gynecol. 2003; 22:609–15.

18. Norderval S, Dehli T, Vonen B. Three-dimensional endoanal ultrasonography: intraobserver and interobserver agreement using scoring systems for classification of anal sphincter defects. Ultrasound Obstet Gynecol. 2009;33:337–43.

19. Voyvodic F, Rieger NA, Skinner S, Schloithe AC, Saccone GT, Sage MR, Wattchow DA. Endosonographic imaging of anal sphincter injury. Does the size of the tear correlate with the degree of dysfunction? Dis Colon Rectum. 2003;46:735–41.

20. Sultan AH, Kamm MA, Hudson CN, Thomas JM, Bartram CI. Anal sphincter disruption during vaginal delivery. N Engl J Med. 1993;329:1905–11.

21. Oberwalder M, Connor J, Wexner SD. Meta-analysis to determine the incidence of obstetric anal sphincter damage. Br J Surg. 2003;90:1333–7.

22. Oberwalder M, Dinnewitzer A, Baig MK, Thaler K, Cotman K, Nogueras JJ, Weiss EG, Efron J, Vernava III AM, Wexner SD. The association between late-onset fecal incontinence and obstetric anal sphincter defects. Arch Surg. 2004;139:429–32.

23. Starck M, Bohe M, Valentin L. The extent of endosonographic anal sphincter defects after primary repair of obstetric sphincter tear increases over time and is related to anal incontinence. Ultrasound Obstet Gynecol. 2006;27:188–97.

24. Scheer I, Thakar R, Sultan AH. Mode of delivery after previous obstetric anal sphincter injuries (OASIS)—a reappraisal. Int Urogynecol J. 2009;20:1095–101.

25. Savoye-Collet C, Savoye G, Koning E, Thoumas D, Michot F, Denis P, Benozio M. Anal endosonography after sphincter repair: specific patterns related to clinical outcome. Abdom Imaging. 1999;24:569–73.

26. Dobben AC, Terra MP, Deutekom M. The role of endoluminal imaging in clinical outcome of overlapping anterior anal sphincter repair in patients with fecal incontinence. AJR Am J Roentgenol. 2007; 189:70–7.

27. de la Portilla F, Vega J, Rada R, Segovia-Gonzáles MM, Cisneros N, Maldonado VH, Espinosa E. Evaluation by three-dimensional anal endosonography of injectable silicone biomaterial (PTQ) implants to treat fecal incontinence: long-term localization and relation with the deterioration of the continence. Tech Coloproctol. 2009;13:195–9.

28. Lienemann A, Anthuber C, Baron A, Kohz P, Reiser M. Dynamic MR colpocystorectography assessing pelvic floor descent. Eur Radiol. 1997;7:1309–17.

29. Kaufman HS, Buller JL, Thompson JR, Pannu HK, DeMeester SL, Genadry RR, Bluemke DA, Jones B, Rychcik JL, Cundiff GW. Dynamic pelvic magnetic resonance imaging and cystocolpoproctography alter surgical management of pelvic floor disorders. Dis Colon Rectum. 2001;44:1575–83.

30. Dvorkin LS, Hetzer F, Scott SM, Williams NS, Gedroyc W, Lunniss PJ. Open-magnet MR defaecography compared with evacuation proctography in the diagnosis and management of patients with rectal intussusception. Colorectal Dis. 2004;6:45–53.

31. Barthet M, Portier F, Heyries L. Dynamic anal endosonography may challenge defecography for assessing dynamic anorectal disorders: results of a prospective pilot study. Endoscopy. 2000;32:300–5.

32. Van Outryve SM, Van Outryve MJ, De Winter BY, Pelckmans PA. Is anorectal endosonography valuable in dyschesia? Gut. 2002;51:695–700.

33. Beer-Gabel M, Teshler M, Schechtman E, Zbar AP. Dynamic transperineal ultrasound vs. defecography in patients with evacuatory difficulty: a pilot study. Int J Colorectal Dis. 2004;19:60–7.

34. Dietz HP, Steensma AB. Posterior compartment prolapse on two-dimensional and three-dimensional pelvic floor ultrasound: the distinction between true rectocele, perineal hypermobility and enterocele. Ultrasound Obstet Gynecol. 2005;26:73–7.

35. Murad-Regadas SM, Regadas FSP, Rodrigues LV, Souza MHLP, Lima DMR, Silva FRS, Filho FSPR. A novel procedure to assess anismus using three-dimensional dynamic ultrasonography. Colorectal Dis. 2006;9:159–65.

36. Murad-Regadas SM, Regadas FSP, Rodrigues LV, Silva FRS, Soares FA, Escalante RD. A novel three-dimensional dynamic anorectal ultrasonography technique (echodefecography) to assess obstructed defecation, a comparison with defecography. Surg Endosc. 2008;22:974–9.

37. Regadas FSP, Haas EM, Jorge JM, Sands D, Melo-amaral I, Wexner SD, Lima DM, Murad-Regadas SM. Prospective multicenter trial comparing echodefecography with defecography in the assessment of anorectal dysfunctions in patients with obstructed defecation. Dis Colon Rectum. 2011;54: 686–92.

38. Murad-Regadas SM, Soares GS, Regadas FSP, Rodrigues LV, Buchen G, Kenmoti VT, Surimã WS, Fernandes GO. A novel three-dimensional dynamic anorectal ultrasonography technique for the assessment of perineal descent, compared with defaecography. Colorectal Dis. 2012;14:740–7.

39. Parks AG, Gordon PH, Hardcastle JD. A classification of fistula-in-ano. Br J Surg. 1976;63:1–12.

40. Buchanan GN, Williams AB, Bartram CI, et al. Potential clinical implications of direction of a trans-sphincteric anal fistula track. Br J Surg. 2003;90:1250–5.

41. Law PJ, Talbot RW, Bartram CI, Northover JMA. Anal endosonography in the evaluation of perianal sepsis and fistula in ano. Br J Surg. 1989;76:752–5.

42. Poen AC, Felt-Bersma RJF, Eijsbouts QA, et al. Hydrogen peroxide-enhanced transanal ultrasound in the assessment of fistula-in-ano. Dis Colon Rectum. 1998;41:1147–52.

43. Deen KI, Williams JG, Hutchinson R, et al. Fistulas in ano: endoanal ultrasonographic assessment assists decision making for surgery. Gut. 1994;35:391–4.

44. Seow-Choen F, Burnett S, Bartram CI, Nicholls RJ. Comparison between anal endosonography and digital examination in the evaluation of anal fistulae. Br J Surg. 1991;78:445–7.

45. Cho DY. Endosonographic criteria for an internal opening of fistola-in-ano. Dis Colon Rectum. 1999; 42:515–8.

46. Santoro GA, Ratto C. Accuracy and reliability of endoanal ultrasonography in the evaluation of perianal abscesses and fistula-in-ano. In: Santoro GA, Di Falco G, editors. Benign anorectal diseases. Milan: Sprinter; 2006. p. 141–57.

47. West RL, Dwarkasing S, Felt-Bersma RJF, et al. Hydrogen peroxide-enhanced three-dimensional endoanal ultrasonography and endoanal magnetic resonance imaging in evaluating perianal fistulas: agreement and patient preference. Eur J Gastroenterol Hepatol. 2004;16:1319–24.

48. Ratto C, Grillo E, Parello A, et al. Endoanal ultrasound-guided surgery for anal fistula. Endoscopy. 2005;37:1–7.

49. Santoro GA, Ratto C, Di Falco G. Three-dimensional reconstructions improve the accuracy of endoanal ultrasonography in the identification of internal openings of anal fistulas. Colorectal Dis. 2004;6 Suppl 2:P214.

50. Buchanan GN, Halligan S, Bartram CI, et al. Clinical examination, endosonography and MR imaging in preoperative assessment of fistula in ano: comparison with outcome-based reference standard. Radiology. 2004;233:674–81.

Endoanal Ultrasonographic Imaging of the Anorectal Cysts and Masses

10

Sthela Murad-Regadas and Giulio A. Santoro

Learning Objectvies

1. To understand the role of 3D-ultrasonography in the assessment of endometriosis
2. To understand the role of 3D-ultrasonography in the assessment of anorectal cysts
3. To understand the role of 3D-ultrasonography in the assessment of anorectal masses

tissues, and vascular structures) require imaging for proper case management. At present, endovaginal ultrasonography and magnetic resonance have become important parts of diagnostic workup of these lesions. This chapter is devoted to discussing the emerging role of three-dimensional endoanal (3D-EAUS) and endorectal (3D-ERUS) ultrasonography particularly with regard to the advantages of these techniques in evaluating the invasion of the rectal layers and adjacent organs.

10.1 Introduction

Anorectal cysts, endometriosis of the rectovaginal septum, and non-mucosal rectal lesions (rare neoplasias of the muscularis propria, connective

S. Murad-Regadas
Department of Surgery, School of Medicine of the Federal University of Ceará, Fortaleza, Ceará, Brazil

Head Pelvic Floor Unit, Clinical Hospital, Federal University of Ceará, Fortaleza, Ceará, Brazil

G.A. Santoro, M.D., Ph.D. (✉)
Head Pelvic Floor Unit, 3rd Division of Surgery, Regional Hospital, Piazzale Ospedale 1, 31100 Treviso, Italy
e-mail: giulioasantoro@yahoo.com

10.2 Endometriosis

Endometriosis is defined by the presence of endometrial glands and stroma outside the endometrial cavity and the myometrium. The most common locations of the ectopic endometriotic implants are found in the pelvis (ovaries and pelvic peritoneum) and followed by deep infiltration sites (uterosacral ligaments, rectosigmoid colon, vagina, and bladder). Imaging techniques have been recommended for the diagnosis and identification of the lesion location [1, 2]. Several reports have demonstrated the accuracy of ultrasonography, performed with different modalities, for the diagnosis of deep infiltrating endometriosis [3–6].

Anorectal ultrasound scanning provides the most detailed view of endometriosis infiltration

S.A. Shobeiri (ed.), *Practical Pelvic Floor Ultrasonography: A Multicompartmental Approach to 2D/3D/4D Ultrasonography of Pelvic Floor*, DOI 10.1007/978-1-4614-8426-4_10, © Springer Science+Business Media New York 2014

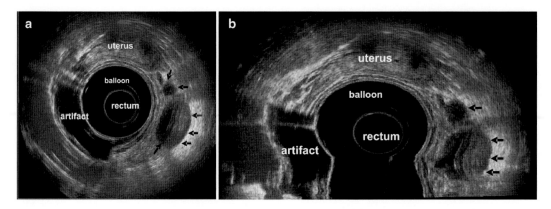

Fig. 10.1 Three-dimensional endorectal ultrasound performed with 2050 transducer (B-K Medical). Endometriosis lesion infiltrating the perirectal fat. The rectal layers are intact. (**a**) Axial plane, (**b**) coronal with axial plane. Two heterogeneous hypoechoic images in the left lateral quadrant compromising the perirectal fat (*arrows*). Mucus in the rectal lumen, outside the lesion site (artifacts)

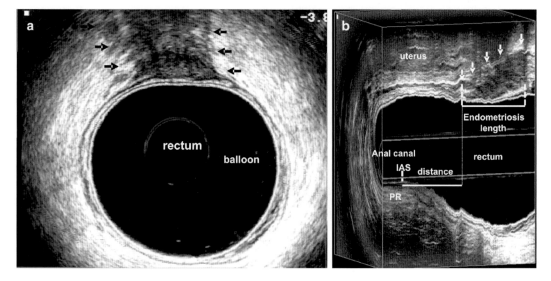

Fig. 10.2 Three-dimensional endorectal ultrasound performed with 2050 transducer (B-K Medical). Endometriosis lesion in the anterior quadrant infiltrating the rectal wall as far as the muscular propria (*arrows*). (**a**) Axial plane. Heterogeneous hypoechoic image compromising 20 % of rectal circumference (*arrows*). (**b**) Sagittal plane. The length of the endometriosis lesion and the distance between the distal infiltration edge and the proximal edge of the sphincter muscles (posterior quadrant) (*arrows*). *IAS* internal anal sphincter, *PR* puborectalis muscle

in the rectum and mesorectal fat. The three-dimensional mode makes it possible to determine the exact circumferential and longitudinal extension of the infiltration into rectal wall or adjacent tissues and the distance between the distal infiltration edge and the proximal edge of the sphincter anal muscles [7], thus providing crucial information for the choice of therapeutic approach. Lesions appear as heterogeneous hypoechoic images mostly located in the recto-vaginal septum, in the mesorectal fat or serosa, and infiltrating into the muscular propria or submucosa layers (Figs. 10.1a, b, 10.2a, b, and 10.3a, b).

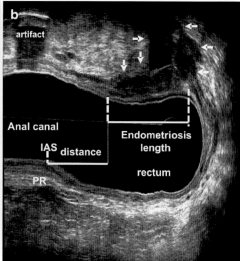

Fig. 10.3 Three-dimensional endorectal ultrasound performed with 2050 transducer (B-K Medical). Endometriosis lesion in the right anterior quadrant infiltrating the rectal wall as far as the muscular propria. (**a**) Axial plane. Heterogeneous hypoechoic image compromising 30 % of rectal circumference (*arrows*). (**b**) Sagittal plane. The length of the endometriosis lesion and the distance between the distal infiltration edge and the proximal edge of the sphincter muscles (posterior quadrant) (*arrows*). Mucus in the rectal lumen, outside the lesion site (artifacts). *IAS* internal anal sphincter, *PR* puborectalis muscle

10.3 Presacral Neoplasia

Perirectal neoplasia is most often located in the retrorectal space and may be of varied etiology. Half the cases are congenital and two thirds are cystic in nature [8, 9]. It tends to affect young female adults but is uncommon in infants. Teratoma is the most frequently observed form in pediatric patients and contains fat or calcifications in 50 % of cases [9, 10].

A wide variety of cystic lesions occur in the retrorectal space, and most are congenital. They are classified as epidermoid cysts, dermoid cysts, enteric cysts (tailgut cysts and cystic rectal duplication), and neurenteric cysts according to their origin and histopathologic features [11]. Anorectal ultrasound may show specific signs and characteristics of the lesion (anechoic area with circular or oval shape, regular margin, and with reinforcement of posterior wall) but the diagnosis remains histopathologic. Ultrasonographic imaging is useful in the evaluation of size, type of lesion (mixed cystic and solid components), and relation with the rectal wall and the sphincter muscles (Figs. 10.4a, b and 10.5a–c).

Perirectal neoplasia appears with different characteristics: as a unilocular or multilocular retrorectal lesion, sometimes a hypoechoic area (cystic) or as an area of mixed echogenicity/heterogeneous image, due to mucoid material or inflammatory debris or solid component, usually with regular outline and not adhering to the rectal wall. In large lesion, an anorectal displacement or stenosis may be visualized due to extrinsic compression. It is important to define the rectal wall invasion or a communication between the cyst and the anorectal lumen (Fig. 10.6a–c).

10.4 Rare Tumors

10.4.1 Rectal Leiomyoma and Leiomyosarcoma

Leiomyoma is a benign mesenchymal neoplasm that usually develops where smooth muscle is present. This lesion is rare, except in the esophagus

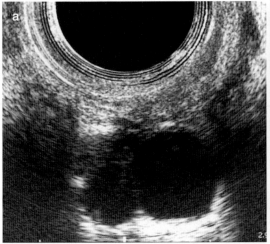 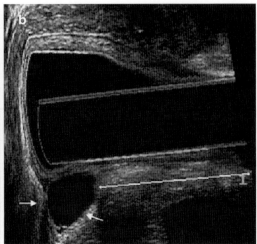

Fig. 10.4 Three-dimensional endorectal ultrasound performed with 2050 transducer (B-K Medical). Female patient. Presacral developmental cyst. The lesion appears as a well-circumscribed, hypoechoic area with posterior reinforcement. The layers of the rectal wall are preserved. (**a**) Axial plane. (**b**) Sagittal plane. Lesion size (longitudinal length and the depth)

and rectum. Only 3 % of these smooth muscle tumors arising from colon are gastrointestinal leiomyomas and constitute about 0.1 % of rectal tumors [12, 13]. In the rectum, most leiomyomas present as small intraluminal polyps and are limited to the muscularis mucosa. Although there are reports of anorectal leiomyomas [14], definitive diagnosis requires anatomical and pathological examination (immunohistochemical staining). Leiomyomas are positive for actin and desmin and negative for CD34 and CD117 [13, 15].

Endorectal ultrasound scanning shows the exact extent of the lesion and relationship with the anatomical structures. Leiomyoma appears as a well-defined, homogeneous hypoechoic mass arising within and confined to the muscularis propria and without invasion of adjacent layers (Fig. 10.7a, b).

Leiomyosarcomas are malignant soft tissue neoplasms arising from smooth muscle tissue located within the muscularis propria and blood or lymphatic vessels. Histologically, leiomyosarcoma features spindle cells with elongated, blunt-ended nuclei in an eosinophilic cytoplasm. Immunohistochemically, these tumors are positive for vimentin, actin, smooth muscle myosin, and desmin. These lesions rarely metastasize through lymphatics and are more likely to spread through the lungs and liver through hematogenous spread.

10.4.2 Gastrointestinal Stromal Tumors

Gastrointestinal stromal tumors (GIST) are the most common mesenchymal tumors of the GI tract but they represent fewer than 1 % of all gastrointestinal (GI) tumors [16]. GIST can occur anywhere along the GI tract, but most often are found in the stomach (60 %) or small intestine (30 %), following rectum (3 %), colon (1–2 %), esophagus (<1 %), and omentum/mesentery (rare) [17].

The clinical presentation and diagnostic of patients with GIST depend on the anatomic location of the lesion and the size and aggressiveness. Small GIST may form solid subserosal, intramural, or less frequently, polypoid intraluminal masses. Large tumors tend to form external masses attached to the outer aspect of the gut involving the muscular layers [18]. The evaluation includes imaging and/or endoscopy but the

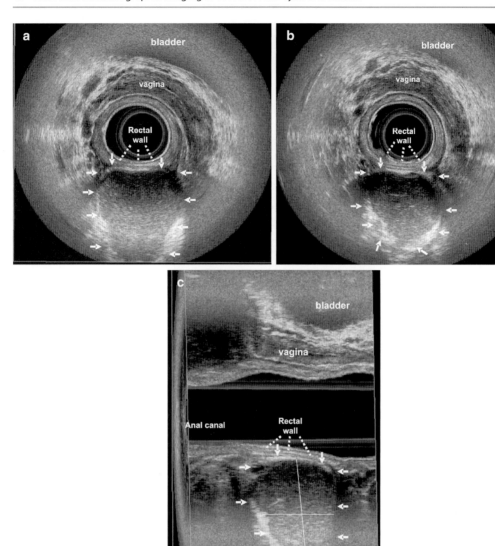

Fig. 10.5 Three-dimensional endorectal ultrasound performed with 2050 transducer (B-K Medical). Female patient. Presacral cystic lesion located at the level of lower rectum with regular outline and without adherence to the rectal wall (*arrows*). The rectal wall is intact. (**a, b**) Axial plane. Mixed echogenicity lesion (*arrows*). (**c**) Sagittal with diagonal planes. A well-circumscribed (hyperechogenic line that surrounds the lesion) and unilocular cystic lesion. Lesion size (longitudinal length and the depth)

pathology and molecular genetics studies are required. Approximately 95 % of GISTs are positive for the CD117 antigen [18].

Anorectal ultrasound scanning provides the most detailed view of lesion and the relationship with the anatomical structures, including perirectal, perianal tissues, anal canal muscles, perirectal wall, and adjacent organs. On ERUS, GIST appears as a well-defined round, homogeneous hypoechoic mass arising from the muscularis propria with an overlying intact mucosa (Fig. 10.8a–c).

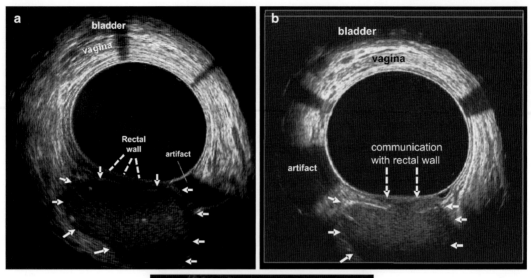

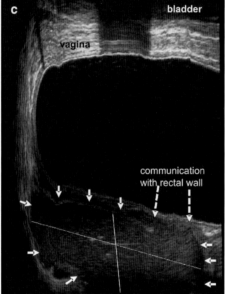

Fig. 10.6 Three-dimensional endorectal ultrasound performed with 2050 transducer (B-K Medical). Female patient. Cystic lesion in the presacral space at the level of lower rectum. There is a contiguous (communication) area with rectal wall. (**a**) Axial plane. In this position, the lesion appears with mixed echogenicity, with regular outline and without adherence to the rectal wall (*arrows*). The rectal wall is intact. (**b**) Axial plane. The image shows the area of the cystic lesion, which communicates with the rectal wall (*interrupted arrows*). (**c**) Sagittal plane. The hyperechogenic line that surrounds the lesion (*arrows*) is interrupted (small area) and there is a communication with rectal wall (*interrupted arrows*). Lesion size (longitudinal length and the depth)

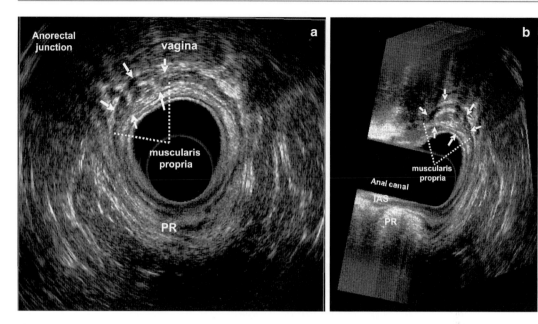

Fig. 10.7 Three-dimensional endorectal ultrasound performed with 2050 transducer (B-K Medical). Small leiomyoma located at the level of the anorectal junction in the right anterior quadrant. The mixed echogenicity lesion expands the outer hypoechoic layer that corresponds to the muscularis propria (*arrows*). (**a**) Axial plane; (**b**) multiplanar: sagittal with diagonal and axial planes. *IAS* internal anal sphincter, *PR* puborectalis muscle

10.4.3 Angiosarcoma

Angiosarcoma accounts for 4 % of all soft tissue malignancies. Tumor originates from vascular and lymphatic walls. It presents as firm, highly vascular lesions. Immunohistochemical stains are often employed to confirm the diagnosis and they include CD 31, CD 34, and BNH 9 (an endothelial marker).

Endorectal ultrasound can demonstrate the presence of vascular structures, appearing as anechoic areas within mixed echogenicity lesion (Fig. 10.9a, b).

10.4.4 Rhabdomyosarcoma

Rhabdomyosarcoma is one of the most common childhood soft tissue tumors, but represents less than 5 % of malignant soft tissue lesions in adult. Anorectal presentation is extremely rare and is seen less than 2 % of cases. It arises from the muscular layer of the bowel. It is described as a grossly uncircumscribed lesion with multiple areas of spherical growth, often resembling a "bunch of grapes" that is soft in consistency. As a result of its mesodermal origin, rhabdomyosarcoma tends to show multiple areas of muscle tissue origin at different stages of development.

This tumor is harder to diagnose in adults, with more advanced disease at presentation and worse prognosis than the younger age groups.

10.4.5 Schwannoma

Schwannoma arises from neural crest cells and can therefore occur in any anatomical region. Grossly these tumors often appear as firm yellow- or brown-colored lesions, which may be pedunculated or sessile. They are almost always restricted to the submucosa and have largely benign slow-growing nature. They are uniformly S-100 positive.

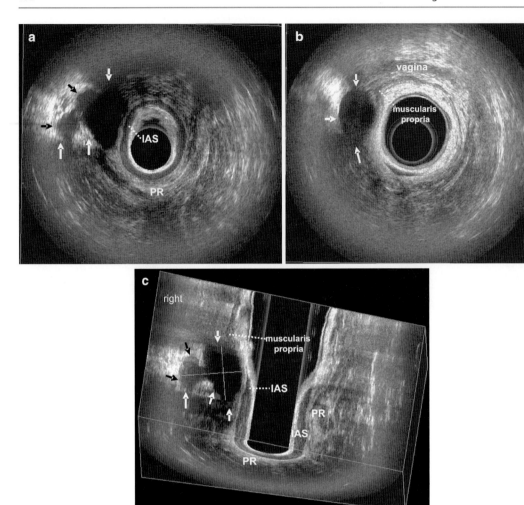

Fig. 10.8 Three-dimensional endorectal ultrasound performed with 2050 transducer (B-K Medical). Female patient. Mixed echogenicity lesion located at the level of lower rectum, anorectal junction, and upper anal canal in the right anterior quadrant. The lesion involved the puborectalis muscle (PR) and the rectal wall. (**a**) Axial plane. Lesion located in the perianal and ischiorectal fat and involving the PR muscle (right anterior quadrant) (*arrows*). The internal anal sphincter (IAS) is intact; (**b**) axial plane. The lesion is located in the perirectal fat and involves the rectal wall as far as the muscular propria (*arrows*); (**c**) coronal plane. Lesion size (longitudinal length and the depth) (*arrows*)

10.5 Conclusions with Future Research

Anorectal cysts, endometriosis of the rectovaginal septum, and non-mucosal rectal lesions (rare neoplasias of the muscularis propria, connective tissues, and vascular structures) are well visualized with 3D endoanal ultrasonography. The lesions are easily available for ultrasound examination to set the course for surgical or non-surgical management. The utilization of this technology largely depends on the availability of the technology to the surgeon.

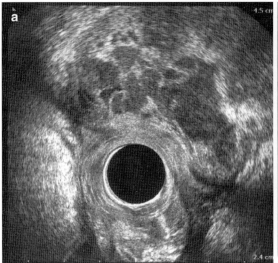 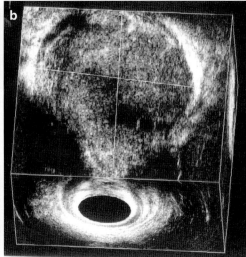

Fig. 10.9 Three-dimensional endorectal ultrasound performed with 2050 transducer (B-K Medical). Female patient. Large mixed echogenicity angiosarcoma with anechoic area inside (vascular structures) located at the level of lower rectum in the anterior quadrant. The lesion is located in the perirectal fat and involves the rectal wall as far as the muscular propria. (**a**) Axial plane; (**b**) coronal plane

References

1. Jenkins S, Olive DL, Haney AF. Endometriosis: pathogenetic implications of the anatomic distribution. Obstet Gynecol. 1986;67:335.
2. Cornillie FJ, Oosterlynck D, Lauweryns JM, Koninckx PR. Deeply infiltrating pelvic endometriosis: histology and clinical significance. Fertil Steril. 1990;53:978–83.
3. Fedele L, Bianchi S, Portuese A, Borruto F, Dorta M. Transrectal ultrasonography in the assessment of rectovaginal endometriosis. Obstet Gynecol. 1998;91:444–8.
4. Bazot M, Malzy P, Cortez A, Roseau G, Amouyal P, Daraï E. Accuracy of transvaginal sonography and rectal endoscopic sonography in the diagnosis of pelvic endometriosis. Ultrasound Obstet Gynecol. 2004;24:180–5.
5. Delpy R, Barthet M, Gasmin M, Berdah S, Shojai R, Desjeux A, Boubli L, Grimaud JC. Value of endorectal ultrasonography for diagnosing rectovaginal septal endometriosis infiltrating the rectum. Endoscopy. 2005;37:357–61.
6. Bahr A, Paredes V, Gadonneix P, Etienney I, Salet-Lizée D, Villet R, Atienza P. Endorectal ultrasonography in predicting rectal wall infiltration in patients with deep pelvic endometriosis: a modern tool for an ancient disease. Dis Colon Rectum. 2006;49:869–75.
7. Regadas FSP, Murad-Regadas SM. 2- and 3-D ultrasonography of endometriosis, pelvic cyst, rectal solitary ulcer, muscle hypertrophy, rare neoplasms. In: Pescatori M, Regadas FSP, Murad-Regadas SM, Zbar AP, editors. Imaging atlas of the pelvic floor and anorectal diseases. Milan: Springer; 2008. p. 159–70.
8. Dozois RR, Chiu LKM. Retrorectal tumours. In: Nicholls RJ, Dozeis RR, editors. Surgery of the colon and rectum. New York: Churchill Livingston; 1997. p. 533–46.
9. Gordon PH. Retrorectal tumours. In: Gordon PH, Nivatvongs S, editors. Principles and practice of surgery for the colon, rectum and anus. St. Louis, MO: Quality Medical Publishers; 1999. p. 427 45.
10. Hjemslad BM, Helwin EB. Tailgut cysts. Report of 53 cases. Am J Clin Pathol. 1988;89:139–47.
11. Levine E, Batnitzky S. Computed tomography of sacral and perisacral lesions. Crit Rev Diagn Imaging. 1984;21:307–74.
12. Chow WH, Kwan WK, Ng WF. Endoscopic removal of leiomyoma of the colon. Hong Kong Med J. 1997;3:325–7.
13. De Palma GD, Rega M, Masone S, Siciliano S, Persico M, Salvatori F, Maione F, Esposito D, Bellino A, Persico G. Lower gastrointestinal bleeding secondary to a rectal leiomyoma. World J Gastroenterol. 2009;15:1769–70.
14. Miettinen M, Furlong M, Sarlomo-Rikala M, Burke A, Sobin LH, Lasota J. Gastrointestinal stromal tumors, intramural leiomyomas, and leiomyosarcomas

in the rectum and anus: a clinicopathologic, immuno-histochemical, and molecular genetic study of 144 cases. Am J Surg Pathol. 2001;25:1121–33.

15. Miettinen M, Sarlomo-Rikala M, Sobin LH. Mesenchymal tumors of muscularis mucosae of colon and rectum are benign leiomyomas that should be separated from gastrointestinal stromal tumors—a clinicopathologic and immunohisto-chemical study of eighty-eight cases. Mod Pathol. 2001;10:950–1.

16. Judson I, Demetri G. Advances in the treatment of gastrointestinal stromal tumours. Ann Oncol. 2007; 18:4–20.

17. AJCC. Gastrointestinal stromal tumor. In: Edge SB, Byrd DR, Compton CC, et al. editors. AJCC cancer staging manual. 7th ed. New York. NY: Springer: 2010. p. 175–180.

18. Corless CL, Heinrich MC. Molecular pathobiology of gastrointestinal stromal sarcomas. Annu Rev Pathol. 2008;3:557–86.

Emerging Imaging Technologies and Techniques

11

S. Abbas Shobeiri and Jittima B. Manonai

Learning Objectives
The complexity of pelvic floor is best appreciated with imaging. Unlike most other parts of the body, pelvic floor anatomy, movement, and function should be evaluated concurrently. In this chapter we review what developments lay on the horizon.

11.1 Introduction

Ultrasound can be considered as a disruptive technology in the medical device arena. A disruptive technology has the potential to break the rules of existing markets. Thanks to its real-time capabilities, its non-ionizing properties, and its cost—much lower than any other medical modality—ultrasound has significantly impacted clinical. It could, in the future, change the rules for screening, and surgery.

S.A. Shobeiri, M.D. (✉)
Female Pelvic Medicine and Reconstructive Surgery,
The University of Oklahoma Health Sciences Center,
WP 2410, 920 Stanton L. Young Boulevard,
Oklahoma City, OK 73104, USA
e-mail: abbas-shobeiri@ouhsc.edu

J.B. Manonai, M.D.
Department of Obstetrics and Gynecology,
Faculty of Medicine Ramathibodi Hospital,
270 Rama VI road, Loong Phayathai, Ratchathewi,
Bangkok 10400, Thailand

In the history of ultrasound, many innovations have been developed since its establishment as a medical imaging device in the 1960s, roughly one or two per decade. The key innovation that launched the modality in the 1960s is the real-time imaging capability through mechanical scanning. Multichannel systems with electronic control of transducer arrays were developed in the 1970s. In the 1980s, flow analysis tools came to maturity through color flow imaging and quantitative Doppler modes (pulse wave Doppler—PWD). In the 1990s significant improvements in image quality were made possible with the introduction of real-time compounding techniques and harmonic imaging. Although many of these concepts were studied in research laboratories years before the commercial dates cited above, it is systematically the maturity of a new technology that triggers the introduction of the innovations on commercially available platforms: for example, real-time imaging was triggered by microprocessors development, Doppler modes were prompted by digital signal processing chips with enough dynamics to detect, at the same time, very weak blood signal and strong tissue echoes. The introduction of low cost analog to digital (A/D) converters has led to fully digital systems, significantly increasing the quality of the information delivered. Harmonic imaging was triggered by large bandwidth transducers, allowing reception of the signal at twice the transmit frequency.

In the first decade of the twenty-first century, technology moved towards extensive miniatur-

S.A. Shobeiri (ed.), *Practical Pelvic Floor Ultrasonography: A Multicompartmental Approach to 2D/3D/4D Ultrasonography of Pelvic Floor*, DOI 10.1007/978-1-4614-8426-4_11,
© Springer Science+Business Media New York 2014

ization leading to the introduction of high performance portable devices. Portable devices have created new markets for ultrasound—the emergency market, for example, underlying again the disruptive potential of the modality. Today portable devices are the primary sources of market growth in the industry and miniaturization can be considered as a global trend of the ultrasound industry: available technologies and innovations are progressively integrated in portable systems.

Today, a new technological breakthrough is ongoing with the advent of massive parallel computing capabilities. This results from the incredible demand in processing and display performances needed in the videogame industry. In addition to multicore architecture CPUs, new graphical processing units (GPU) allow parallel processing on thousands of channels simultaneously. This technology is available for the ultrasound industry and is the enabler to full software-based architecture systems [1].

In the area of pelvic floor imaging, 2D abdominal transducers were used for pelvic floor imaging [2–4]; transducers designed for 3D fetal imaging were adapted for pelvic floor disorders opening a new area of investigation and discovery [5–7]. Adaptation of 3D endoanal probes [8, 9] for use in pelvic floor imaging opened another area of investigation [10, 11]. Investigations from this adaptation have produced logarithmic publications in the area of pelvic floor disorders [12–20].

In this chapter we introduce some advances in imaging technologies in general and introduce new ultrasound uses and forthcoming advances in pelvic floor imaging.

11.2 Operative Pelvic Floor Ultrasonography

Although clinical examination and urodynamic study are the basic methods in the diagnostics of incontinent women recently more often significance of transperineal ultrasound (TPUS) is mentioned in many publications as the method enabling the assessment of the position of the urethra, its anatomical relations, mobility, and hyperrotation. TPUS is a very simple diagnostic method, which may be performed by every clinician involved in pelvic floor diagnostics; it does not require special transducers and sophisticated scanners. The equipment used for TPUS is widely accessible in obstetrics, radiology, gynecology, urology, surgery, and other specialties; thus the access is easy and no extra investment is needed. Ultrasound has been used in the office or the operating room for drainage of hematomas and seromas. This anatomical access however does not allow for getting full information about complex anatomy of the urethra and its relations to the bladder, elements of levator ani, and vaginal walls including pubocervical fascia. The interesting observation is that with knowledge comes the ability to detect cause of problems that have eluded us and invent different ways of correcting root cause of these problems.

Recent applications of botulinum toxin A have included treatment of refractory pelvic pain and pelvic floor spasm [21–23]. There has been reported variability in patient response with this treatment approach, and response rates may vary due to anatomic variations of the pelvic musculature. 3D endovaginal ultrasound guided-injection to the levator ani is a novel application of injecting botulinum toxin A in patients with levator ani spasm. Using the 2052 probe, the needle is readily visualized in real time and injections can be performed in a directed fashion. The potential advantages of this method are many, and include direct visualization of adjacent anatomical structures, direct visualization of the targeted muscle, with the possibility of repositioning the needle in cases of misdistribution or distortion of anatomy, and avoidance of potential intravascular injections. The long-term efficacy of this approach is currently the subject of an ongoing study. The technique for needle localization is reported in the literature [24].

Another interesting area of investigation has been how do we repair the levator ani muscles and does this make a difference (Fig. 11.1). Levator ani muscle repair has been reported and it is known to be a technically challenging surgery. Dietz and colleagues have reported on repair of these muscles in the labor and delivery suite [25]. The same group reported on 20 levator repairs using a mesh patch in 17 women (three

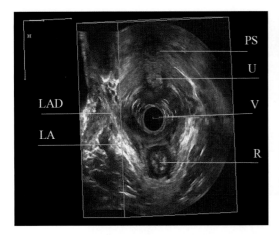

Fig. 11.1 3D EVUS of the pelvic floor of a patient with bilateral levator ani separation from the pubic bone. BK 8838 probe is used for imaging. *PS* pubic symphysis, *U* urethra, *V* vagina, *R* rectum, *LAD* levator ani defect, *LA* levator ani. *Source*: Shobeiri. Surgical repair of bilateral levator ani muscles. IUGJ 2012

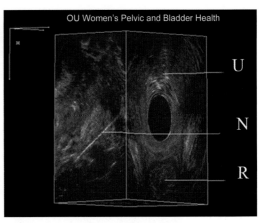

Fig. 11.2 J-hook needle in the puborectalis muscle by endovaginal 360° ultrasound. *U* urethra, *N* needle, *R* rectum. *Source*: Shobeiri. Surgical repair of bilateral levator ani muscles. IUGJ 2012

bilateral). Six patients complained of symptoms of recurrent prolapse, three of de novo dyspareunia, and four of pain related to the repair site on palpation. There were two mesh erosions, one of which healed with estrogen treatment. Prolapse recurrence beyond the hymen was observed in five patients. The mean hiatal area on Valsalva was reduced from 36.84 to 30.71 cm^2 ($P=0.001$) [26]. Looking at the pictures published in the article, it seems that the authors were in the vicinity of the puboperinealis muscles. It can be concluded that mesh usage in this area has a high complication rate. The authors concluded that the effect of surgery on prolapse recurrence and hiatal dimensions is relatively disappointing [26].

A direct repair technique has been described with a "bridging" method using fascia lata [27]. This surgery is technically difficult and not easily adaptable. A recent report documents the implementation of needle-guidance and 3D endovaginal ultrasound for the surgical repair of levator ani muscle defects (Fig. 11.2) [24]. As described, the technique involves an intraoperative 3D endovaginal ultrasound (using the 8838 probe), and under ultrasound guidance, the detached levator muscles are tagged with J-hook needles (MPM Medical, Elmwood Park, NJ, USA). The authors describe the ability to manipulate the needle in order to identify the torn ends of the muscles.

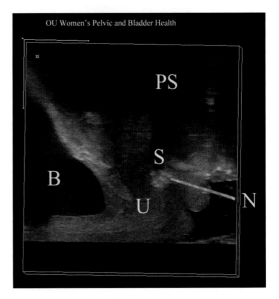

Fig. 11.3 During surgery, in cases where the sling is not palpable, a needle is inserted into the sling which facilitates location and division of the sling. *B* bladder, *PS* pubic symphysis, *S* sling, *N* needle, *U* urethra. *Source*: Shobeiri. Transvaginal sling release with intraoperative ultrasound guidance. JPMS 2013

Further longitudinal follow-up in a series of patient will be needed to determine the success of this approach.

A useful utilization of 3D endovaginal ultrasound is that of clear visualization of synthetic implants, such as midurethral sling materials (Fig. 11.3). Surgical removal of these synthetic

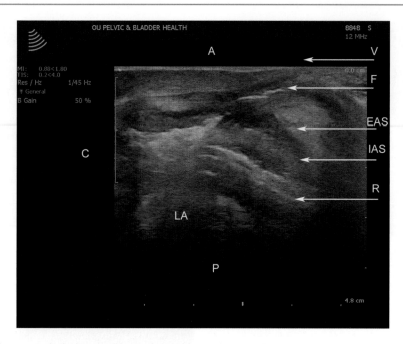

Fig. 11.4 The transvaginal ultrasound image in a mid-sagittal orientation with full visualization of the fistula tract after hydrogen peroxide injection. *A* anterior, *C* cephalad, *EAS* external anal sphincter, *F* fistula tract, *IAS* internal anal sphincter, *LA* levator ani muscle, *P* posterior, *R* rectum, *V* vagina. *Source*: © Shobeiri

materials can be challenging in nature, especially when performed in patients remote from surgery. 3D endovaginal ultrasound provides real-time visualization of the midurethral sling material. It allows for visualization of the precise location of the synthetic, relative to the urethrovasical junction, as an adjunct to surgical planning, or allows for real-time needle localization of the location of the material, just prior to surgical prepping [28].

Ultrasonography can also be used for localization of rectovaginal fistula tracts while patient is under anesthesia. To view small complex fistulas, injection of hydrogen peroxide into the fistula tract may be required (Fig. 11.4).

11.3 Functional Imaging

11.3.1 Manometry

Currently, the best functional imaging may be afforded by the magnetic resonance imaging (MRI) because of its extended field of view. However, pelvic organ prolapse staging with the use of POP-Q, dynamic MR imaging, and perineal ultrasonography only correlates in the anterior compartment and has poor correlation in central and posterior compartments [29]. MRI has been useful for creating finite element models to evaluate mechanisms of pelvic floor injury [30, 31]. What have been missing in functional evaluation are manometric measurements. Manometry has been used in years for evaluation of the anal sphincter complex [32]. Vaginal pressure is a key measure of the strength of the pelvic floor muscles. Kegel was the first to use a pneumatic resistance chamber to measure vaginal pressure and perform biofeedback therapy using his device to improve the strength of pelvic floor muscle. Since then, several investigators have used various types of devices to measure vaginal pressure/force as a measure of the pelvic floor strength. Pressures in general are directionless and should be symmetrical on all sides. However, such is not the case in various sphincters or high-pressure zones (HPZs) of the body because these

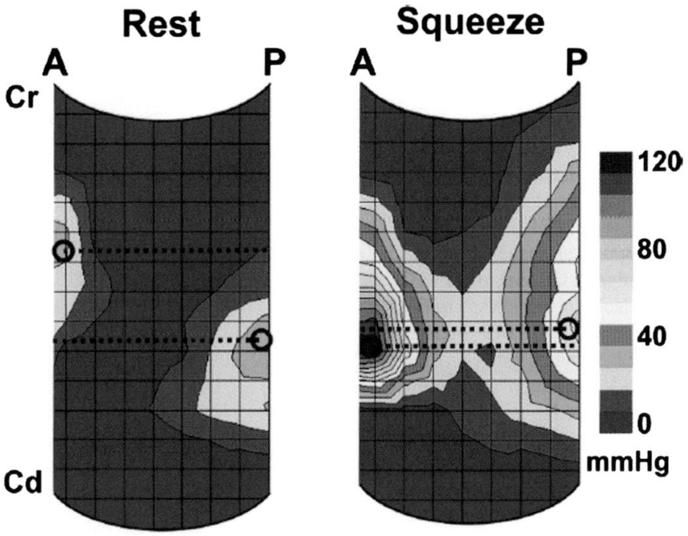

Fig. 11.5 Sagittal view of the HDM plots at rest and during squeeze, demonstrating the location of the peak pressure in the anterior (*A*) and posterior (*P*) *midline* (*n* = 11). *Black circle* marks the location, and *broken line* depicts the level of peak pressures. With pelvic floor con-traction, the distance (Δ = delta) between the peak pressures decreases from 1.0 to 0.2 cm. *Cd* caudal end, *Cr* cranial end, *HDM* high definition manometry. *Source: Raizada. HDM, US, and MRI of pelvic floor muscles. Am J Obstet Gynecol 2010*

are contact and not the cavity or fluid pressures. Using a side-hole infusion manometry technique that can measure contact pressure at a point location, we found that there is a HPZ in the distal part of the vagina that shows axial and circumferential asymmetry of the contact pressures both at rest and during contraction. Furthermore, the contact pressures increase significantly during pelvic floor contraction. Static and dynamic characteristics of vaginal HPZ using a novel, tactile pressure-sensing technology (i.e., high definition manometry—HDM) have been investigated [33]. To further understand the characteristics of vaginal HPZ revealed by HDM, the authors recorded dynamic, two-dimensional (2D) US images of the pelvic floor muscles. Additionally, dynamic magnetic resonance (MR) imaging of the pelvis and pelvic floor muscles was performed to study the anatomical relationship between vaginal HPZ and the adjacent pelvic floor structures [33]. Their data showed the following results. First, HDM plots revealed that, in the vaginal HPZ, the contact pressures are distributed asymmetrically in different quadrants, with lateral contact pressures being significantly smaller than the anterior and posterior ones. During pelvic floor contraction, there is significant increase in the contact pressure in all quadrants of the vaginal HPZ, but the major increase occurs in the anterior and posterior directions. Second, with pelvic floor contraction, there is significant cranial movement of the posterior contact pressure cluster in relationship to the anterior contact pressure cluster. In fact, anterior and posterior contact pressure clusters come axially (along the probe) closer to each other. Third, 2D US and MR images showed that the anorectal angle moves in the ventral and cranial directions during pelvic floor contraction. The cranial movement of the anorectal angle, as revealed by US images and MR images, is of the same magnitude as that of the vertical movement of the posterior contact pressure cluster on the HDM probe. Fourth, MR images with a collapsible bag in the vagina showed the location of vaginal HPZ in relationship to the pubic symphysis, urethra, anal canal, and other pelvic floor structures (Fig. 11.5) [33]. The investigators proposed that using HDM probe one may investigate whether it is possible to divide pelvic floor disorders into disorders of elevator (pubovisceralis)

Fig. 11.6 Sagittal image of the high definition anal manometry pressure plot at rest and squeeze. A *line* connecting the peak pressure in the anterior and posterior *midline* shows movements of the peak posterior pressure in the cranial direction with squeeze. The change in the angle of the above *line* is similar to the change in angle measured in the magnetic resonance images and reflects the elevator function of the pelvic floor muscle. *Cd* caudal end, *Cr* cranial end, *HDM* high definition manometry. *Source*: *Raizada. Functional morphology of anal sphincter complex, Neurogast & mobility, 2011*

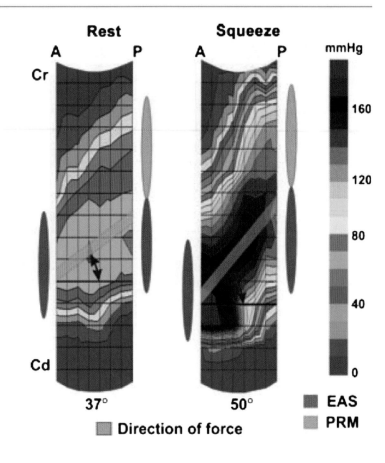

and constrictor (puborectalis) functions. Using the same technology, the same group reported on functional morphology of the anal sphincter complex (Fig. 11.6). They concluded that by high definition anal manometry (HDAM) plots the anal canal pressures are highly asymmetric in the axial and circumferential direction. Anal canal length determined by the 3D US images is slightly smaller than that measured by HDAM. The external anal sphincter (EAS) (1.9±0.5 cm long) and PRM (1.7±0.4 cm long) surround distal and proximal parts of the anal canal, respectively. With voluntary contraction, anal canal pressures increase in the proximal (PRM) and distal (EAS zone) parts of anal canal. Posterior peak pressure in the anal canal moves cranially in relation to the anterior peak pressure, with squeeze. Similar to the movement of peak posterior pressure, MR images show cranial movement of anorectal angle with squeeze [34].

11.3.2 MR Imaging

A major shortcoming of the above manometric studies is that HDM can be used to measure pressures and MRI and TPUS are used to image the pelvic floor, and then the correlation is made. In the search for an improved three-dimensional (3D) imaging modality that simultaneously looks at anatomy and function, recently the use of diffusion tensor imaging (DTI) with fiber tractography was proposed for the visualization of the normal female pelvic floor using MRI [35]. The enhanced 3D visualization with DTI and fiber tractography might have the potential to both visualize and quantify abnormal pelvic floor support in patients with prolapse. Zijta and colleagues performed a study to examine the clinical application of DTI and fiber tractography of the pelvic floor support, by prospectively evaluating and comparing the fiber tract outcomes and basic

DTI parameters of women with pelvic organ prolapse with those of women with pelvic floor symptoms but without pelvic organ prolapse, and with those of asymptomatic nulliparous women. We also intended to investigate the degree of inter-rater reliability. Their findings were as follows: anatomical representation of the puboviceral muscle in 34 % (19/56); puborectal muscle in 13 % (7/56); superficial transverse perineal muscle in 27 % (15/56); ischiocavernosus muscle in 54 % (30/56); bulbospongiosus muscle in 43 % (12/28); and urethral sphincter complex in 29 % (8/28) of the datasets, respectively. No perceptible differences in tractability or nontractability were found in per-group distributions. The iliococcygeus muscle was rated non-satisfactory in all datasets (56/56). The following anatomical structures were identified in most of the DTI datasets: perineal body 100 % (28/28), anal sphincter complex 93 % (26/28), and internal obturator muscle 100 % (56/56) (Fig. 11.1). Despite the overall non-satisfactory visualization of the global appearance of the puboviceral muscle in the datasets (37/56), analyses of its subdivisions resulted in a satisfactory visualization of the puboperineal muscle in 23 of the 28 subjects. Both the pubovaginal and puboanal subdivision could not or only insufficiently be tracked. Substantial overall inter-rater agreement was found for the independent qualitative scores. The overall weighted kappa for all muscle assessments was 0.71 (95 % CI 0.63–0.78). Qualitative inter-observer agreement for the anatomical structures which met the criteria for quantification was also substantial (PABAK 0 0.76). The authors concluded that DTI permits 3D visualization and quantification of part of the pelvic floor anatomy, with reliable high-quality tractability of the anal sphincter complex, perineal body, and the puboperineal muscle [35]. The authors state DTI and fiber tractography are feasible noninvasive tools to assess in vivo pelvic floor anatomy, which exceed the resolution of frequently applied conventional MR techniques and might provide complement information in pelvic floor disorders (Fig. 11.7) [36].

11.3.3 Endocavitary Ultrasound and Real-Time Elastography (RTE)

Ultrasound real-time elastography (RTE) is a rather new imaging modality based on differences in radiofrequency signals following endogenous/exogenous compression due to different elastic properties of the targeted tissues or organs. This may yield additional image information and, therefore, enhance diagnostic accuracy and potentially improve clinical management [37]. Elastography is a term referring to imaging techniques that aim to assess tissue elasticity. All approaches that have been introduced to date are based on a common three-step methodology:

1. Generate a low frequency vibration in tissue to induce shear stress.
2. Image the tissue with the goal of analyzing the resulting stress.
3. Deduce from this analysis a parameter related to tissue stiffness elastography, which uses ultrasound to assess tissue differences in ultrasound imaging and provides both morphological (gray-scale images) and functional imaging (flow imaging) of soft tissue. Using ultrafast capabilities, a third dimension can be added to ultrasound: pathophysiological information through the assessment of tissue viscoelasticity. Ultrafast imaging can be used to capture phenomena that have never been imaged on commercial ultrasound devices: transient shear waves propagating in soft tissue. Shear wave imaging leads to quantification of tissue mechanical properties. Once properly generated and imaged, a transient shear wave can provide many insights on the mechanical properties of the imaged tissue.

Elastography technology is similar to DTI and tractography comprising enhanced MRI techniques that enable the three-dimensional visualization of anisotropic tissue, such as muscle fibers, and provide a quantitative description of tissue organization and integrity [36]. MR imaging utilizes (monochromatic) vibration. Stationary waves induced in the body are analyzed to deduce tissue elasticity. Dynamic elastography is well suited for MR systems as the

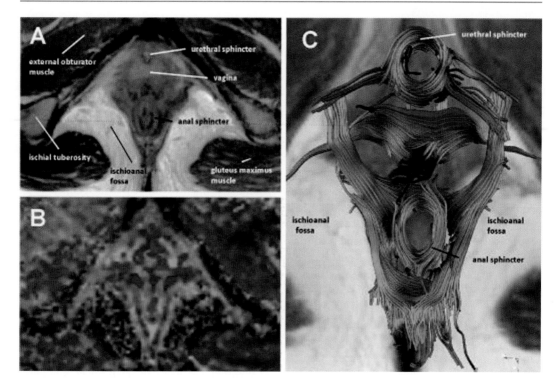

Fig. 11.7 Axial T2-weighted image of a 26-year-old nullipara (**a**) with corresponding directionally coded FA map (**b**). The pervoxel vector values are color coded as follows: *green* (anteroposterior direction), *blue* (craniocaudal direction), and *red* (mediolateral direction). Fiber tractography (**c**) demonstrates the multidirectional organization of the complex pelvic floor anatomy with a clear visualization of circularly orientated fibers at the level of the urethral and anal sphincter complex. *Source*: Zijta, Diffusion Tensor Imaging and Fiber Tractography, Clinical anatomy 2013

vibration pattern is not time-dependent but must be assessed in a volume. It is a quantitative approach but suffers from the usual MR drawbacks: high cost, limited availability, and lack of real-time imaging. The elastographic pictures registered simultaneously with conventional gray-scale B-mode images during sonography or endosonography can be assumed to better help distinguish malignant from inflamed areas and thus facilitate the diagnostic work-up [38]. In other important conditions, such as pelvic floor disorders, this technology remains untested.

Endocavitary ultrasound with RTE can be performed using multifunctional ultrasound equipment (Fig. 11.8) (Hi vision Preirus; Hitachi Aloka, Wallingford, USA). The Hi vision 8500 includes the innovative sonoelastography option, which provides a new set of information by measuring the relative stiffness of tissue and overlaying that information onto the standard B-mode

image as a traditional color map. The system also features multi-angle compound imaging, adaptive noise reduction, and four modes of tissue harmonics. It allows users to adjust the imaging parameters of a frozen image. Use of a high-frequency probe R54 (Fig. 11.9) will allow a circular view (frequency spectrum: 5–10 MHz). The R54 is similar to BK 2052 transducer. The probe can show images in a four-window view (Fig. 11.10). The images with this transducer appear rendered and with soft edges since the software adapted for its use is same as the one used for fetal imaging. This makes differentiation between different levator ani subdivisions rather difficult. The probe is not automatic and must be hand-drawn to produce a 3D data volume. As such, one can assume that the volume and area measurements may not be accurate. On the positive side the data volume produced is simple to manipulate like BK's software (Fig. 11.11).

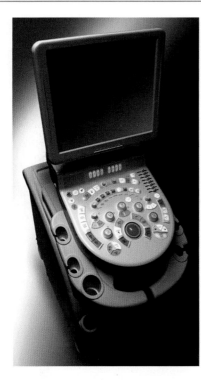

Fig. 11.8 Hitachi Aloka Preirus Hi Vision 8500, an LCD monitor, and control panel are incorporated as a unit, which can be moved vertically and horizontally together by means of a flexible arm. The operator can perform examinations in the best position whether he/she is standing or sitting

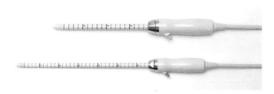

Fig. 11.9 Hitachi Aloka R54 probe: Frequency band: 5.0–10.0 MHz. Radius/sector angle: 6 mm/270°. Depth of field of view: 30–170 mm. Display modes: B-Mode, M-Mode, PW, CFM, CFA. Probe length: 190 and 330 mm, adaptable with rectoscope

On the negative side, the Hitachi Aloka software does not have a PC platform and can be manipulated only on the ultrasound machine. This lack of PC/Apple specific software makes storing data volumes for clinical or investigational use difficult. The Hitachi Aloka R54 probe targets the colorectal audience and has a smaller diameter compared to BK's 2052 or 8838. The smaller

diameter may be an issue for endovaginal imaging since probe–tissue contact will require ample ultrasound gel. Additional probes used for pelvic floor imaging are EUP-C524 (Fig. 11.12) which can be used for 3D transperineal imaging just like the GE or Phillips transducers. The C524 probe can be used for 2D functional imaging of the pelvic floor (Fig. 11.13). By placing the probe on the perineal area, a 3D volume is obtained which can be manipulated on the ultrasound machine (Fig. 11.14a, b). There is also a EUP-U533 probe (Fig. 11.15) which is similar to BK's 8848 probe. EUP-U533 obtains excellent mid-sagittal views of the bladder and the anorectum useful for functional imaging.

For endoanal RTE, the balloon at the tip of the probe should be repeatedly filled with water (10 mL/s, maximum volume 20 mL) under strictly controlled dynamic strain conditions as indicated on a graded scale located at the right margin of the elastogram with monitoring of color distribution within the region of interest (ROI). In a study of anal sphincter by Allgayer and colleagues, in 43 patients sufficiently reproducible color distribution patterns were obtained with the desired strain range as indicated by the built-in strain indicator equaling three (four) points on the seven-point scale [39]. In that study, particular care was taken to ensure that the morphology and diameter of the inner anal sphincter (IAS) and EAS as judged from the simultaneous gray-scale 2D image remained as constant as possible compared to baseline conditions and that the probe remained centrally positioned. The procedure was repeated at least three times and recorded by taking consecutive single-frame pictures and cine-loop images. A 180° ROI sector view was used at the level where the IAS and EAS structures on the simultaneous gray-scale image could best be distinguished, this area being in most cases the ventral view of the transition level between the IAS and EAS (Fig. 11.16). It was assumed that the distribution of the elastographically obtained color areas within predefined structures of the IAS and EAS reflects elastic properties, red areas representing soft, green intermediate, and blue hard tissue or organ elastic properties. For a semiquantitative assessment, the

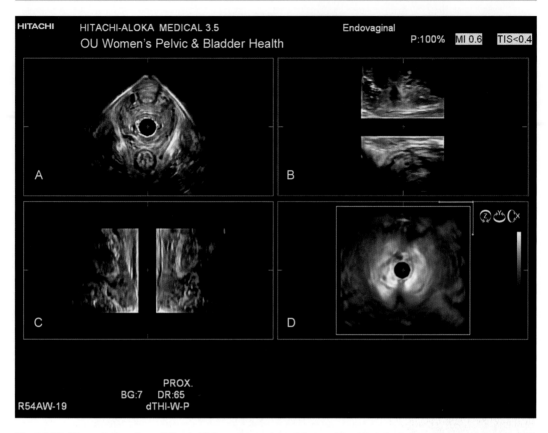

Fig. 11.10 Four-window view of Hitach Aloka software: (**a**) axial view, (**b**) mid-sagittal view, (**c**) coronal view, and (**d**) 3D volume. © Shobeiri

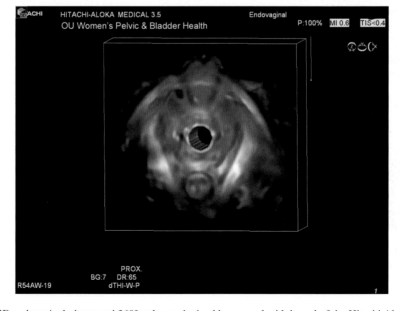

Fig. 11.11 3D endovaginal ultrasound 360° volume obtained by manual withdrawal of the Hitachi Aloka R54 probe. Notice the rendered appearance of the 3D volume. © Shobeiri

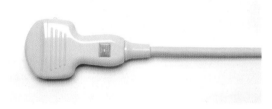

Fig. 11.12 Hitachi Aloka 3D abdominal convex probe EUP-C524 used for transperineal imaging. Frequency band: 3.5–7.5 MHz. Radius/angle: 40 mm/70°. Depth of field of view: 40–210 mm. Display modes: B-Mode, M-Mode, PW, CFM, CFA, dTHI, WPI

elastogram distribution of red, green, or colors within the IAS and EAS structures was estimated using a graded visual scale ranging from 0 to 3.0. Three points indicated that >70 % of the total IAS and EAS area consisted of the corresponding color, two points indicated a percentage range from 30 to 70 %, one point a percentage range from 10 to 30 %, and zero points a percentage of <10 %. For each analysis, three consecutive single frames obtained under identical conditions from each patient were taken. In summary, the main finding was that the IAS differed

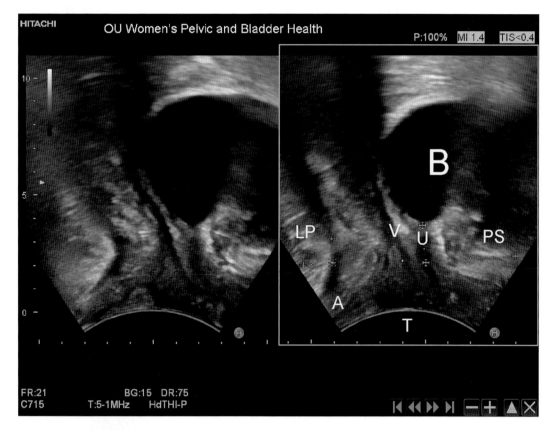

Fig. 11.13 2D transperineal view obtained by Hitachi Aloka EUP-C524 probe. *B* bladder, *PS* pubic symphysis, *U* urethra, *V* vagina, *T* transducer, *LP* levator plate, *A* anus. © Shobeiri

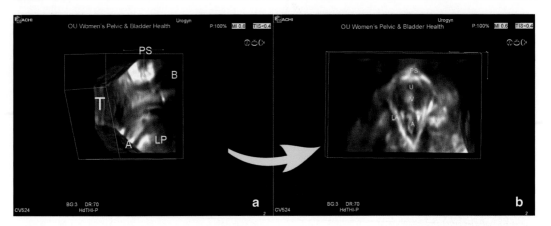

Fig. 11.14 (**a**) The 3D data pelvic floor volume obtained by Hitachi Aloka 3D abdominal convex probe EUP-C524. (**b**) The volume is rotated (the *yellow arrow*) to face the axial plane and advanced cephalad to reach the levator ani muscles. *B* bladder, *LP* levator plate, *PS* pubic symphysis, *A* anus, *T* transducer, *U* urethra, *V* vagina, *LA* levator ani. © Shobeiri

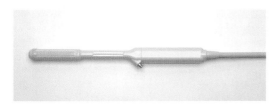

Fig. 11.15 Hitachi Aloka linear/convex endocavitary EUP-U533 probe. Frequency band: 5.0–10.0 MHz linear, 5.0–9.0 MHz radial. Linear length/radius/sector angle: 64 mm/10 mm/200°. Depth of field of view: 30–170 mm. Display modes: B-Mode, M-Mode, PW, CFM, CFA, dTHI, WPI

significantly from the EAS with regard to elastogram color distribution. There were no significant correlations with clinical and functional parameters. There was, however, a nonsignificant increase in the percentage of blue (hard) areas in the IAS in patients neoadjuvantly irradiated for rectal or cervical cancer compared to nonirradiated patients, which was accompanied by a significant decrease in the resting sphincter pressure ($p < 0.009$). The authors concluded that the IAS, a smooth muscle, and the EAS, a striated muscle, have different elastogram color distributions, probably reflecting their different elastic properties. The absence of significant correlations with the major clinical and functional parameters sug-

gests that in routine clinical practice ultrasound RTE may not yield additional information in patients with fecal incontinence. There may be exceptions, particularly in irradiated patients [39].

Elastography is intended to yield additional visual and clinically valuable information compared to conventional gray-scale B-mode images. There remain important questions such as the problem of appropriately quantifying elastographic information in terms of elastic tissue properties, the underlying structural substrate for the observed elastographic differences between different muscles, and, finally, the clinical relevance of elastography in patients with pelvic floor weakness [39].

11.4   Conclusions and Future Research

Elastography in ultrasound and DTI in MRI are two advancements that bring us one step closer to true 3D functional imaging that may help with investigation of underlying causes of pelvic floor disorders. Although the elastic properties of the pelvic floor tissue are important for

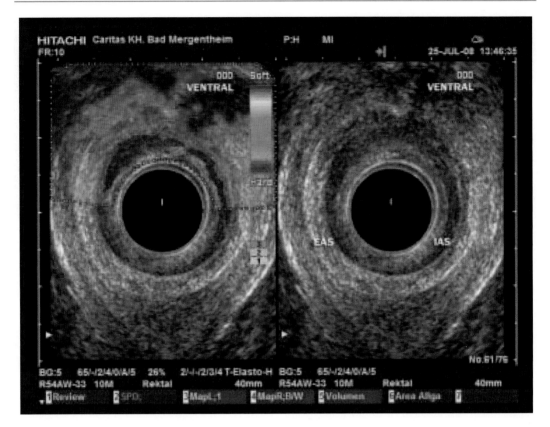

Fig. 11.16 Simultaneous elastogram (*left*) and gray-scale B-mode single-frame image (*right*) from a 64-year-old patient with partial fecal incontinence following lower anterior resection for rectal cancer. Gray-scale B-mode image shows normal IAS and EAS morphology. The computerized analysis of the color distribution yielded 47.8 % *red* (soft), 47.4 % *green* (intermediate), and <5.0 % *blue* (hard) areas within the IAS; corresponding values for the EAS were 41.6 % *blue* (hard), 58.5 % *green* (intermediate), and *no red* (soft) areas. The strain level was three on the seven-point graded scale. *Source*: Allgayer, Endosonographic elastography of the anal sphincter. Scandinavian Journal of Gastroenterology, 2010

pelvic organ support and labor and delivery, elastography of pelvic floor remains untested (Fig. 11.17). The ultimate solution would be an endocavitary probe that has the 3D capability of the high resolution manometry. Although both MRI and 3D endovaginal ultrasound can image the levator ani muscles reasonably well, neither can easily assess the integrity of the connective tissues of pelvic floor support such as the utero-sacral cardinal ligament complex, perineal membrane, and the pubocervical fibromuscularis and the rectovaginal tissue. With advancing technology, reliable and reproducible 3D/4D ultrasound technologies may contribute to unlocking mysteries of pelvic floor disorders that plague us today.

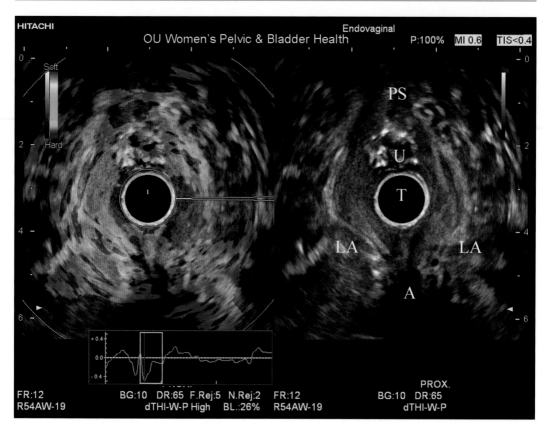

Fig. 11.17 Simultaneous elastogram (*left*) and gray-scale B-mode single-frame image (*right*) from a patient with normal muscle morphology. The computer shows a complex mixture of hard and soft tissues. *LA* levator ani, *A* anus, *T* transducer, *U* urethra, *PS* pubic symphysis. © Shobeiri

References

1. Bercoff J. Ultrafast ultrasound imaging. O. Minin, editor. Croatia: INTECH OPEN ACCESS. http://www.intechopen.com/books/ultrasound-imaging-medical-applications/ultrafast-ultrasound-imaging. Ultrafast Ultrasound Imaging. 2011; 2–24. doi: 10.5772/19729

2. Dietz HP, Wilson PD. Anatomical assessment of the bladder outlet and proximal urethra using ultrasound and videocystourethrography. Int Urogynecol J Pelvic Floor Dysfunct. 1998;9(6):365–9. PubMed PMID: 9891957. English.

3. Dietz HP, Wilson PD, Clarke B. The use of perineal ultrasound to quantify levator activity and teach pelvic floor muscle exercises. Int Urogynecol J Pelvic Floor Dysfunct. 2001;12(3):166–8. discussion 8–9. PubMed PMID: 11451004. English.

4. Shobeiri SA, Nolan TE, Yordan-Jovet R, Echols KT, Chesson RR. Digital examination compared to trans-perineal ultrasound for the evaluation of anal sphincter repair. Int J Gynaecol Obstet. 2002;78(1):31–6. PubMed PMID: 12113968.

5. Dietz HP, Jarvis SK, Vancaillie TG. The assessment of levator muscle strength: a validation of three ultrasound techniques. Int Urogynecol J Pelvic Floor Dysfunct. 2002;13(3):156–9. discussion 9. PubMed PMID: 12140708. English.

6. Dietz HP, Steensma AB, Hastings R. Three-dimensional ultrasound imaging of the pelvic floor: the effect of parturition on paravaginal support structures. Ultrasound Obstet Gynecol. 2003;21(6):589–95. PubMed PMID: 12808677. English.

7. Kruger JA, Dietz HP, Murphy BA. Pelvic floor function in elite nulliparous athletes. Ultrasound Obstet Gynecol. 2007;30(1):81–5. PubMed PMID: 17497753. English.

8. Santoro GA, Fortling B. The advantages of volume rendering in three-dimensional endosonography of the anorectum. Dis Colon Rectum. 2007;50(3):359–68. PubMed PMID: 17237912. English.

9. Dal Corso HM, D'Elia A, De Nardi P, Cavallari F, Favetta U, Pulvirenti D'Urso A, et al. Anal endo-

sonography: a survey of equipment, technique and diagnostic criteria adopted in nine Italian centers. Tech Coloproctol. 2007;11(1):26–33. PubMed PMID: 17357863. English.

10. Shobeiri SA, Leclaire E, Nihira MA, Quiroz LH, O'Donoghue D. Appearance of the levator ani muscle subdivisions in endovaginal three-dimensional ultrasonography. Obstet Gynecol. 2009;114:66–72. PubMed PMID: 19546760.

11. Rostaminia G, White D, Hegde A, Quiroz LH, Davila GW, Shobeiri SA. Levator ani deficiency and pelvic organ prolapse severity. Obstetrics and Gynecology. 2013;121(5):1017–24. doi: 10.1097/AOG.0b013e31828ce97d.

12. Santoro GA, Wieczorek AP, Dietz HP, Mellgren A, Sultan AH, Shobeiri SA, et al. State of the art: an integrated approach to pelvic floor ultrasonography. Ultrasound Obstet Gynecol. 2011;37:381–96.

13. Santoro GA, Wieczorek AP, Shobeiri SA, Mueller ER, Pilat J, Stankiewicz A, et al. Interobserver and interdisciplinary reproducibility of 3D endovaginal ultrasound assessment of pelvic floor anatomy. Int Urogynecol J Pelvic Floor Dysfunct. 2011;22:53–9.

14. Wieczorek AP, Wozniak MM, Stankiewicz A, Santoro GA, Bogusiewicz M, Rechberger T, et al. Quantitative assessment of urethral vascularity in nulliparous females using high-frequency endovaginal ultrasonography. World J Urol. 2011;29(5):625–32. PubMed PMID: 21796481.

15. Wieczorek AP, Wozniak MM, Stankiewicz A, Santoro GA, Bogusiewicz M, Rechberger T. 3-D high-frequency endovaginal ultrasound of female urethral complex and assessment of inter-observer reliability. Eur J Radiol. 2012;81(1):e7–12. PubMed PMID: 20970275. Epub 2010/10/26. eng.

16. Shobeiri SA, Rostaminia G, Shobeiri H. Endoanal Phantom. J Ultrasound Med. 2013;32(8):1393–6. doi: 10.7863/ultra.32.8.1393. PubMed PMID: 23887948.

17. Rostaminia G, White DE, Quiroz LH, Shobeiri SA. Visualization of periurethral structures by 3D endovaginal ultrasonography in midsagittal plane is not associated with stress urinary incontinence status. Int Urogynecol J. 2013;24(7):1145–50. PubMed PMID: 23179501.

18. Shobeiri MS, Rostaminia G, White D, Quiroz L. The determinants of minimal levator hiatus and their relationship to the puborectalis muscle and the levator plate. BJOG. 2013;120(2):205–11. PubMed PMID: 23157458.

19. Shobeiri SA, White D, Quiroz LH, Nihira MA. Anterior and posterior compartment 3D endovaginal ultrasound anatomy based on direct histologic comparison. Int Urogynecol J. 2012;23(8):1047–53. PubMed PMID: 22402641. Epub 2012/03/10. eng.

20. Rostaminia G, White D, Hegde A, Quiroz LH, Davila GW, Shobeiri SA. Levator ani deficiency and pelvic organ prolapse severity. Obstet Gynecol. 2013;121(5):1017–24.

21. Abbott JA, Jarvis SK, Lyons SD, Thomson A, Vancaille TG. Botulinum toxin type A for chronic pain and pelvic floor spasm in women: a randomized controlled trial. Obstet Gynecol. 2006;108(4):915–23. PubMed PMID: 17012454.

22. Ghazizadeh S, Nikzad M. Botulinum toxin in the treatment of refractory vaginismus. Obstet Gynecol. 2004;104(5 Pt 1):922–5. PubMed PMID: 15516379.

23. Park AJ, Paraiso MF. Successful use of botulinum toxin type a in the treatment of refractory postoperative dyspareunia. Obstet Gynecol. 2009;114(2 Pt 2):484–7. PubMed PMID: 19622971.

24. Rostaminia G, Shobeiri SA, Quiroz LH. Surgical repair of bilateral levator ani muscles with ultrasound guidance. Int Urogynecol J. 2013;24(7):1237–9. PubMed PMID: 22885726. Epub 2012/08/14. Eng.

25. Dietz HP, Gillespie AVL, Phadke P. Avulsion of the pubovisceral muscle associated with large vaginal tear after normal vaginal delivery at term. Aust N Z J Obstet Gynaecol. 2007;47(4):341–4. PubMed PMID: 17627693. English.

26. Dietz HP, Shek KL, Daly O, Korda A. Can levator avulsion be repaired surgically? A prospective surgical pilot study. Int Urogynecol J. 2013;24(6):1011–5. PubMed PMID: 23152050. Epub 2012/11/16. Eng.

27. Shobeiri SA, Chimpiri AR, Allen A, Nihira MA, Quiroz LH. Surgical reconstitution of a unilaterally avulsed symptomatic puborectalis muscle using autologous fascia lata. Obstet Gynecol. 2009;114(2 Pt 2):480–2. PubMed PMID: 19622969.

28. Mukati M, Shobeiri SA. Transvaginal sling release with intraoperative ultrasound guidance. Female Pelvic Med Reconstr Surg. 2013;19(3):184–5.

29. Broekhuis SR, Kluivers KB, Hendriks JC, Futterer JJ, Barentsz JO, Vierhout ME. POP-Q, dynamic MR imaging, and perineal ultrasonography: do they agree in the quantification of female pelvic organ prolapse? Int Urogynecol J Pelvic Floor Dysfunct. 2009;20(5):541–9. PubMed PMID: 19221680.

30. Chen L, Ashton-Miller JA, DeLancey JO. A 3D finite element model of anterior vaginal wall support to evaluate mechanisms underlying cystocele formation. J Biomech. 2009;42(10):1371–7. PubMed PMID: 19481208. Pubmed Central PMCID: Source: NLM. NIHMS117052. Source. NLM. PMC2744359.

31. Hsu Y, Summers A, Hussain HK, Guire KE, Delancey JOL. Levator plate angle in women with pelvic organ prolapse compared to women with normal support using dynamic MR imaging. Am J Obstet Gynecol. 2006;194(5):1427–33. PubMed PMID: 16579940. Pubmed Central PMCID: Source: NLM. NIHMS10238. Source: NLM. PMC1479225.

32. Sultan AH, Kamm MA. Relationship between parity and anal manometry. Dis Colon Rectum. 1993;36(8):783–4. PubMed PMID: 8348872. English.

33. Raizada V, Bhargava V, Jung S-A, Karstens A, Pretorius D, Krysl P, et al. Dynamic assessment of the vaginal high-pressure zone using high-definition manometery, 3-dimensional ultrasound, and magnetic resonance imaging of the pelvic floor muscles. Am J Obstet Gynecol. 2010;203(2):172.e1–8. PubMed PMID: 20462564. Pubmed Central PMCID: NIHMS182519 [Available on 08/01/11]. PMC2910785 [Available on 08/01/11]. English.

34. Raizada V, Bhargava V, Karsten A, Mittal RK. Functional morphology of anal sphincter complex unveiled by high definition anal manometery and three dimensional ultrasound imaging. Neurogastroenterol Motil. 2011;23(11):1013–9. e460. PubMed PMID: 21951657. Pubmed Central PMCID: 3190080.

35. Zijta FM, Lakeman MM, Froeling M, van der Paardt MP, Borstlap CS, Bipat S, et al. Evaluation of the female pelvic floor in pelvic organ prolapse using 3.0-Tesla diffusion tensor imaging and fibre tractography. Eur Radiol. 2012;22(12):2806–13.

36. Zijta FM, Froeling M, Nederveen AJ, Stoker J. Diffusion tensor imaging and fiber tractography for the visualization of the female pelvic floor. Clin Anat. 2013;26(1):110–4. PubMed PMID: 23168612.

37. Saftoiu A, Vilman P. Endoscopic ultrasound elastography—a new imaging technique for the visualization of tissue elasticity distribution. J Gastrointestin Liver Dis. 2006;15(2):161–5. PubMed PMID: 16802011. English.

38. Kamoi K, Okihara K, Ochiai A, Ukimura O, Mizutani Y, Kawauchi A, et al. The utility of transrectal real-time elastography in the diagnosis of prostate cancer. Ultrasound Med Biol. 2008;34(7):1025–32. PubMed PMID: 18255215. English.

39. Allgayer H, Ignee A, Dietrich CF. Endosonographic elastography of the anal sphincter in patients with fecal incontinence. Scand J Gastroenterol. 2010;45(1):30–8. PubMed PMID: 20001748.

Post-Test Questions

For the following questions, there is only one right answer to each question.

1. Looking at the below 3D volume please circle which one is Anterior?

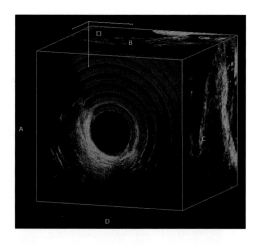

[A]

[B]

[C]

[D]

2. Looking at the below 3D volume please circle which one is Cephalad?

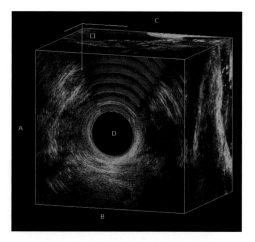

[A]

[B]

[C]

[D]

3. Looking at the below 3D volume please circle which one is the vagina?

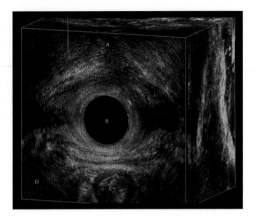

[A]

[B]

[C]

[D]

4. Looking at the below 3D volume please circle which one is the superficial transverse perinei muscle?

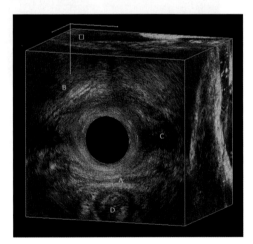

[A]

[B]

[C]

[D]

5. Which probe was used to obtain these images?

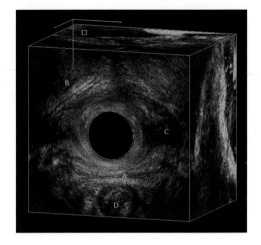

[A] BK 2052 360° probe

[B] BK 8848 Convex probe

[C] BK 8848 Linear probe

[D] BK 8802 Transperineal probe

6. Looking at the below 3D volume please circle which one is the puboperinealis muscle?

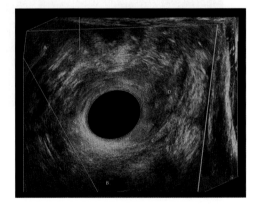

[A]

[B]

[C]

[D]

7. Looking at the below 3D volume please circle which one is the puboanalis muscle?

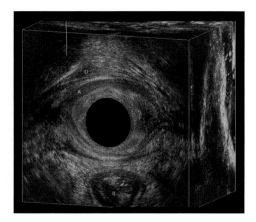

[A]

[B]

[C]

[D]

8. Looking at the below 3D volume please circle which one is the puborectalis muscle?

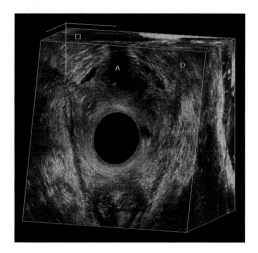

[A]

[B]

[C]

[D]

9. Looking at the below 3D volume please circle which one is the iliococcygeous muscle?

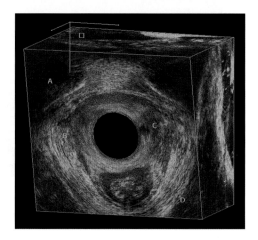

[A]

[B]

[C]

[D]

10. The view demonstrated here is

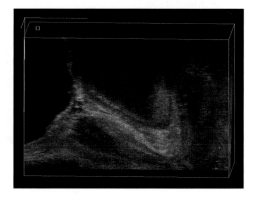

[A] Sagittal

[B] Coronal

[C] Axial

[D] Cephalad

11. Which probe is used to acquire this image?

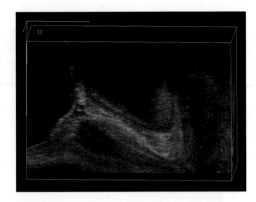

[A] BK 2052 360° probe

[B] BK 8848 Convex probe

[C] BK 8848 Linear probe

[D] BK 8802 Transperineal probe

12. Looking at the below 3D volume where is anterior?

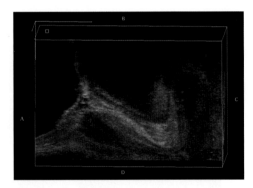

[A]

[B]

[C]

[D]

13. Looking at the below 3D volume please indicate where the pubic arch is

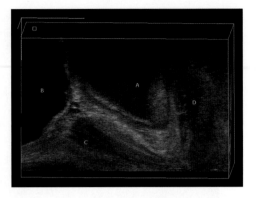

[A]

[B]

[C]

[D]

14. Looking at the below 3D volume please circle which layer is trigone?

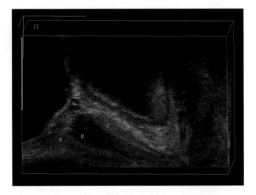

[A]

[B]

[C]

[D]

15. Looking at the below 3D volume please circle which layer is the urethral lumen?

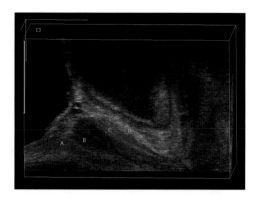

[A]

[B]

[C]

[D]

16. Looking at the below 3D volume please circle which layer is longitudinal/circular smooth muscle layer?

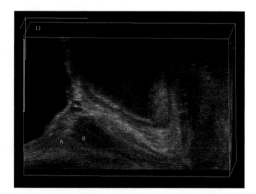

[A]

[B]

[C]

[D]

17. Looking at the below 3D volume please circle which layer is the striated muscle layer (Rhabdomyosphincter)?

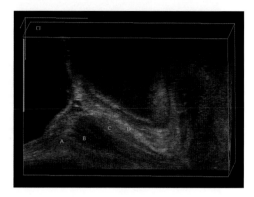

[A]

[B]

[C]

[D]

18. The view demonstrated here is

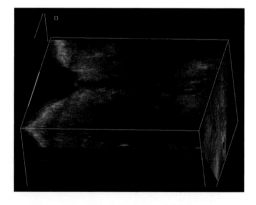

[A] Sagittal view of the anorectum

[B] Coronal view of the urethra and the bladder

[C] Axial view of the anus

[D] Cephalad view of the levator ani

19. Which probe is used to obtain this image?

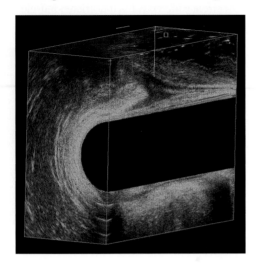

[A] BK 2052 360° probe

[B] BK 8848 Convex probe

[C] BK 8848 Linear probe

[D] BK 8802 Transperineal probe

20. Looking at the below 3D volume please circle which one is the external anal sphincter?

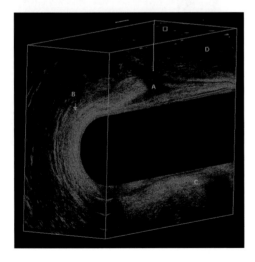

[A]

[B]

[C]

[D]

21. Looking at the below 3D volume please circle which one is the levator plate?

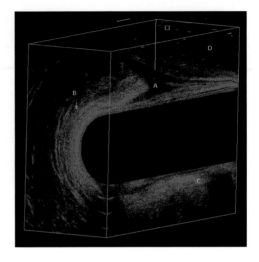

[A]

[B]

[C]

[D]

22. Looking at the below 3D volume please circle where is the internal anal sphincter?

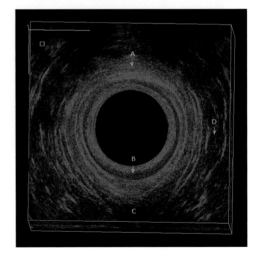

[A]

[B]

[C]

[D]

23. Looking at the below 3D volume please circle where is the external anal sphincter?

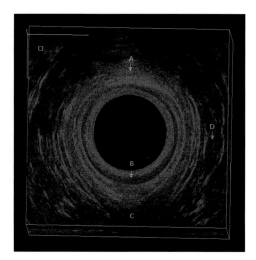

[A]

[B]

[C]

[D]

24. Looking at the below 3D volume please circle where is posterior?

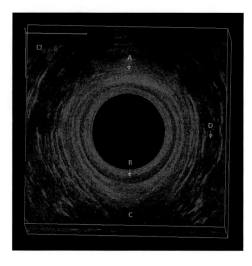

[A]

[B]

[C]

[D]

25. The view demonstrated here is

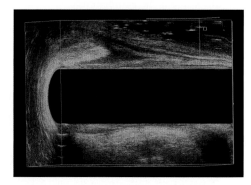

[A] Sagittal view of the anorectum

[B] Coronal view of the urethra and the bladder

[C] Axial view of the anus

[D] Cephalad view of the levator ani

26. Looking at the below 3D volume please circle where is the perineal body?

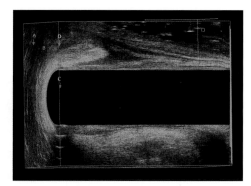

[A]

[B]

[C]

[D]

27. Looking at the below 3D volume please circle where is the anorectum?

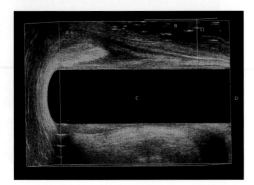

[A]

[B]

[C]

[D]

28. Looking at the below 3D volume please circle where is the vagina?

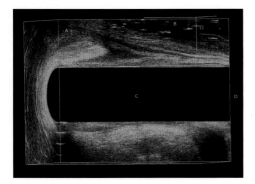

[A]

[B]

[C]

[D]

29. Looking at the below 3D volume please circle where is cephalad?

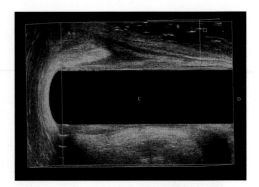

[A]

[B]

[C]

[D]

30. Looking at the below 3D volume please circle where is the internal anal sphincter?

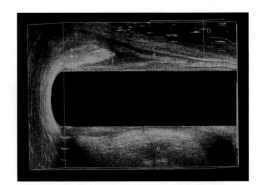

[A]

[B]

[C]

[D]

31. Looking at the below 3D volume please circle where is the external anal sphincter?

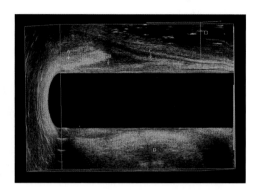

[A]

[B]

[C]

[D]

32. Looking at the below 3D volume please circle where is the levator plate?

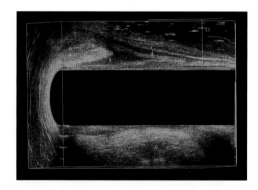

[A]

[B]

[C]

[D]

33. Looking at the below 3D volume please circle where is the rectovaginal fascia?

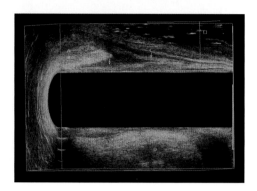

[A]

[B]

[C]

[D]

34. Which probe is used to acquire this image?

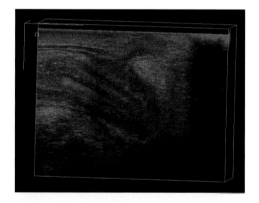

[A] 2052 360° probe

[B] 8848 Convex probe

[C] 8848 Linear probe

[D] 8802 Transperineal probe

35. The view demonstrated here is

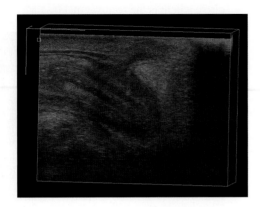

[A] Sagittal view of the anorectum

[B] Coronal view of the urethra and the bladder

[C] Axial view of the anus

[D] Cephalad view of the levator ani

36. Looking at the below 3D volume please identify where the vagina would be?

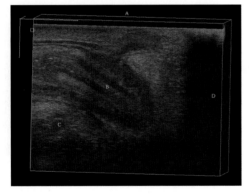

[A]

[B]

[C]

[D]

37. Looking at the below 3D volume please identify the anorectum

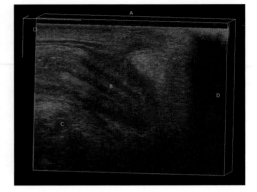

[A]

[B]

[C]

[D]

38. Looking at the below 3D volume please identify the external anal sphincter muscle

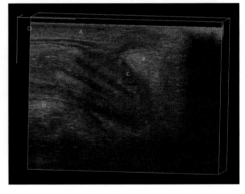

[A]

[B]

[C]

[D]

39. Looking at the below 3D volume please identify the levator plate

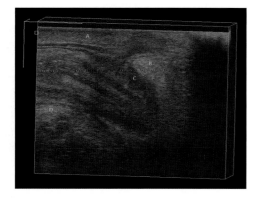

[A]

[B]

[C]

[D]

40. Looking at the below 3D volume please identify the internal anal sphincter muscle

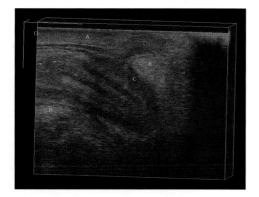

[A]

[B]

[C]

[D]

41. Which probe is used to acquire this image?

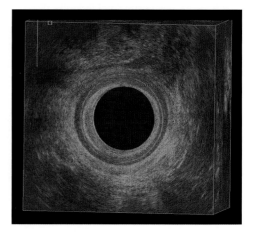

[A] 2052 360° probe

[B] 8848 Convex probe

[C] 8848 Linear probe

[D] 8802 Transperineal probe

42. The view demonstrated here is

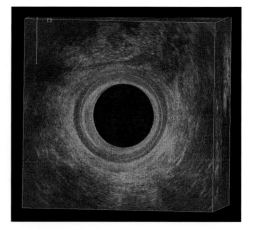

[A] Sagittal view of the anorectum

[B] Coronal view of the urethra and the bladder

[C] Axial view of the anus

[D] Cephalad view of the levator ani

43. Looking at the below 3D volume please identify where the vagina would be?

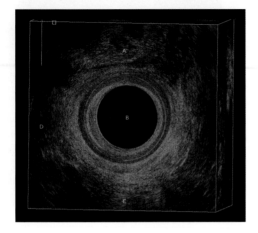

[A]
[B]
[C]
[D]

44. Looking at the below 3D volume please identify the anorectum

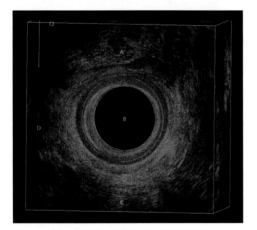

[A]
[B]
[C]
[D]

45. Looking at the below 3D volume please identify the "defect," or a structure that you would not expect to see here

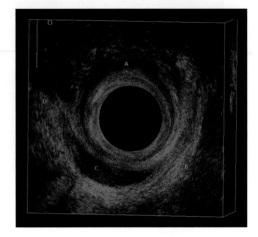

[A]
[B]
[C]
[D]

46. The view demonstrated here is

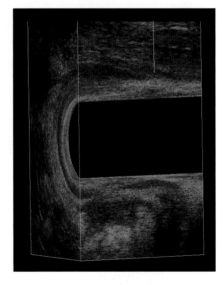

[A] Sagittal view of the anorectum

[B] Coronal view of the urethra and the bladder

[C] Axial view of the anus

[D] Cephalad view of the levator ani

47. Looking at the below 3D volume please identify the anorectum

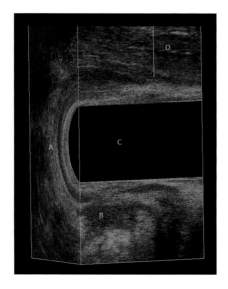

[A]
[B]
[C]
[D]

48. Looking at the below 3D volume please identify the external anal sphincter

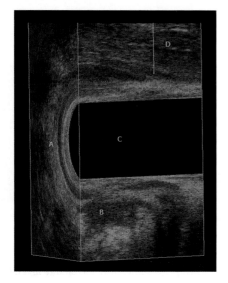

[A]
[B]
[C]
[D]

49. Looking at the below 3D volume please identify the "defect" or a structure that you do not expect to see here

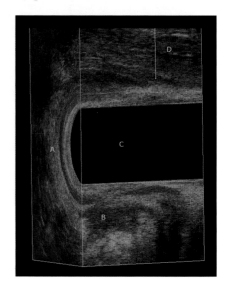

[A]
[B]
[C]
[D]

50. Which probe is used to acquire this image?

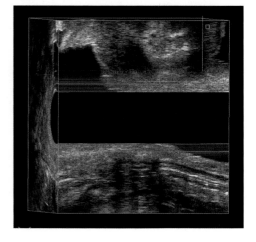

[A] 2052 360° probe
[B] 8848 Convex probe
[C] 8848 Linear probe
[D] 8802 Transperineal probe

51. The view demonstrated here is

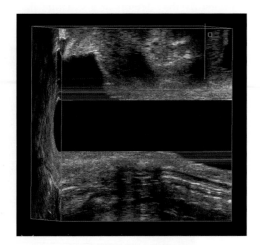

[A] Sagittal view of the anorectum

[B] Coronal view of the urethra and the bladder

[C] Axial view of the anus

[D] Cephalad view of the levator ani

52. Looking at the below 3D volume please identify the vagina

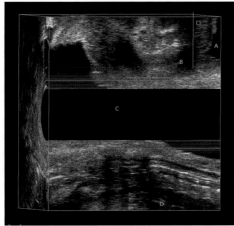

[A]

[B]

[C]

[D]

53. Looking at the below 3D volume please identify the anorectum

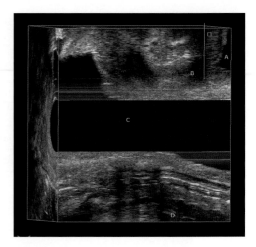

[A]

[B]

[C]

[D]

54. Looking at the below 3D volume please identify the urethra

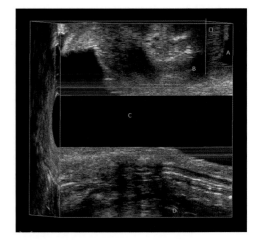

[A]

[B]

[C]

[D]

55. Looking at the below 3D volume please identify the bladder

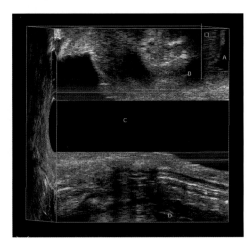

[A]

[B]

[C]

[D]

56. Looking at the below 3D volume please identify the posteriorly implanted pig tissue

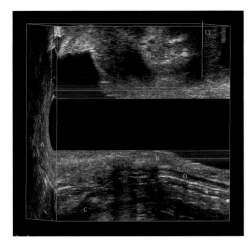

[A]

[B]

[C]

[D]

57. The view demonstrated here is

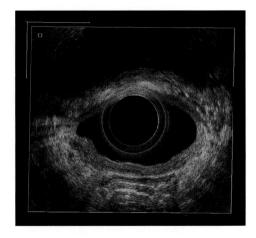

[A] Sagittal view of the anorectum

[B] Coronal view of the urethra and the bladder

[C] Axial view of the vagina

[D] Cephalad view of the levator ani

58. Looking at the below 3D volume please identify the vagina

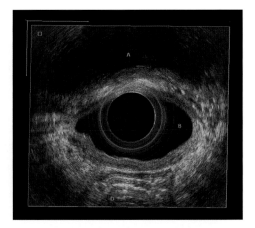

[A]

[B]

[C]

[D]

59. Looking at the below 3D volume please identify the bladder

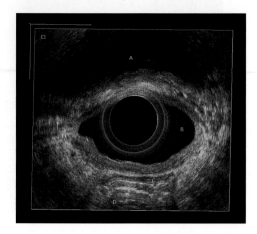

[A]
[B]
[C]
[D]

60. Looking at the below 3D volume please identify the posteriorly implanted pig tissue

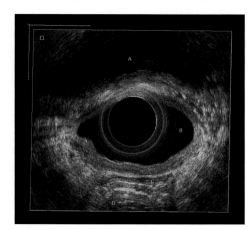

[A]
[B]
[C]
[D]

Post-Test Key

1. [B]

2. [C]

3. [B]

4. [A]

5. [A]

6. [C]

7. [C]

8. [C]

9. [B]

10. [A]

11. [C]

12. [B]

13. [A]

14. [A]

15. [B]

16. [C]

17. [D]

18. [B]

19. [A]

20. [B]

21. [C]

22. [B]

23. [A]

24. [C]

25. [A]   43. [A]

26. [D]   44. [B]

27. [C]   45. [C]

28. [B]   46. [A]

29. [D]   47. [C]

30. [B]   48. [A]

31. [A]   49. [B]

32. [D]   50. [A]

33. [C]   51. [A]

34. [C]   52. [C]

35. [A]   53. [D]

36. [A]   54. [B]

37. [B]   55. [A]

38. [B]   56. [D]

39. [D]   57. [C]

40. [C]   58. [B]

41. [A]   59. [A]

42. [C]   60. [C]

Index

A
Aging
  Bland Altman plot, 83
  MLH and LPA, 83–87
Anal sphincter damage
  anal canal assessment, 166
  EAUS, 167
  FI, 170, 171
  fibroelastic component, 165
  fistula surgery, 178, 179
  hypoechoic layer, 164
  measurement, 167
  ODS, 172–174, 176
  pelvis, 163
  scanning, 168
  shape, 167
Angiosarcoma, 191, 193
Anismus
  activation, 121
  evaluation, 123, 126
  levator ani trauma, 123
  stage 2 prolapse, 121
Anorectal angle (ARA) measures
  pelvic floor dyssynergy, 119, 126
  sagittal plane, 117, 119
Anorectal cysts and masses
  description, 185
  endometriosis, 185 187
  presacral neoplasia (see Presacral neoplasia)
  rare tumors (see Rare tumors)
Anorectum and 3D EVUS
  assessment, posterior compartment disorders,
    130–131
  defecography, 130
  description, 115
  imaging
    endovaginal (see Endovaginal ultrasound,
      anorectum)
    transperineal, 115–116
  limition, 130

prolapse evaluation, 130
techniques and literature
  endovaginal ultrasound (see Endovaginal
    ultrasound, anorectum)
  translabial ultrasound (see Transperineal
    ultrasonography (TPUS))
  and TPUS, 130
ARA measures. See Anorectal angle (ARA) measures
Arcus
  pararectal defect, 9
  pubocervical fibromuscularis, 3
  tendineus fascia pelvis, 6–7

B
Bartholin cyst
  3D endovaginal ultrasound, 154
  duct, 154
  glands, 154
  gonococcal infection, 154
  treatment, 154
Biologic grafts, POP surgery
  apical–anterior and apical–posterior wall repair, 146
  augmentation, 145
  behavior, 145–146
  composite kit, 145
  3D EVUS, 146
  FDA recommendatin, 145
  InteXen LP graft, 145
  material, 146
  non-cross-linked porcine dermis, 146
  synthetic tape, 146
BK 3D Viewer Software
  annotation and arrow icon, 25
  endovaginal frame, 25, 27
  measurement icon, 25, 26
  multiple functions, 28, 29
  screen view, 24
  sculpting icon, 25, 26
  structure, axial, sagittal/coronal planes, 28, 29

S.A. Shobeiri (ed.), *Practical Pelvic Floor Ultrasonography: A Multicompartmental Approach to 2D/3D/4D Ultrasonography of Pelvic Floor*, DOI 10.1007/978-1-4614-8426-4,
© Springer Science+Business Media New York 2014